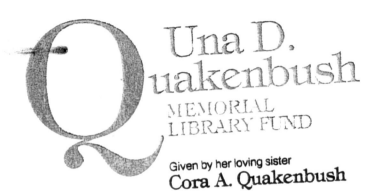

Hormone Replacement Therapy *and* Cardiovascular Disease

The Current Status of Research and Practice

Hormone Replacement Therapy *and* Cardiovascular Disease

The Current Status of Research and Practice

Edited by

A. R. Genazzani

President of the International Menopause Society
and
Chairman of the Division of Obstetrics and Gynecology
University of Pisa, Italy

**Published under the auspices of
the International Menopause Society**

The Parthenon Publishing Group

International Publishers in Medicine, Science & Technology

NEW YORK

LONDON

Library of Congress Cataloguing-in-Publication Data

Data available on request

British Library Cataloguing in Publication Data
Hormone replacement therapy and cardiovascular
disease : the current status of research and practice
  1. Cardiovascular system – Diseases
  2. Cardiovascular system – Diseases – Sex
  differences 3. Cardiovascular system –
  Diseases – Endocrine aspects
  I. Genazzani, Andrea
616.1

ISBN 1-84214-038-8
ISSN 1474-3930

Published in the USA by
The Parthenon Publishing Group Inc.
One Blue Hill Plaza
PO Box 1564, Pearl River
New York 10965, USA

Published in the UK and Europe by
The Parthenon Publishing Group Limited
Casterton Hall, Carnforth
Lancs. LA6 2LA, UK

Copyright © 2001 The Parthenon Publishing Group

Typeset by AMA DataSet, Preston, UK

Printed and bound by Butler & Tanner Ltd.
Frome and London, UK

Contents

Section III Cardiovascular effects of available hormone replacement therapy

Section IV Clinical effects of hormone replacement therapy: primary and secondary prevention of cardiovascular disease

List of principal contributors

P. Collins
The National Heart & Lung Institute
Imperial College of Science
Royal Brompton Hospital
London SW3 6NP
UK

D. Crook
Formerly Department of Cardiovascular
    Biochemistry
St. Bartholomew's and The Royal London
    School of Medicine
Charterhouse Square
London EC1M 6BQ
UK

S. Curtis Hewitt
NIEHS MD E4 01
111 TW Alexander Dr
PO Box 12233
Research Triangle Park
North Carolina 27709
USA

P. de Vane
Wyeth-Ayerst Pharmaceuticals
555 East Lancaster Avenue
St. Davids
Pennsylvania 19087
USA

K. E. Friday
1430 Tulane Avenue, SL53
New Orleans
Louisiana 70112
USA

A. R. Genazzani
University of Pisa
Division of Obstetrics and Gynecology
Via Roma 35
56126 Pisa
Italy

F. Grodstein
Channing Laboratory
181 Longwood Avenue
Boston
Massachusetts 02115
USA

J.-Å. Gustafsson
Department of Biosciences
Karolinska Institute
Novum
14186 Huddinge
Sweden

E. G. Lakatta
Laboratory of Cardiovascular Science
Gerontology Research Center
Intramural Research Program
National Institute on Aging
5600 Nathan Shock Drive
Baltimore
Maryland 21224
USA

P. M. Mannucci
Department of Internal Medicine
Università degli Studi di Milano
Via Pace 9
20122 Milan
Italy

M. E. Mendelsohn
New England Medical Center
750 Washington Street, Box 80
Boston
Massachusetts 02111
USA

L. Mosca
New York Presbyterian Hospital
Columbia and Cornell Universities
ICCR PH 10-203 D
622 West 168th Street
New York
New York 10032-3784
USA

E. Moscarelli
Women's Health Business Unit
Eli Lilly Italia Spa
Via Gramsci 731
50019 Sesto Fiorentino
Florence
Italy

B. W. O'Malley
M613, Department of Molecular & Cellular
   Biology
Baylor College of Medicine
One Baylor Plaza
Houston
Texas 77030
USA

F. Parazzini
Laboratorio di Epidemiologia Analitica
Istituto di Ricerche Farmacologiche 'Mario
   Negri'
Via Eritrea 62
20157 Milan
Italy

G. M. C. Rosano
Department of Internal Medicine, Cardiology
San Raffaele – Roma
Via della Pisana 235
00163 Rome
Italy

J. Rosing
Department of Biochemistry
Maastricht University
PO Box 616
6200 MD Maastricht
The Netherlands

A. Salvetti
Department of Internal Medicine
Università degli Studi di Pisa
Via Roma 67
56127 Pisa
Italy

R. Sitruk-Ware
Contraceptive Development
Center for Biomedical Research
The Population Council
1230 York Avenue
New York
New York 10021
USA

J. C. Stevenson
Endocrinology and Metabolic Medicine
Mint Wing
St. Mary's Hospital
Praed Street
London W2 1NY
UK

M. J. Tikkanen
Department of Medicine
Helsinki University Central Hospital
00290 Helsinki
Finland

Y. Tsouderos
Institut de Recherches Internationales Servier
6, Place des Pléiades
92415 Courbevoie Cedex
France

C. Varas-Lorenzo
Novartis Spain Global Epidemiology
Gran Via de la Cortez Catalana 764
Barcelona 08013
Spain

J. K. Williams
Wake Forest University School of Medicine
Winston-Salem
North Carolina 27157-1040
USA

Introduction

It is for me a pleasure to present this volume, which brings together the presentations given during the Expert Workshop on *Hormone Replacement Therapy and Cardiovascular Disease*, organized by the International Menopause Society, and held in London on October 13–16, 2000 at the Royal Society of Medicine. This meeting is the first of a series of Expert Workshops that our Society is planning on Controversial Issues in Climacteric Medicine. The next workshop will be held in Pisa on the subject of *Hormone Replacement Therapy and Cancer*.

Climacteric medicine is a reality in modern western society. Women now live one-third to one-half of their lives after menopause. A large body of evidence on estrogen action, the consequences of estrogen loss, and the comprehensive benefit/risk ratio of menopausal hormone replacement has been accumulated in recent years. The menopause can be seen as a time of positive change, provided that women can understand and their physicians can individualize their health care. It should be emphasized that climacteric medicine is not only hormone replacement therapy. The use of hormone replacement is an individual decision, which must take into account symptoms, risk factors and the woman's preferences and needs. Alternatives should also be care-fully considered. Hormone replacement therapy can be used for short-term treatment of symptoms at the lowest dosage that will adequately control hot flushes or vaginal dryness or dyspareunia. The use of hormone replacement therapy is not necessarily a long-term commitment, and there should be flexibility in prescribing, since there is no ideal regimen for every woman.

The aim of our Workshops on Controversial Issues in Climacteric Medicine is to provide updated overviews of the real impact of menopause, hormone replacement therapy and, when applicable, therapeutic alternatives on specific debatable topics, in order to assist health-care providers involved in the management of menopausal health in making appropriate recommendations.

I hope that this volume, together with the Position Paper that was published in the December, 2000 issue of *Climacteric*, the Official Journal of the International Menopause Society, can fully describe and make clear the complex effect of menopause and hormone replacement therapy on cardiovascular disease, providing new and important information on which to reflect in order to assist our patients.

Andrea R. Genazzani
President of the IMS

Trends in mortality rates for cardiovascular and cerebrovascular diseases in developed countries

F. Parazzini, C. La Vecchia, F. Levi, F. Lucchini and E. Negri

INTRODUCTION

Over the last five decades, significant changes have been observed in mortality rates for cardio- and cerebrovascular diseases in developed countries. For cardiovascular disease, mainly coronary heart disease, substantial and generalized upward trends in mortality rates were registered during the first six decades of the last century, followed by levelling off and declines in more recent decades[1,2]. The declines started early in the USA, and in a few other countries such as Australia, but were observed only more recently in western European countries such as the UK, Scandinavia, France, Germany and Italy.

For cerebrovascular diseases, in most developed countries, with the main exception of eastern Europe, major declines in mortality rates have been registered during the most recent four decades[3].

Despite these generally decreasing trends, marked differences in mortality rates for cardiovascular and cerebrovascular diseases are still present among developed countries. The World Health Organization (WHO) mortality database includes death certification data from the early 1950s onwards for most developed countries. We have analyzed the trends in mortality rates for cardio- and cerebrovascular diseases between 1955 and 1989 in selected European and North American countries[4]. Differences between countries in cardiovascular mortality rates have relevant implications for evaluating the impact on a population of hormone replacement therapy (HRT) in the prevention of cardiovascular disease.

MATERIALS AND METHODS

Information included in the analysis was derived from the WHO database which contains data on mortality rates and populations for about 100 countries. During the period 1955-89, four different revisions of the International Classification of Diseases (ICD) were used[5-8]. Classifications of all deaths in the period considered were therefore revised according to the Ninth Revision of the International Classification of Diseases (ICD-9). This meant that, for the purpose of the present analysis, deaths from all cerebrovascular diseases were considered in a single group. Also, for deaths from all ischemic heart diseases, only data registered in the period 1968-89 were considered, due to major changes in the classification which occurred in 1968.

Estimates of the resident populations, generally based on official censuses, were obtained from the same WHO database. From the matrices of certified deaths and resident populations, age-specific mortality rates for each standardized 5-year calendar period were computed. Age-standardized rates were based on the world standard population[9].

In a few countries, data were missing for part of one or more 5-year calendar periods. When a single year was missing, data were interpolated linearly from the previous and subsequent calendar years. No extrapolation was made for missing data at the beginning or the end of the calendar period considered, or when no data were available for a 5-year period.

RESULTS

Ischemic heart diseases

In the period 1968–69, the highest overall mortality rates for all ischemic heart diseases within Europe were registered in northern countries. Ischemic heart disease mortality rates were lower in southern Europe (65/100 000 females in Italy; < 50/100 000 females in all other southern European countries), France, Poland and Romania. The highest mortality rate registered (Denmark) was more than six-fold higher than the lowest rate registered (Poland) (Table 1).

Over the last three decades, two different general patterns were observed. In western Europe, rates were generally stable until the mid-1970s, but consistent declines were registered thereafter. In eastern Europe, consistent and steady upward trends were observed up to the most recent 5-year period. In the late 1980s, the highest rate was only four-fold higher than the lowest rate, indicating a levelling of differences across Europe. The differ-

ent trends observed in western and eastern Europe are probably due to complex modifications of risk factors.

In North American countries, mortality rates in the late 1960s for ischemic heart disease were 166/100 000 females in the USA and 131/100 000 females in Canada. Thereafter, mortality rates for ischemic heart disease declined by one-half over two decades.

Cerebrovascular diseases

Overall age-standardized mortality rates for cerebrovascular diseases in the late 1950s were between 40 and 100/100 000 females in most European countries. The lowest rates were observed in Poland (33.4/100 000) (Table 1). Over the following three decades, in all western European countries except Greece and Portugal (data not shown)[4], substantial declines were observed in overall cerebrovascular disease mortality rates, and in the late 1980s, rates ranged

Table 1 Mortality rates for cardiovascular and cerebrovascular diseases

	Rates/100 000 women*							
	1955–59		1965–69		1975–79		1985–89	
	IHD	CVD	IHD	CVD	IHD	CVD	IHD	CVD
North America								
USA	—	79.3	166.0	66.8	124.0	46.2	86.3	31.4
Canada	—	80.2	130.7	59.3	108.2	44.5	76.8	29.8
Europe								
Belgium	—	—	63.6	74.7	56.9	65.0	42.5	44.2
Czechoslovakia	—	76.6	63.7	84.4	66.7	108.5	72.1	96.9
Denmark	—	82.3	121.9	61.5	111.7	42.5	92.3	37.7
France	—	75.1	27.9	64.1	29.4	52.1	26.5	34.6
East Germany	—	—	—	—	54.3	37.3	66.1	49.3
West Germany	—	116.6	39.5	96.2	39.7	72.2	32.4	48.7
Greece	—	—	28.6	81.1	34.4	84.2	33.0	81.2
Italy	—	94.5	65.2	80.2	64.7	67.5	39.6	54.7
Norway	—	44.6	93.4	37.8	77.6	26.0	71.1	18.8
Poland	—	33.4	21.6	30.4	38.9	43.4	38.3	41.7
Romania	—	58.1	49.8	105.2	61.8	105.5	—	—
Spain	—	84.8	23.3	86.3	35.4	83.1	28.6	58.0
Sweden	—	90.0	115.7	59.7	113.8	46.7	84.8	37.2
UK (England and Wales)	—	96.1	104.0	84.7	104.0	68.8	91.9	52.3
Former Yugoslavia	—	—	37.6	68.7	49.7	71.0	40.9	80.0

*Age-standardized rates based on the world standard population[9]. IHD, ischemic heart disease; CVD, cerebrovascular disease

between 30 and 60/100 000 females in most countries. In several countries these declines became steeper in the most recent calendar periods.

Cerebrovascular disease mortality rates increased in all eastern European countries, including both countries with low rates in the 1950s (Poland and East Germany). The rate for Bulgaria (data not shown)[4] was > 125/100 000 females in 1985–89 (the highest on a worldwide scale). There is therefore a clear distinction between trends in cerebrovascular disease mortality rates in western and eastern Europe.

In the USA and Canada, overall age-standardized mortality rates for cerebrovascular diseases were around 80/100 000 in the late 1950s, declining steadily to about 30/100 000 in 1985–89.

COMMENTS

Despite marked changes in the overall mortality rates for cardiovascular and cerebrovascular diseases observed over the last five decades in Europe and North American countries, marked differences between countries are still present. The data presented in this report consider the period 1955–1989. However, the trends observed in that period (i.e. declining trends in the North American and western European countries, increasing trends in the eastern European countries) are still largely present in the late 1990s[10].

To explain these trends is not easy and beyond the scope of this discussion. However, the reasons for the trends in ischemic heart diseases probably involve improved diet, reduced smoking, more efficient control of hypertension, improved physical activity and improved treatment of the conditions[2,11,12]. Since hypertension is the main determinant of cerebrovascular disease, this would suggest that inadequate control of hypertension on a population level is still widespread in eastern Europe[13]. Additional risk factors, including smoking, alcohol consumption and diet (including salt used in food processing and preservation) may also have had some role.

It is interesting to note that the marked differences in the mortality rates for (and probably incidences of) cardiovascular diseases among countries may have relevance for the impact of hormone replacement therapy (HRT) on life expectancy. Considering the potential protective effect of HRT against cardiovascular disease and related mortality[14], and the possible increased risk of breast cancer[15], the risk/benefit balance for HRT on a population scale should be positive (i.e. live-saving) in countries characterized by higher mortality rates for cardiovascular disease than for breast cancer (in particular in the perimenopausal group aged 50–60 years), but should be negative in the countries with higher mortality rates for breast cancer than for cardiovascular disease[16].

Finally, considering the trends observed in mortality rates for cardiovascular disease over recent decades, and considering the expected reduction in mortality rates for cardiovascular disease in most developed countries over the next few decades, the impact of HRT on public health should take into account these expected changes, as well as the risks of mortality from breast cancer[17].

References

1. Uemura K, Pisa Z. Trends in cardiovascular disease mortality in industrialized countries since 1950. *World Health Stat Q* 1988;41:155–78
2. Ragland KE, Selvin S, Merrill DW. The onset of decline in ischemic heart disease mortality in the United States. *Am J Epidemiol* 1988;127:516–31
3. Whisnant JP. The decline of stroke. *Stroke* 1984;15:160–8
4. La Vecchia C, Levi F, Lucchini F, Negri E. Trends in mortality from cardiovascular and cerebrovascular disease. *Soz Praventivmed* 1993;1:S3–S71

5. World Health Organization. *International Classification of Disease: 6th Revision*. Geneva: World Health Organization, 1950

6. World Health Organization. *International Classification of Disease: 7th Revision*. Geneva: World Health Organization, 1957

7. World Health Organization. *International Classification of Disease: 8th Revision*. Geneva: World Health Organization, 1967

8. World Health Organization. *International Classification of Disease: 9th Revision*. Geneva: World Health Organization, 1977

9. Doll R, Smith PG. Comparison between registries: age-standardized rates. In Waterhouse JAH, Muir CS, Shanmugaratnam K, Powell J, eds. *Cancer Incidence in Five Continents*, Vol. IV. Lyon: International Agency for Research on Cancer, 1982:671–5

10. Levy D, Kannel WB. Searching for answers to ethnic disparities in cardiovascular risk. *Lancet* 2000;356:266–7

11. Rose G. Causes of the trends and variations in CHD mortality in different countries. *Int J Epidemiol* 1989;18:S174–S179

12. Gramenzi A, Gentile A, Fasoli M, Negri E, Parazzini F, La Vecchia C. Association between certain foods and risk of acute myocardial infarction in women. *Br Med J* 1990;300:771–3

13. Ostfeld AM. A review of stroke epidemiology. *Epidemiol Rev* 1980;2:136–52

14. Colditz GA, Hankinson SE, Hunter DJ, *et al*. The use of estrogens and progestins and the risk of breast cancer in postmenopausal women. *N Engl J Med* 1995;332:1589–93

15. Collaborative Group on Hormonal Factors in Breast Cancer. Breast cancer and hormone replacement therapy: collaborative reanalysis of data from 51 epidemiological studies of 52705 women with breast cancer and 108411 without breast cancer. *Lancet* 1997;350:103–5

16. Panico S, Galasso R, Cementano E, Ciardullo AV, Frova L, Capocaccia R, Trevisan M, Berrino F. Large-scale hormone replacement therapy and life expectancy: results from an international comparison among European and North American populations. *Am J Public Health* 2000;90:1397–1402

17. Richards MA, Stockton D, Babb P, Coleman MP. How many deaths have been avoided through improvements in cancer survival? *Br Med J* 2000;320:395–8

Cardiovascular aging in women and men in the absence of clinical disease

2

E. G. Lakatta

INTRODUCTION

The exponential increases in so-called 'degenerative vascular diseases', such as arterio- and atherosclerosis and hypertension, associated with advanced age reach epidemic proportions among older people, leading to heart failure and stroke. Quantitative information on age-associated alterations in cardiovascular structure and function in health is essential. This is in order to define and target the specific characteristics of the cardiovascular aging process that render age the major risk factor for these diseases, and for the heart failure and strokes that ensue. However, because it is difficult to separate the effects of aging from those of different lifestyles, such as lack of physical activity or smoking, it is difficult to define the effects of aging on cardiovascular structure and function. Over the past few decades, a sustained effort has been applied to characterization of how aging in health modifies cardiovascular structure and function in women and men who participate in the Baltimore Longitudinal Study on Aging (BLSA). These community-dwelling women and men are rigorously screened to detect both clinical and occult cardiovascular disease and categorized with respect to lifestyle, particularly exercise habits, in an attempt to partially deconvolute the interactions noted above (Figure 1). Some aspects of how cardiovascular structure and function vary with age in this population are described in this paper.

VASCULAR STRUCTURE AND FUNCTION IN HEALTHY MEN AND WOMEN

Between the ages of 20 and 90 years the large elastic arteries of healthy male and female subjects in the BLSA become dilated and the artery walls become thicker (Figures 2a and 2b). The vascular intima thickens during aging (Figure 2b), and exhibits some features that resemble strikingly those that occur during early atherosclerosis[1]. These composite vascular alterations are accompanied by arterial stiffening (Figure 2c), which leads to an enhanced pulse wave velocity (Figure 2d) and to early reflected pulse waves (Figure 2e), that produce a late augmentation in central systolic arterial pressure. As a result, arterial systolic (Figure 2f) and pulse pressures increase with aging. After the fifth decade, the diastolic pressure reaches a plateau or declines, due to conduit artery stiffening (Figure 2g). In general, changes with aging in resistance vessels in healthy individuals appear to be less marked than those in the large, elastic arteries. The increase in total peripheral vascular resistance is relatively less than the reduction in compliance in larger arteries in men and women (Figure 2h). These age-associated vascular changes and, as observed in other populations, an age-associated impairment of endothelial function detected in healthy men years before it occurs in women[6], are presently considered to be below the 'clinical disease threshold'. Rather, these vascular changes that accompany aging, somewhat surprisingly, have been characterized as 'normal' by today's standards and guidelines for disease prevention have not generally been offered by the medical community. However, emerging evidence indicates that arterial stiffening, increases in arterial wall thickness and increases in arterial pressure, even within the 'normal' range, are independent risk factors for subsequent clinical vascular disease.

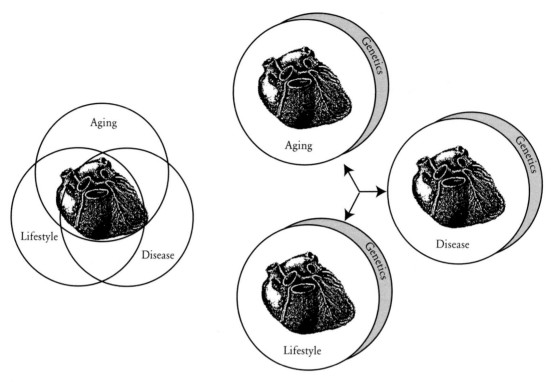

Figure 1 Interactions between age, lifestyle and disease, and genetic modulation of these factors, determine cardio-vascular structure and function. Reprinted from reference 1

CARDIAC STRUCTURE AND FUNCTION IN HEALTHY MEN AND WOMEN

Structure and resting function

The left ventricle (LV) wall thickness increases with age in both women and men in the BLSA (Figure 3a). The early LV filling rate decreases with age (Figure 3b). Structural changes and hetero-geneity of myocardial relaxation occurring among different regions of the LV of older persons may also contribute to this reduction in peak LV filling rate. Left atrial enlargement and an enhanced atrial contribution to ventricular filling measured via M-mode echocardiography increase with age (Figure 3c). The ratio of early to late LV filling therefore decreases dramatically with aging (Figure 3d).

Left ventricular systolic function was studied with the use of radionuclide ventriculography, in a subset of healthy community-dwelling men ($n = 121$) and women ($n = 79$) in the BLSA,

distributed evenly across a broad age range (22–86 years) and carefully screened to exclude latent coronary artery disease. Since heart performance varies with body size, various cardiac performance indices require adjustment for body surface area. In this study, average weight and body surface area were greater in men than in women (80.7 ± 12.5 vs. 63.6 ± 9.9 kg, and 1.98 ± 0.17 vs. 1.69 ± 0.14 m^2, respectively). Although body weight declined by an average of 10% and surface area by an average of 7% over six decades in men, neither variable was significantly related to age in women. Total body muscle mass, measured as 24-h urinary creatinine excretion, was greater in men than in women (1501 ± 355 vs. 925 ± 212 mg), and declined with age in both sexes. Heart performance also varies with the level of physical conditioning. To mini-mize differences in physical activity habits across age ranges and between sexes, subjects who regularly engaged in endurance training activities (≥ 3 times/week) and whose peak aerobic capacity exceeded the normal age-adjusted sedentary mean

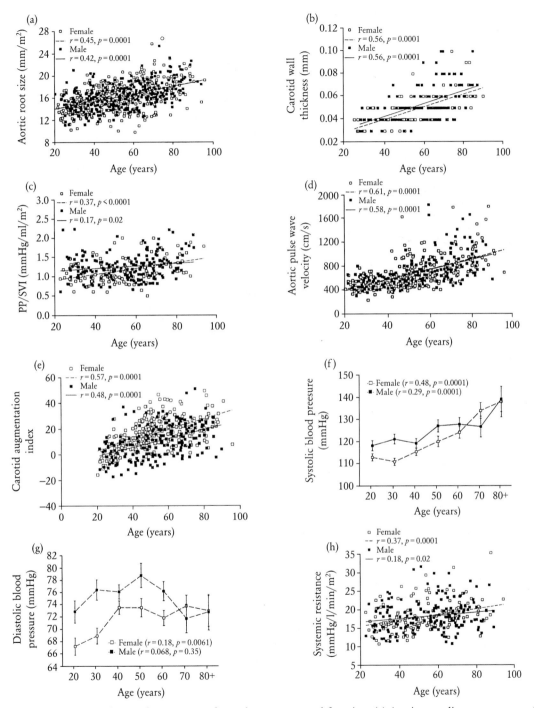

Figure 2 Variation with age of parameters of vascular structure and function. (a) Aortic root diameter, measured by M-mode echocardiography[2]. (b) Carotid intimal–medial wall thickness measured by echo Doppler techniques[3]. (c) Pulse pressure (PP)/stroke volume index (SVI) ratio at seated rest in healthy volunteers from the Baltimore Longitudinal Study on Aging (BLSA)[4]. (d) Aortic pulse wave velocity, an index of aortic stiffness[5]. (e) Augmentation index of the carotid pulse pressure due to a late peak in systolic pressure. This late augmentation of systolic pressure in older individuals is attributable to early reflected pulse waves caused by the increased stiffness of large vessels. (f) Systolic and (g) diastolic blood pressure in healthy subjects from the BLSA[4]. (h) Total vascular resistance at seated rest in healthy volunteers from the BLSA[4]

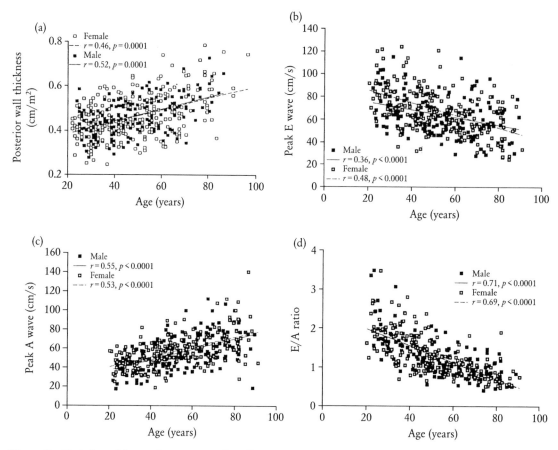

Figure 3 Variation with age of parameters of cardiac structure and function. (a) The left ventricular posterior wall thickness, measured by M-mode echocardiography, increases with age in healthy men and women from the Baltimore Longitudinal Study on Aging (BLSA)[2]. There are also age-associated changes in (b) the early (E) diastolic left ventricular filling, (c) the atrial (A) contribution to filling, and (d) the ratio of early filling and atrial filling[7]

values of the larger BLSA cohort by > 1 SD were excluded. In this BLSA study subset, the average aerobic capacity, measured as VO_{2max}, the international standard estimate of cardiorespiratory fitness, was higher in men than women (35.8 ± 8.7 vs. 28.9 ± 6.3 ml/kg/min) and declined with age in both groups (by about 1% per decade). Total physical activity time per day was nearly identical in men and women (34.0 ± 4.8 and 37.3 ± 4.0 min/day, respectively) and declined weakly but nonsignificantly with age in both men and women. Thus, routine physical activity in this sedentary BLSA subset was well maintained with age, and no age-gender interactions were observed for any of the above variables.

Changes in hemodynamic variables with age, measured in the sitting position before exercise,

are presented in Figures 4–6. In both sexes, heart rate (HR) declined significantly (Figure 4a) and systolic brachial blood pressure (SBP) (Figure 4b) and mean blood pressure (MBP) (data not shown) increased with age. Women had higher HR and lower SBP than did men across the age span. The cardiac index (CI), the cardiac output normalized for body surface area, declined by 16% between the third and eighth decades in women (Figure 4c). The total systemic vascular resistance (TSVR) (Figure 4d), derived from the CI and MBP, increased by 46% in women. In contrast, neither variable was age-related in men. The resting end diastolic volume index (EDVI), end systolic volume index (ESVI) and stroke volume index (SVI) (Figure 5a) increased by approximately 20% across the full age range in men but not in women.

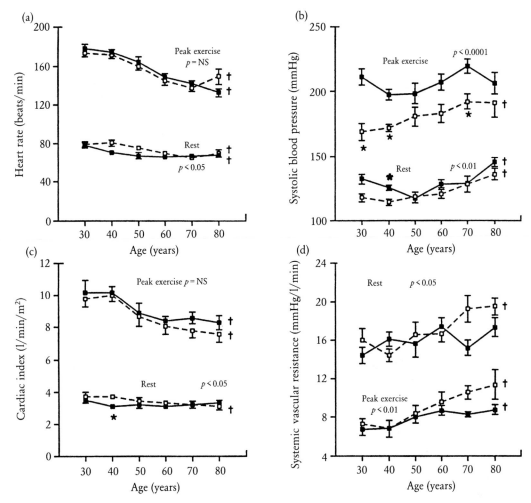

Figure 4 Systemic hemodynamic variables plotted by age at rest and at peak exercise in males (solid lines) and females (dashed lines): (a) heart rate; (b) systolic blood pressure; (c) cardiac index; (d) systemic vascular resistance. [†]Significant age regressions within gender at rest or peak effort. The p values shown indicate gender differences by analysis of variance. NS, not significant.[*] Significant gender differences for individual decades, adjusted for multiple comparisons. Regression equations and gender comparisons by covariance analysis at peak effort are given in Table 1[4]

Gender differences in resting EDVI and ESVI are thus most prominent in later decades. Resting indices of LV systolic pump performance are shown in Figure 5. The LV ejection fraction (EF) was not age-related in either sex, but was consistently higher in women across the full age range (Figure 6a). The SBP/ESVI ratio, an index of myocardial contractility, increased by 37% with age in women but did not change in men (Figure 6b), whereas the stroke work index (SWI), the product of stroke volume and brachial systolic pressure, increased with age in both sexes (Figure 6c).

A prominent gender difference observed at seated rest was therefore that EDVI and SVI increased with age in men but not women. As the resting HR declined with age in both sexes, the augmented SVI in older men prevented an age-associated decline in resting CI, whereas in women a substantial decline in CI and an increase in TSVR occurred between the third and ninth decades. The lower resting HR in men than in women may be related to the higher aerobic capacity and peak work rate in men (Figure 7), even though all men and women in the present study were sedentary by

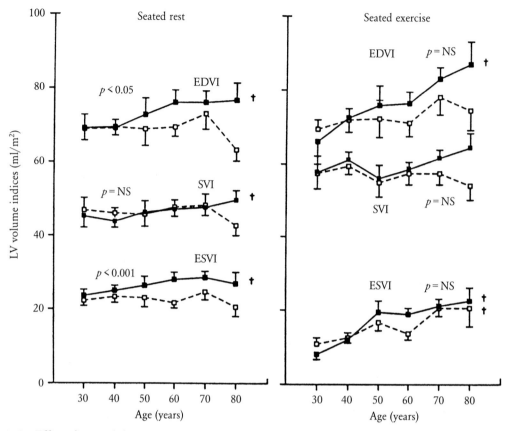

Figure 5 Effect of age on left ventricular (LV) volume indices (end diastolic volume index, EDVI; stroke volume index, SVI; end systolic volume index, ESVI) at rest (left panel) and peak exercise (right panel) in males (solid lines) and females (dashed lines). The statistical analyses and symbols are identical to those used in Figure 4. Regression equations and gender comparisons by covariance analysis at peak effort are given in Table 1[4]

clinical criteria. It is therefore likely that differences in aerobic capacity within a typical ambulatory non-endurance-trained population influence the hemodynamic profile at rest in a direction similar to that caused by endurance training.

A unified interpretation of age-associated changes in cardiac structure and resting function (Figures 3–6) suggests that these are, in part at least, adaptive, i.e. they occur in response to aging of the arterial system (Figure 8). The chronic augmentation in arterial pressure with advancing age in humans causes an enhanced mechanical load in the heart, leading to left ventricular wall thickening. The increase in LV wall thickness moderates the increase in LV wall tension occurring secondary to increased vascular loading. A prolonged myocardial contraction maintains a normal ejection time and ejection function in the presence

of the late augmentation of aortic impedance due to early reflected pulse waves. Otherwise, the increase in the vascular loading of the myocardium in late systole would lead to premature closure of the aortic valve. A disadvantage of prolonged contractile activation is that myocardial relaxation at the time of the mitral valve opening is relatively more incomplete in older than younger individuals. This is one factor that causes the early LV filling rate to be reduced in older individuals (Figure 3). Structural changes and heterogeneity of myocardial relaxation occurring within different regions of the LV of older persons may also contribute to this reduction in peak LV filling rate. However, concomitant adaptations – left atrial enlargement[2] and an enhanced atrial contribution to ventricular filling (Figure 4d) – compensate for the reduced early diastolic filling (Figure 3c). Thus,

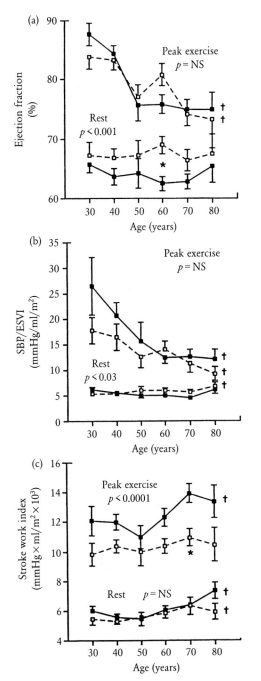

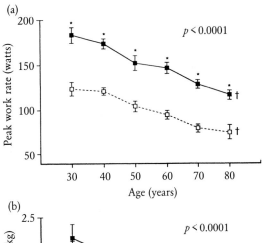

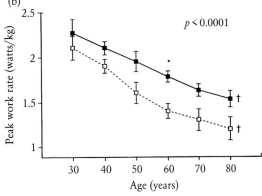

Figure 7 Relationship between peak cycle work rate and age in males (■) and females (□), (a) before and (b) after adjustment for body weight.[†]$p < 0.001$. By analysis of variance, peak work rate was higher in men, both before ($p < 0.0001$) and after ($p < 0.0001$) weight adjustment. *$p < 0.05$ for gender difference at specific age decades, after Bonferroni adjustment for multiple comparisons[4]. Definition of symbols and p values as for Figure 4

Figure 6 Hemodynamic variables indicative of left ventricular performance plotted by age at rest and at peak effort in males (solid lines) and females (dashed lines), using statistical analyses and symbols identical to those used in Figure 4. (a) Ejection fraction; (b) systolic blood pressure (SBP)/end systolic volume index (ESVI) ratio; (c) stroke work index. Regression equations and gender comparisons by covariance analysis at peak effort are given in Table 1[4]

overall systolic cardiac pump function at rest in clinically normotensive, sedentary, community-dwelling men and women is not substantially altered by age, although some specific gender differences are noted in arterial pressure, cardiac volumes and ejection fraction (Figures 1, 4 and 5).

Cardiovascular reserve capacity

As anticipated, the peak work rate achieved during upright cycle exercise in the sitting position was higher in men than in women (148.6 ± 36.5 vs. 101.9 ± 27.4 W) and declined with age by about 36% and 42% in men and women, respectively (Figure 7a). When peak work rate was normalized

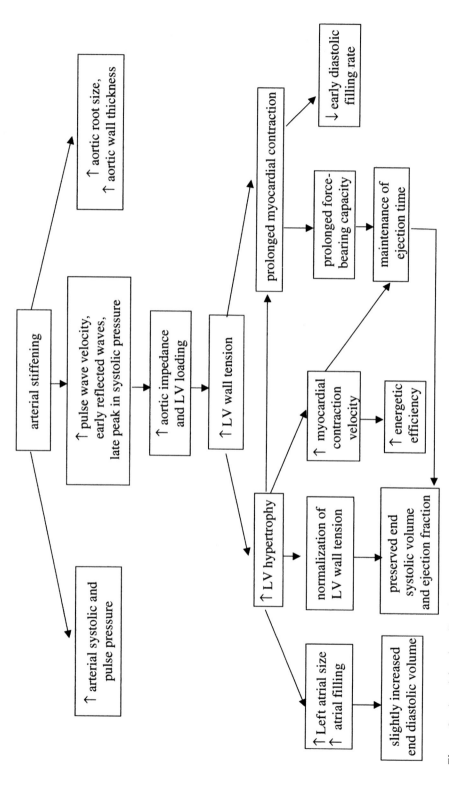

Figure 8 Arterial and cardiac changes that occur with aging in healthy humans. One interpretation is that vascular changes lead to cardiac structural and functional alterations that maintain cardiac function. LV, left ventricle. Reprinted from reference 8

for body weight, an age-associated decline was still observed (Figure 7b).

Age regressions for hemodynamic variables at peak effort are listed in Table 1, and plots of these variables at peak effort against age are shown in Figures 4-6. Concordance between age regressions (Table 1) and per decade analyses (Figures 4-6) was generally quite strong. Peak HR declined by approximately 25% across the full age range in both sexes (Figure 4a). Although diastolic blood pressure (DBP) and MBP at exhaustion increased significantly with age in both sexes (data not shown), peak SBP (Figure 4b) increased with age only in women. All arterial pressures were higher in men than in women by covariance analyses. Peak CI decreased with age in both sexes by approximately 25% across the full age range (Figure 4c), and TSVR at peak effort (Figure 4d) was higher with age in both sexes, although the increase was steeper in women than in men (56 vs. 30%). However, SVI was maintained with age in both sexes. That SVI is preserved with age in both men and women at peak effort in this BLSA cohort is in disagreement with results of several prior studies using cycle[9,10] and treadmill exercise[11]. In prior cycle ergometry studies[9,10], stroke volumes of older men were reduced by 10-14% and peak cardiac outputs were reduced by 26-30%, compared to younger men. Because these earlier studies preceded the availability of thallium scintigraphy, their samples were likely to have inadvertently included older individuals with silent coronary artery disease, which increases dramatically with age[12]. Because these earlier studies used invasive dye dilution techniques to derive stroke volume, methodological differences may also account, in part, for the discrepancy between their findings and those in Figures 4-6 and Table 1. In addition, no screening for physical conditioning status was employed in those prior studies. Deconditioning in some of their older subjects or inclusion of younger subjects with vigorous exercise habits might have caused such a result, since deconditioning is associated with a reduction of blood volume and stroke volume as well as aerobic capacity, whereas endurance training has opposite effects.

Studies using cardiac output estimates derived from regression equations[13] and acetylene rebreathing[11] during peak treadmill exercise have also suggested age-associated decreases in SVI in both sexes. Noteworthy differences between those studies and the BLSA are their much higher peak HR, especially in the older subjects. The higher HR attained during treadmill exercise compared with cycle exercise results in shorter diastolic filling periods, which when coupled with the greater orthostatic stress of walking might favor less use of the Frank-Starling mechanism. Those studies

Table 1 Hemodynamic parameters at peak effort: linear regression on age

Parameter	Males				Females			
	Intercept	Slope	r	p	Intercept	Slope	r	p
Heart rate (beats/min)	208.1	−1.02	−0.74	0.001	194.6	−0.77	−0.63	0.0001
SBP (mmHg)*	194.9	0.23	0.15	NS	160.0	0.41	0.29	0.01
DBP (mmHg)*	87.4	0.21	0.24	0.01	78.1	0.29	0.33	0.004
MAP (mmHg)*	124.9	0.19	0.21	0.02	105.0	0.34	0.41	0.0003
Cardiac index (l/min/m²)	11.5	−0.05	−0.38	0.0001	11.2	−0.05	−0.43	0.0001
TSVR (mmHg/l/min)*	5.19	0.05	0.41	0.0001	4.44	0.09	0.51	0.0001
EDVI (ml/m²)	57.7	0.38	0.36	0.0001	66.4	0.12	0.14	NS
ESVI (ml/m²)**	2.35	0.29	0.49	0.0001	8.22	0.14	0.29	0.008
SVI (ml/m²)	56.3	0.07	0.10	NS	58.1	−0.02	−0.03	NS
Ejection fraction (%)	93.2	−0.28	−0.50	0.0001	86.9	−0.15	−0.29	0.009
SBP/ESVI (mmHg/ml/m²)*	30.2	−0.28	−0.43	0.0001	21.9	−0.17	−0.34	0.004
SWI (mmHg/ml/m²)*	10 600.4	37.2	0.20	0.04	9593.0	14.5	0.10	NS

SBP, systolic blood pressure; DBP, diastolic blood pressure; MAP, mean arterial pressure; TSVR, total systemic vascular resistance; EDVI, end diastolic volume index; ESVI, end systolic volume index; SVI, stroke volume index; SWI, stroke work index; p value are for age regressions within each sex; NS, not significant; *gender difference $p < 0.05$; **age-gender interaction $p < 0.05$; from reference 4

also included very few subjects > 70 years old, which could have limited their ability to detect age-associated cardiac dilatation during exercise.

The EDVI increased over six decades in men by about 35% but not in women (Figure 5b). The ESVI increased nearly three-fold with age in men and two-fold with age in women. Figure 5 and Table 1 suggest that, with advancing age, men make greater use of the Frank–Starling mechanism than do women, both at rest and during exercise. To further illustrate this point, SVI is plotted as a function of EDVI in younger and older men and women at rest and across common external work rates (Figure 9). In subjects < 40 years old (Figure 9a), this relationship followed a nearly identical pattern in both sexes. However, for individuals > 60 years old (Figure 9b), at rest and for any given work rate the SVI and EDVI were both higher in men than in women. Furthermore, a comparison of Figures 9a and 9b, which are plotted with identical axis scales, indicates that the coordinates for older women during exercise resemble those for both younger groups, whereas those for older men lie upward and rightward of the other three groups. Thus, whether examined across relative effort levels or fixed external work rates, older men utilize the Frank–Starling relationship to a greater extent than do older women, a gender difference not present in young adults.

In comparing Figures 9a and 9b, it is noteworthy that these EDVI and SVI values in the older men also exceeded those of both younger groups, as found in an earlier study in a predominantly male BLSA cohort[14], although this earlier study did not measure absolute cardiac volumes or compare gender responses. A prior study in another cohort[15] also observed higher end-diastolic counts in older than younger men across fixed external submaximal cycle work rates. The lack of a gender difference in cardiac volumes across fixed work rates in a prior study[16] may reflect the relative youth of the subjects (mean age 38 years, with very few individuals > 60 years).

Because the absolute level of any given hemodynamic variable during exercise is determined in part by the resting value for that variable, a useful concept for examining the hemodynamic response to exercise is that of cardiovascular reserve, i.e. the

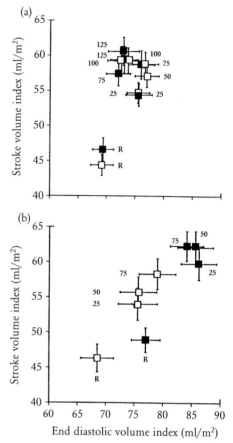

Figure 9 Relationship between stroke volume index and end-diastolic volume index in younger (< 40 years) and older (> 60 years) males (■) and females (□) across common external work rates. The numbers in bold signify work rates in watts. Values represent the mean ± SEM. (a) There is no gender difference in young subjects from rest (R) through to 125 watts, a work rate achieved by 41/43 men and 21/31 women. (b) In older subjects, at rest (R) and at each work rate through to 75 watts, a level achieved by 39/40 men and 17/21 women, the data points for older men lie upward and rightward of those for older women, indicating greater utilization of the Frank–Starling mechanism in older men[4].

difference between peak exercise and resting values. In the BLSA, the HR reserve (Figure 10a) declined with age in both sexes, but the rate of decline was greater in men than in women. The SVI reserve (Figure 10b) was unrelated to age. The reduction in ESVI from the resting level (Figure 10b) was blunted with age in both sexes, with men demonstrating greater ESVI reserve (i.e. greater reduction in ESVI) at any age. The EDVI reserve

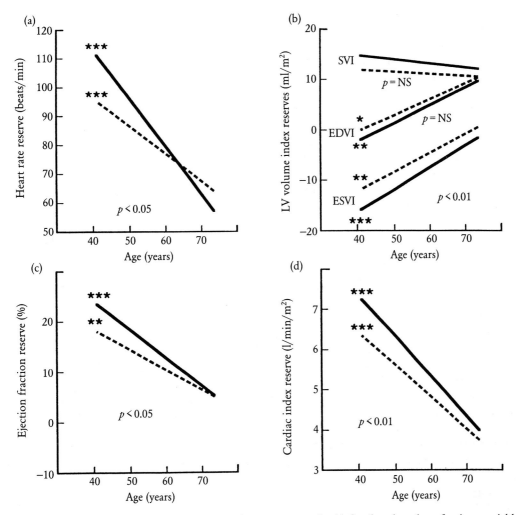

Figure 10 Linear regression analysis of cardiovascular reserve capacity (defined as the value of a given variable at peak effort minus the value at rest) as a function of age in males (—) and females (- - -). (a) Heart rate; (b) left ventricular (LV) volume indices (stroke volume index, SVI; end diastolic volume index, EDVI; end systolic volume index, ESVI); (c) ejection fraction; (d) cardiac index. There are significant age relationships within gender: *$p < 0.05$; ** $p < 0.01$; ***$p < 0.001$. The p values shown indicate gender differences by covariance analysis[4]. NS, not significant

(Figure 10b) was similar in men and women, with each sex augmenting EDVI by almost 2ml per decade from rest to peak effort. The gender differences in the absolute EDVI-age relationship at peak exercise (Table 1 and Figure 5) and in the SVI-EDVI relationship (Figure 9b) are therefore attributable to a greater resting heart size in older men than in women.

Ejection fraction (EF) (Figure 6a) and the SBP/ESVI ratio (Figure 6b) demonstrated a similar age-associated blunting in both sexes. The SWI rose by 19% with age in men but not women (Table 1)

and was higher in men than women across the full age range (Figure 6c). In a prior study[17], age-associated increases in EDVI and ESVI and declines in EF, HR and CI were observed which were similar to our present results, but the study found no gender difference except for a greater EF response in men. These results differ from those in another study population[18], which reported a 30% increase in end-diastolic counts from rest to peak effort in a small sample of women aged 32-68 years, but no change in men of similar age during a peak upright cycle protocol similar to our own.

That study also observed no gender difference in stroke counts because of a greater EF response in the men. However, a more recent study by these investigators in a larger cohort aged 20–70 years revealed no gender difference in either LV volumes or EF at peak effort[16], which is similar to the findings presented here for the BLSA. The age-associated increase in EDVI from rest to peak effort in both sexes may be a compensatory mechanism for the diminished ability of the older heart to empty completely, shown by the smaller exercise-induced reduction in ESVI and the resulting lesser augmentation of EF. This increase in EDVI allows SVI reserve and peak SVI to be successfully maintained across the adult age span, at least through to the eighth decade. Whether this age difference in hemodynamics is due to reduced myocardial reserve or to increased impedance to ejection in older subjects[19] cannot be resolved using the present data. Both myocardial reserve and aortic impedance during exercise are modulated by β-adrenergic tone, which declines with age[19].

That women exhibit a higher resting EF than do men across the full age span, but that women and men have a similar EF at peak effort (Figure 6), indicates that women display a lesser augmentation of EF from rest to peak effort than do men (Figure 10c), consistent with several prior studies[16,18,20,21]. Our results extend this finding across a very broad age range in highly screened subjects, indicating that at any age the increase in EF reserve with exercise is lower in women. Because of the age-associated decline in EF augmentation in both sexes, this physiological finding has practical diagnostic implications. If a normal exercise EF response is defined as an increase of ≥ 5 points from rest, approximately 50% of normal women > 60 years old but only 30% of older men will be misclassified as abnormal[4].

Estrogen status and cardiac hemodynamics

To determine whether supplemental estrogen administration might alter the hemodynamic response to exercise, we compared the six premeno-pausal women receiving oral contraceptives with their age peers not taking these drugs. No differences were observed in hemodynamic variables between the two groups at rest or at peak effort, or in the cardiovascular reserve (all $p > 0.2$). Similarly, the 10 women aged > 60 years receiving estrogen replacement therapy were compared with their unmedicated age peers. At rest and at peak effort, all hemodynamic variables were similar in the two groups. Only the change in ESVI from rest to peak effort differed between groups, with a decrease of 5.9 ± 3.5 ml/m^2 in unsupplemented women compared with 1.0 ± 4.2 ml/m^2 in estrogen users ($p < 0.02$).

Summary of cardiac findings in healthy men and women

To summarize our findings, normal aging in a sedentary, carefully screened subset of both sexes of the BLSA cohort was associated with significant attenuation of peak aerobic capacity, HR, EF and CI, and attenuation of the reductions in ESVI and TSVR that accompany exhaustive upright cycle exercise. The SVI, however, was well maintained across the age range in both men and women. Older age and male sex were associated with higher blood pressure responses to peak as well as sub-maximal effort. EDVI increased with age only in men both at rest and at peak effort. The relationship between SVI and EDVI was shifted upward and rightward in older men at fixed external workloads, providing evidence of greater utilization of the Frank–Starling mechanism to enhance exercise cardiac performance. Women demonstrated a greater HR response to exercise than men at all relative work rates, as well as a less prominent age-associated reduction in HR reserve. When hemodynamics were expressed as the change from rest to peak effort, both sexes showed age-associated increases in EDVI and ESVI and reductions in EF, HR and CI. However, the exercise-induced reduction in ESVI and the increase in EF, CI and SWI from rest were larger in men. These results indicate gender differences in the mechanisms for augmenting cardiac performance during upright exercise, particularly in older subjects.

CARDIAC SYMPATHETIC MODULATION

When results from various studies, including measurements of stress response in intact humans and studies of subcellular biochemistry in animal models, are integrated, it is found that a diminished responsiveness to β-adrenergic modulation and augmented vascular afterload are among the most notable changes that occur in the cardiovascular system to limit cardiovascular reserve with advancing age.

The essence of sympathetic modulation of the cardiovascular system is to (a) ensure that the heart beats faster, (b) ensure that the heart retains a small size, by reducing the diastolic filling period, reducing LV afterload, and augmenting myocardial contractility and relaxation, and (c) redistribute blood to working muscles and to skin so as to dissipate heat. All of the factors that have been identified as playing a role in deficient cardiovascular regulation with aging (heart rate filling time, cardiac and vascular afterload, myocardial contractility, and redistribution of blood flow) exhibit a deficient sympathetic modulatory component.

Apparent deficits in sympathetic modulation of these functions occur with aging in the presence of exaggerated neurotransmitter levels. Plasma levels of norepinephrine and epinephrine, during any perturbation from the supine basal state, increase to a greater extent in older vs. younger healthy humans. The age-associated increase in plasma levels of norepinephrine probably results, in part, from an increased spillover into the circulation and reduced plasma clearance. An age-associated increase in neurotransmitter spillover into the circulation during acute stress implies a greater receptor occupancy by these substances. Experimental evidence indicates that this leads to desensitization of the post-synaptic signaling components of sympathetic modulation. Indeed, multiple lines of evidence support the idea that the efficiency of post-synaptic β-adrenergic signaling declines with age[22].

One line of evidence stems from the observation that acute β-adrenergic receptor blockade changes the exercise hemodynamic profile of younger persons to resemble that of older persons.

The age-associated differences in LV early diastolic filling rate both at rest and during exercise (Figure 11a) are abolished by acute β-adrenergic blockade. The heart rate reduction during exercise in the presence of acute β-adrenergic blockade is greater in younger vs. older subjects (Figure 11b) and significant β-adrenergic blockade-induced LV dilatation occurs only in younger subjects (Figure 11c). Note, however, that the β-adrenergic blockade shown in Figure 11 causes the SVI to increase to a greater extent in younger individuals than in older ones, suggesting that mechanisms other than deficient β-adrenergic regulation compromise LV ejection. One potential mechanism is an age-associated decrease in maximum intrinsic myocardial contractility. Another likely mechanism is enhanced vascular afterload due to the structural changes in compliance arteries, and possibly also due to impaired vasorelaxation during exercise. Other evidence for a diminished efficacy of synaptic β-adrenergic receptor signaling is the fact that cardiovascular responses at rest to β-adrenergic agonist infusions decrease with age.

CARDIOVASCULAR AGING IN HEALTH AND THE ASSOCIATED RISK OF CARDIOVASCULAR DISEASE

In the USA, cardiovascular diseases (coronary artery disease, myocardial infarction, stroke and heart failure) are the leading causes of mortality, accounting for over 40% of deaths in those aged 65 years and above. Over 80% of all cardiovascular deaths occur in this age group. Thus age is the major risk factor for cardiovascular disease. Figure 12 depicts how the clinical manifestations and the prognoses of these cardiovascular diseases worsen with age, because in older individuals the specific pathophysiological mechanisms are superimposed on heart and vascular substrates that are modified by aging. The horizontal line separating the lower and upper parts of Figure 12 represents the clinical practice 'threshold' for disease recognition. Above the line, cardiovascular changes are classified as 'diseases' that lead to heart and brain failure. Changes presently thought to occur as a result of the 'normal' or 'physiologic' aging process are depicted below the line.

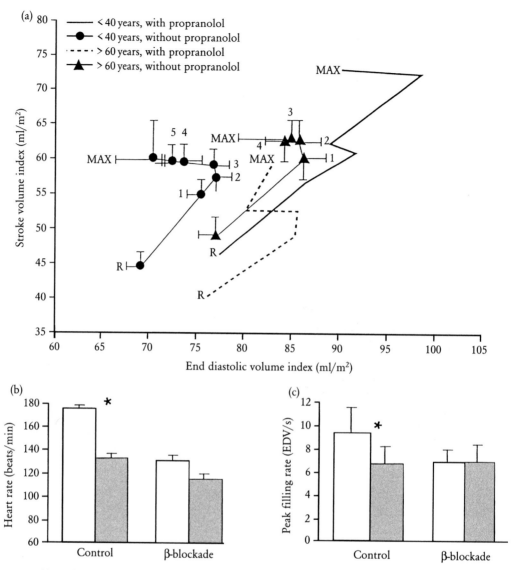

Figure 11 (a) Stroke volume index as a function of end diastolic volume index at seated rest (R) and during graded cycle workloads (1-5, MAX) in the upright seated position in healthy men in the presence and absence of β-adrenergic blockade (propranolol). Note that in the absence of propranolol the data points for older men (—▲—) are shifted rightward of those for younger men (—●—). This indicates that the left ventricle (LV) of older men in the sitting position compared to that of younger men operates from a greater preload both at rest and during submaximal and maximal exercise. Propranolol markedly shifts the data points rightward in younger men (——), but does not markedly shift the data points in older men (- - -). Thus, with respect to this assessment of ventricular function, β-adrenergic blockade with propranolol makes younger men appear like older ones. The abolition of the age-associated differences in the LV function curve after administration of propranolol is accompanied by a reduction or abolition of the age-associated reduction in heart rate at maximum effort (b). (c) The age-associated reduction in peak LV diastolic filling rate at maximum effort in healthy subjects is abolished during exercise in the presence of β-adrenergic blockade with propranolol[24]. Blank columns, men aged < 40 years; shaded columns, men aged > 60 years; *$p < 0.05$, age effect

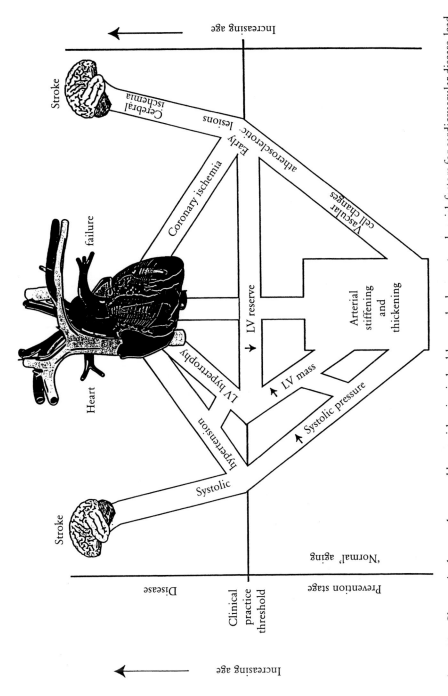

Figure 12 Changes in the vasculature and heart with aging in health may also be construed as risk factors for cardiovascular disease, leading to heart and brain disorders in older age (see text for details). LV, left ventricle. Reprinted from reference 25

These age-associated changes in cardiac and vascular properties alter the substrate upon which cardiovascular disease is superimposed in several ways (Table 2). First, they lower the extent of disease severity required to cross the threshold that results in clinically significant signs and symptoms. For example, mild ischemia-induced relaxation abnormalities may be asymptomatic in a younger individual but may cause dyspnea in an older individual, who, by virtue of age alone, has pre-existing slowed and delayed early diastolic relaxation. Age-associated changes may also alter the manifestations and presentation of common cardiac diseases. This usually occurs in patients with acute infarction in whom the diagnosis is delayed because of atypical symptoms, resulting in

Table 2 Relationship of cardiovascular human aging in health to cardiovascular diseases[26]

Age-associated changes	Plausible mechanisms	Possible relation to human disease
Cardiovascular structural remodeling		
Increase in vascular intimal thickness	increased migration of and increased matrix production by VSMC, possible derivation of intimal cells from other sources	early stages of atherosclerosis
Increase in vascular stiffness	elastin fragmentation, increased elastase activity, increased collagen production by VSMC and increased cross-linking of collagen, altered growth factor regulation/tissue repair mechanisms	systolic hypertension, left ventricular wall thickening, stroke, atherosclerosis
Increase in LV wall thickness	increased LV myocyte size with altered Ca^{2+} handling, decreased myocyte number (necrotic and apoptotic death), altered growth factor regulation, focal matrix collagen deposition	retarded early diastolic cardiac filling, increased cardiac filling pressure, lower threshold for dyspnea, increased likelihood of heart failure with relatively normal systolic function
Increase in left atrial size	increased left atrial pressure/volume	increase in prevalence of lone atrial fibrillation and other atrial arrhythmias
Cardiovascular functional changes		
Altered regulation of vascular tone	decreased NO production/effects	vascular stiffening, hypertension, early atherosclerosis
Reduced threshold for cell Ca^{2+} overload	changes in gene expression of proteins that regulate Ca^{2+} handling; increased ω6 : ω3 polyunsaturated fatty acids ratio in cardiac membranes	lower threshold for atrial and ventricular arrhythmia, increased myocyte death, increased fibrosis, reduced diastolic and systolic function
Decrease in cardiovascular reserve	increased vascular load, decreased intrinsic myocardial contractility, increased plasma levels of catecholamines, decreased β-adrenergic modulation of heart rate myocardial contractility and vascular tone due to post-synaptic signaling deficits	lower threshold for, and increased severity of heart failure
Reduced physical activity		
	learned lifestyle	exaggerated age changes in some aspects of cardiovascular structure and function, negative impact on atherosclerotic vascular disease, hypertension and heart failure

VSMC, vascular smooth muscle cells; LV, left ventricle; NO, nitric oxide

increased time to onset of therapy. Age-associated changes, including those in β-adrenergic responsiveness and in vascular stiffness, also influence the selection of therapeutic interventions in older individuals with cardiovascular disease. Processes presently considered to reflect 'normal' or 'physiologic' aging therefore perhaps ought to be construed as specific risk factors for the diseases that they relate to, and thus might be targets for interventions designed to decrease the occurrence and/or manifestations of cardiovascular disease at later ages. Such a strategy would thus advocate the treating of 'normal' aging. However, additional studies of the specific risks of each 'normal' age-associated change and the effectiveness of treatment regimens to delay or prevent each change are required for this strategy to be put into practice.

CAN RISKY ASPECTS OF CARDIOVASCULAR AGING BE REDUCED OR PREVENTED?

There is some evidence to indicate that diet and exercise habits affect both the heart and blood vessels of older individuals. Physical conditioning appears to lessen the vascular stiffening associated with aging[27,28] (Figure 13a), and the augmentation of the late systolic peak in arterial pressure, an index of arterial stiffness, is inversely related to aerobic capacity in sedentary individuals[5]. Endothelial function in older persons also improves following exercise conditioning, and allows the maximum LV ejection fraction to approach that in younger persons[30]. Some age-associated vascular changes in humans, depicted in Figure 2, also occur in rodents[31], and are dramatically retarded by chronic angiotensin-converting enzyme inhibition. Novel agents that break non-enzymatic cross-links reduce the magnitude of measures of arterial stiffness in rodents, dogs and non-human primates[27,32,33], and are presently under study with respect to their efficacy in reducing arterial stiffness in humans.

Physical conditioning can improve the aerobic capacity of older individuals. The improvement is generally attributable to increases in both maximum cardiac output and O_2 utilization. Exercise conditioning improvements in cardiac output are derived only from increases in stroke volume (SV), as the age-associated reduction in the maximum heart rate persists following conditioning (Figure 13b). The improvement in SV derived from conditioning is due largely to an increase in the ability to eject blood from the heart, as reflected in a reduction of ESV (Figure 13b) and an increase in ejection fraction. This appears to be attributable to an augmentation in intrinsic myocardial contractility and a reduction in vascular afterload. The impaired communication between the brain and heart with aging (i.e. diminished effects of β-adrenergic stimulation) appears not to change with exercise conditioning.

These preventive lifestyle or pharmacological strategies can be undertaken to some extent even now, but additional studies of the specific risks of each 'normal' age-associated change are required. Future genetic characterization of individuals will allow person-specific stratification with respect to risk, efficacy and cost-effectiveness of preventive measures. Finally, an elucidation of the age-associated cardiovascular changes at the cellular and molecular levels may also make gene therapy very plausible for healthy people as they age.

SUMMARY

In summary, there is an age-associated increase in vascular afterload on the heart which is due to arterial stiffening and is reflected in the age-associated modest increase in systolic blood pressure at rest. In healthy individuals, these vascular changes are compensated for, in large part, by the age-associated changes in the architecture and contractile properties of the heart which, despite reductions in aortic distensibility, allow the aged heart to pump a normal quantity of blood at rest. In the seated upright position at rest, the heart rate decreases with aging in men, and the ventricular preload (diastolic volume) increases modestly, although the early rapid filling rate is slowed. The fraction of end-diastolic volume ejected with each beat (ejection fraction) does not decline with age. Major age-associated alterations in the cardiovascular response to exercise are evident. There is a striking age-associated decrease in the maximum heart rate, but the maximum stroke volume in older individuals is preserved via

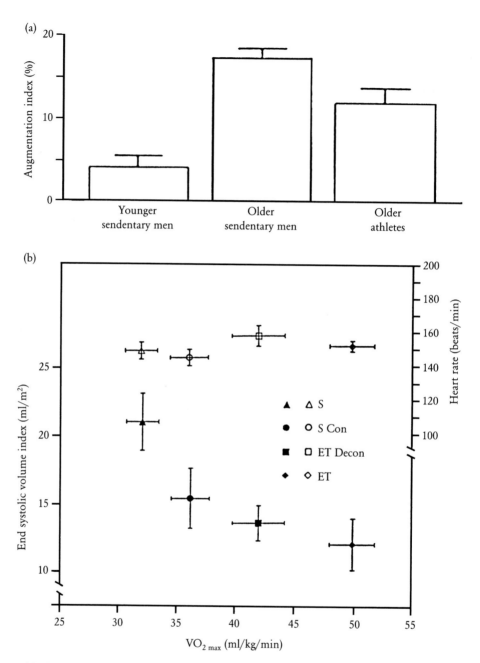

Figure 13 (a) The increase in carotid augmentation index in highly trained older men (60–85 years) is only about half of that expected on the basis of age[5]. (b) Heart rate (empty symbols) and end systolic volume (filled symbols) across a broad range of aerobic capacity in healthy males who have been exercise conditioned or deconditioned[29]. S, sedentary; SCon, sedentary after conditioning; ETDecon, exercise trained but stopped for study to become detrained/deconditioned; ET, exercise trained

the Frank-Starling mechanism. The extent to which the end-systolic volume is reduced and the ejection fraction increases at peak exercise are reduced with aging, and these deficits probably result from deficient intrinsic myocardial performance, and from an augmented afterload, both due, in part, to a deficiency in β-adrenergic stimulation to enhance myocardial contractility or reduce the pulsatile components of vascular afterload. A decrease in the maximum capacity for physical work with ageing is due to both diminished cardiac (heart rate) and peripheral factors. Some of the cardiovascular deficits that accompany aging in health can be retarded by physical conditioning. Alterations in cardiac function that exceed the identified limits for changes in healthy elderly individuals are most likely to be manifestations of the interaction between excessive physical deconditioning and cardiovascular disease, which is unfortunately so prevalent within economically developed populations. Finally, many of the 'normal' aging changes described herein in apparently healthy men and women should not be considered to be 'normal' but rather as major risk factors for cardiovascular diseases. These age-associated changes in cardiac structure and function are likely to be the major reason why age is in itself the major risk factor for cardiovascular disease. The next decade will hopefully witness interventions to retard or prevent these age-associated cardiovascular changes.

ACKNOWLEDGEMENT

The author wishes to thank Christina R. Link for her editorial assistance in preparing this manuscript.

References

1. Lakatta EG. Cardiovascular aging: perspectives from humans to rodents. *Am J Geriatr Cardiol* 1998;7:32–45
2. Gerstenblith G, Frederiksen J, Yin FCP, Fortuin NJ, Lakatta EG, Weisfeldt ML. Echocardiographic assessment of a normal adult aging population. *Circulation* 1977;56:273–8
3. Nagai J, Metter EJ, Earley CJ, Kemper MK, Becker LC, Lakatta EG, Fleg JL. Increased carotid artery intimal-medial thickness in asymptomatic older subjects with exercise-induced myocardial ischemia. *Circulation* 1998;98:1504–9
4. Fleg JL, O'Connor F, Gerstenblith G, Becker LC, Clulow J, Schulman SP, Lakatta EG. Impact of age on the cardiovascular response to dynamic upright exercise in healthy men and women. *J Appl Physiol* 1995;78:890–900
5. Vaitkevicius PV, Fleg JL, Engel JH, O'Connor FC, Wright JG, Lakatta LE, Yin FCP, Lakatta EG. Effects of age and aerobic capacity on arterial stiffness in healthy adults. *Circulation* 1993;88:1456–62
6. Celermajer DS, Sorensen KE, Spiegelhalter DJ, Georgapoulos D, Robinson J, Deanfield JE. Aging is associated with endothelial dysfunction in healthy men years before the age-related decline in women, *J Am Coll Cardiol* 1994;24:471–6
7. Swinne CJ, Shapiro EP, Lima SD, Fleg JL. Age-associated changes in left ventricular diastolic performance during isometric exercise in normal subjects. *Am J Cardiol* 1992;69:823–6
8. Lakatta EG. Cardiovascular regulatory mechanisms in advanced age. *Physiol Rev* 1993;73:413–65
9. Granath A, Jonsson B, Strandell T. Circulation in healthy old men studied by right heart catheterization at rest and during exercise in supine and sitting positions. *Acta Med Scand* 1964;176: 425–46
10. Julius S, Amery A, Whitlock LS, Conway J. Influence of age on the hemodynamic response to exercise. *Circulation* 1967;36:222–30
11. Ogawa T, Spina RJ, Mahia WH III, Kohrt WM, Schechtman KB, Holloszy JO, Ehsani AA. Effects of aging, sex and physical training on cardiovascular responses to exercise. *Circulation* 1992; 86:494–503
12. Fleg JL, Gerstenblith G, Zonderman AB, Becker LC, Weisfeldt ML, Costa PT, Lakatta EG. Prevalence and prognostic significance of exercise-induced silent myocardial ischemia detected by thallium scintigraphy and electrocardiography in asymptomatic volunteers. *Circulation* 1990;81:428–36
13. Hossack KF, Bruce RA. Peak cardiac function in sedentary normal men and women: comparison of age-related changes. *J Appl Physiol* 1982;53:799–804
14. Rodeheffer RJ, Gerstenblith G, Becker LC, Fleg JL, Weisfeldt ML, Lakatta EG. Exercise cardiac output is maintained with advancing age in healthy human subjects: cardiac dilatation and increased stroke volume compensate for a diminished heart rate. *Circulation* 1984;69:203–13

15. Mann DL, Denenberg BS, Gash AK, Makler PT, Bove AA. Effects of age on ventricular performance during graded supine exercise. *Am Heart J* 1986;111:108–15

16. Sullivan MJ, Cobb FR, Higginbotham MB. Stroke volume increases by similar mechanism during upright exercise in normal men and women. *Am J Cardiol* 1991;67:1405–12

17. Younis LT, Melin JA, Robert AR, Detry JMR. Influence of age and sex on left ventricular volumes and ejection fraction during upright exercise in normal subjects. *Eur Heart J* 1990;11:916–24

18. Higginbotham MB, Morris KG, Coleman RE, Cobb FR. Sex-related differences in the normal cardiac response to upright exercise. *Circulation* 1984;70:357–66

19. Yin FCP, Weisfeldt ML, Milnor WR. Role of aortic input impedance in the decreased cardiovascular response to exercise with aging in dogs. *J Clin Invest* 1981;68:28–38

20. Adams KF, Vincent LM, McAllister SM, El-Ashmawy H, Sheps DS. The influence of age and gender on left ventricular response to supine exercise in asymptomatic normal subjects. *Am Heart J* 1987;113:732–40

21. Kuo LC, Billi R, Thornby J, Roberts R, Verani MS. Effects of exercise tolerance, age and gender on the specificity of radionuclide angiography: sequential ejection fraction analysis during multistage exercise. *Am Heart J* 1987;113:1130–89

22. Xiao RP, Spurgeon HA, O'Connor F, Lakatta EG. Age-associated changes in β-adrenergic modulation on rat cardiac excitation–contraction coupling. *J Clin Invest* 1994;94:2051

23. Fleg JL, Schulman S, O'Connor FC, Becker LC, Gerstenblith G, Clulow JF, Renlund DG, Lakatta EG. Effects of acute β-adrenergic receptor blockade on age-associated changes in cardiovascular performance during dynamic exercise. *Circulation* 1994;90:2333–41

24. Schulman SP, Lakatta EG, Fleg JL, Lakatta L, Becker LC, Gerstenblith G. Age-related decline in left ventricular filling at rest and exercise. *Am J Physiol* 1992;263:H1932–H1938

25. Lakatta EG, Weisfeldt ML, Gerstenblith G. The aging heart: structure, function and disease. In Braunwald E, ed. *Heart Disease. A Textbook of Cardiovascular Medicine*, 5th edn. Philadelphia: W.B. Saunders, 1996: 1687–1703

26. Lakatta EG. Research agenda for cardiovascular aging - humans to molecules. *Am J Geriatr Cardiol* 2000;9:1–13

27. Vaitkevicius PV, Lane M, Spurgeon H, Ingram DK, Roth GS, Egan JJ, Vasan S, Wagle DR, Ulrich P, Brines M, Wuerth JP, Cerami A, Lakatta EG. A cross-link breaker has sustained effects on arterial and ventricular properties in older rhesus monkeys. *Proc Natl Acad Sci USA* 2001;in press

28. Tanaka H, DeSouza CA, Seals DR. Absence of age-related increase in central arterial stiffness in physically active women. *Arterioscler Thromb Vasc Biol* 1998;18:127–32

29. Schulman SP, Fleg JL, Busby-Whitehead J, Goldberg AP, Hagberg JM, O'Connor FC, Gerstenblith G, Becker LC, Lakatta LE, Lakatta EG. Continuum of cardiovascular performance across a broad range of fitness levels in healthy older men. *Circulation* 1996;94:359–67

30. Rywik TM, Blackman MR, Yataco AR, Vaitkevicius PV, Zink RC, Cottrell EH, Wright JG, Katzel LI, Fleg JL. Enhanced endothelial vasoreactivity in endurance trained older men. *J Appl Physiol* 1999;87:2136–42

31. Michel JB, Heudes D, Michel O, *et al*. Effect of chronic ANGI-converting enzyme inhibition on aging processes: II. Large arteries. *Am J Physiol* 1994;267:R124

32. Wolfenbuttel BHR, Boulanger CM, Crijns FRL, Huijberts MSP, Poitevin P, Swennen GMN, Vasan S, Egan JJ, Ulrich P, Cerami A, Levy B. Breakers of advanced glycation end products restore large artery properties in experimental diabetes. *Proc Natl Acad Sci USA* 1998;95:4630–4

33. Asif M, Egan J, Vasan S, Jyothirmayi G-N, Masurekar M-R, Lopez S, Willams C, Torres R-L, Wagle D, Ulrich P, Cerami A, Frines M, Regan T-J. An advanced glycation endproduct cross-link breaker can reverse age-related increases in myocardial stiffness. *Proc Natl Acad Sci USA* 2000;97:2809–13

Lipid metabolism

3

J. C. Stevenson

INTRODUCTION

The processes by which exogenous and endogenous lipids are transported and metabolized in the body are complex and finely tuned. Abnormalities in these processes can lead to significant health problems. The role of lipids in coronary heart disease, which is potentially life-threatening, is important and should not be understated. This chapter reviews the transport, structure, function and classification of lipids in the body and assesses the roles of lipoproteins and other lipids in coronary heart disease. Also discussed are the effects of the menopause on lipid profile and risk factors for coronary heart disease.

LIPID TRANSPORT

Cholesterol, triglycerides and other lipids are solubilized and transported in the circulation by lipoproteins, which are microscopic, plasma-soluble complexes of protein molecules with lipid. Lipoproteins have a hydrophobic core of cholesterol esters and triglycerides surrounded by a shell of phospholipids, non-esterified cholesterol and lipoprotein-specific proteins (apolipoproteins). The main functions of lipoproteins are to solubilize highly hydrophobic lipids and to regulate the movement of particular lipids into and out of specific target cells and tissues. The circulation of lipoproteins enables the transport of lipids to the body tissues, where they are used as fuel (triglycerides are an essential fuel with their storage in adipose tissue providing the body's principal energy store) and to provide cholesterol for the cell manufacturing process (cholesterol is an essential component of cell membranes and is also a precursor for steroid hormones).

PROTEIN COMPONENT OF LIPOPROTEINS

The type of protein in the lipoprotein determines the class of lipoprotein. The major protein components (apolipoproteins) of lipoproteins are shown in Table 1.

Apolipoprotein (apo) AI is the principal protein component of high-density lipoproteins (HDL). The HDL subfractions HDL_2 and HDL_3 contain apo AI (it is the principal protein in HDL_2) and HDL_3 also contains a significant amount of apo AII. Apo B_{100} is the main protein in low-density lipoproteins (LDL) and very-low-density lipoproteins (VLDL); it is also present in lipoprotein(a). Another apo B protein, apo B_{48}, is present in chylomicrons, and apo(a) is present in lipoprotein(a).

This list is by no means complete. There are many other protein components that will not be discussed in this review, such as apo C and its subclasses, and apo E, which may be important in cholesterol transfer.

CLASSIFICATION OF LIPOPROTEINS

Lipoproteins are classified according to size and density (Figure 1).

Table 1 Major protein components of lipoproteins

Apolipoprotein	Present in
Apo AI	HDL_2 and HDL_3
Apo AII	HDL_3
Apo B_{100}	LDL, VLDL and lipoprotein(a)
Apo B_{48}	chylomicrons
Apo(a)	lipoprotein(a)

Apo, apolipoprotein; HDL, high-density lipoprotein; LDL, low-density lipoprotein; VLDL, very-low-density lipoprotein

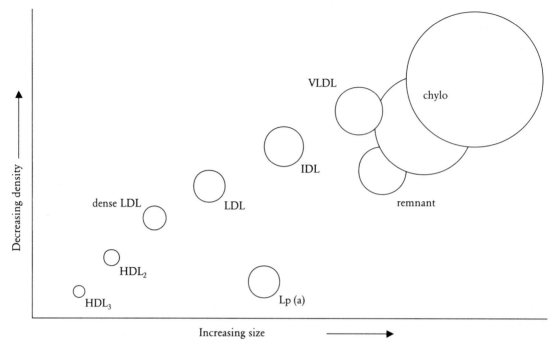

Figure 1 Classification of lipoproteins. Adapted from Segrest JP. Non-LDL lipid risk factors: HDL; triglycerides; small, dense LDL; and Lp(a). *Clin Rev* 2000; Spring: 23–8. Reproduced with permission from Southern Association for Primary Care

Chylomicrons and chylomicron remnants

Chylomicrons are large particles (80–500 nm in diameter) that enable the fat from the diet to be absorbed. They have a low density (< 0.94 g/cm³) because they are rich in triglycerides and have a protein content of less than 2%. Chylomicrons transport the lipids that are obtained from the diet (i.e. exogenous lipids) from the intestine to the liver and adipose tissue.

The products of digested fat after a meal or snack (i.e. triglycerides, phospholipids and cholesterol esters) are taken up by the gastrointestinal enterocytes, where they are combined with an apolipoprotein (apo B₄₈) to form chylomicrons and then secreted into the lymph. Chylomicrons enter the blood system from the lymphatic system via the thoracic duct. Once in the circulation, chylomicrons are combined with apo C, which comes from HDL. This activates the enzyme lipoprotein lipase, which is found in various tissues and organs in the body, particularly in the vascular endothelium. Lipoprotein lipase hydrolyzes and releases the triglycerides from the

chylomicrons; the released triglycerides can then be used as fuel. The chylomicrons, therefore, transfer and transport energy from ingested food to the cells in the body in the form of triglycerides.

The release of triglycerides from chylomicrons leaves cholesterol-rich residues known as chylomicron remnants. These are cleared in the liver by specific chylomicron remnant receptors and by the apo B receptors, which also clear LDL (these receptors recognize the apo B₄₈ component of chylomicron remnants). Chylomicron remnants are atherogenic, so it is important to clear them from the blood as quickly as possible. The rate of clearance of these and other atherogenic particles is increased by sex steroids.

Very-low-density lipoproteins

Exogenous triglycerides are transported from ingested food to the cells in the body to provide energy. As food intake is not continuous, and there are times of fasting (e.g. during the night), there is also need for an endogenous energy transport system. VLDL are synthesized and secreted by the liver to transport endogenous triglycerides to the tissues.

VLDL contain apo B_{100} and are very rich in triglycerides and cholesterol. The free cholesterol in VLDL is transferred to HDL, where it is esterified to produce cholesterol esters. Cholesterol ester transfer protein (CETP) then transfers the cholesterol esters back to VLDL in exchange for triglycerides via an active transport mechanism. Triglycerides are released from VLDL in the circulation mainly by lipoprotein lipase. The removal of triglycerides from VLDL produces intermediate-density lipoproteins (IDL), then LDL, and finally small dense LDL.

Exogenous versus endogenous triglycerides

The particles carrying exogenous and endogenous triglycerides differ in the type of apoprotein present (chylomicrons contain apo B_{48} and VLDL contain apo B_{100}). This fundamental difference could be used to distinguish between these particles; however, apo B_{48} is difficult to measure. Development of a sensitive method for the measurement of apo B_{48} would enable easier differentiation between the particles transporting exogenous and endogenous triglycerides.

Low-density lipoproteins

LDL are derived from VLDL (via IDL) and contain apo B_{100}. LDL cross the vascular endothelium and enter the tissue fluid, thereby providing a source of cholesterol to the cells. After delivery of cholesterol, LDL are cleared from the circulation, primarily by apo B_{100} receptors. LDL are regarded as the 'bad' type of cholesterol because they are particularly associated with the development of atherosclerotic plaques and CHD.

LDL cross the vascular endothelium and continuously drift in and out of the subendothelial space, without causing harm. Damage only occurs when LDL are present in excess and become lodged in the subendothelial space. Unfortunately, in humans, LDL circulate in concentrations near to the saturation point of the apo B_{100} receptors that clear these lipoproteins; therefore, only a small increase in circulating LDL will overwhelm the system for their removal. When the apo B_{100} receptors are saturated, excess LDL are removed by non-receptor membrane binding and scavenger mechanisms, such as macrophage receptor binding.

Triglyceride levels and lipoprotein metabolism

It has recently been shown that the metabolism of LDL is linked to the level of endogenous triglycerides[1,2]. Increased triglyceride levels are associated with the formation of triglyceride-rich VLDL and LDL. The hydrolysis and release of triglycerides from these lipoproteins by lipoprotein lipase cause increased production of small dense LDL, which are the most atherogenic LDL, with the possible exception of lipoprotein(a). Small dense LDL are highly atherogenic because they are more readily cleared through scavenger mechanisms (e.g. via macrophages) and are more likely to become lodged in the arterial wall, where they are more susceptible to oxidative damage; this increases the likelihood of atheroma.

Small dense LDL are a major risk factor and a risk marker for CHD, particularly in females. The levels of small dense LDL showed a greater increase in female patients with CHD compared with male patients[3].

LDL ingested in food are not necessarily harmful, particularly if LDL are cleared rapidly from the circulation in an undamaged form. Problems arise when clearance is affected because the apo B_{100} receptors are saturated, defective (e.g. familial hypercholesterolaemia, see later) or malfunctioning, and/or the LDL is oxidatively damaged.

There is a significant, negative relationship between the level of fasting (i.e. endogenous) serum triglycerides and the size of the LDL. The higher the triglyceride level, the smaller and denser are the LDL particles.

There is a similar relationship between VLDL triglyceride content and the size of LDL. The more triglyceride-rich the VLDL, the more it is metabolized into the smaller, denser LDL particles.

Lipoprotein(a)

Lipoprotein(a) is larger and denser than LDL (Figure 1) and contains apo B_{100} and apo(a). Apo(a) is a structural mutant of plasminogen. It comprises plasminogen repeated many times with repeated cringles in the domain (the type of lipoprotein(a) is determined by the number of cringles within the apo(a) component).

Lipid retention and atherogenesis

Lipoprotein(a) binds avidly to arterial proteoglycans; this retains the lipoprotein in the subendothelial space, where it is susceptible to oxidative damage. The presence of proteoglycans in the artery is often related to shear stresses and turbulent blood flow, so the physical characteristics of the artery determine the proteoglycan content. The presence of proteoglycan-bound lipoprotein(a) in the artery enhances the binding and retention of LDL in the subendothelial space, thereby increasing the susceptibility of LDL to oxidation. Oxidized LDL is a chemoattractant to smooth muscle cells and macrophages, which then develop into foam cells. These steps are considered to be key in the development of atheroma (Figure 2)[4].

Lipoprotein(a) and LDL retention are therefore potentially important factors in atherogenesis.

Lipoprotein(a) and LDL levels

As lipoprotein(a) is a mutant of plasminogen, it has been postulated that it may compete with plasminogen and inhibit fibrinolysis, thereby encouraging clot formation and propagation. This has not been proven. Increased levels of lipoprotein(a) are known to be associated with an increase in coronary heart disease, and lipoprotein(a) has been used as an independent lipoprotein risk marker for coronary heart disease; however, it is not that simple.

We have previously shown that young women with endometriosis (a relatively common gynecological disorder in which endometrial tissue is found outside the lining of the uterine cavity), have very high levels of lipoprotein(a). Yet this is not a group who have an increased risk for coronary heart disease, probably because they have very low levels of LDL cholesterol[5]. Certain populations in Africa have also been shown to have high lipoprotein(a) levels, but extremely low LDL cholesterol levels and no coronary heart disease[6]. This implies that lipoprotein(a) is an important

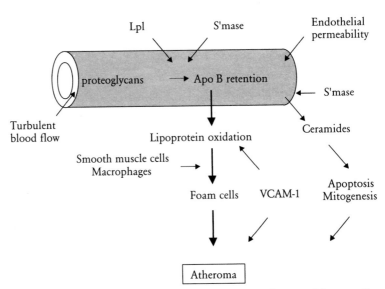

Figure 2 Lipid retention and atherogenesis. Lpl, lipoprotein lipase; S'mase, sphingomyelinase. Adapted from reference 4

risk factor for coronary heart disease only in the presence of pre-existing high levels of LDL.

High-density lipoproteins

HDL are produced by the liver and the gut and take up free cholesterol by reverse cholesterol transport. After uptake by HDL, cholesterol is esterified by lecithin : cholesterol acyl transferase (LCAT) and then removed from the lipoprotein by hepatic lipase, or transferred to VLDL in exchange for triglycerides. HDL are catabolized by hepatic lipase. The activity of this enzyme is increased in obesity, and by androgens. Obese people and users of androgenic steroids, therefore, usually have lower levels of HDL. Provided there is no sex steroid effect, HDL is normally inversely related to the level of triglycerides. The HDL subfraction HDL_2 is thought to be the most important lipoprotein subfraction in terms of cardiovascular protection; higher levels of HDL_2 are associated with lower coronary heart disease risk. HDL_3 is a precursor of HDL_2. It is not clear whether the HDL_3 subfraction has any further role.

The importance of the apolipoprotein component of HDL in atherogenesis has been assessed in animal models in which a sort of 'atheroma' is induced. Mice that are genetically manipulated to overexpress apo AI (the major apoprotein in HDL_2) had reduced atheroma compared with non-manipulated controls[7]. In contrast, mice that overexpress apo AII (which is mainly found in HDL_3) had increased atheroma[8,9]. Apo AI (and HDL_2) therefore seems to be more beneficial for protection against atheroma.

Although high levels of HDL are considered to be cardioprotective, reducing HDL cholesterol may not necessarily be detrimental if it is mainly the HDL_3 subfraction (and therefore the apo AII) that is reduced. There is no clinical evidence to suggest that reducing overall HDL levels reduces reverse cholesterol transport.

Data from healthy postmenopausal women have shown that there is a negative relationship between the levels of triglycerides and HDL_2 (i.e. the higher the triglyceride level, the lower the HDL_2 subfraction), but there is no relationship between triglycerides and HDL_3 [10].

Triglycerides

Triglycerides are a major energy source and are stored in the adipose tissue. They provide much more energy than glucose, and are utilized in preference to glucose by the myocardium. Fuel, as triglycerides, is constantly supplied to the cells via chylomicrons (exogenous triglycerides) and VLDL (endogenous triglycerides). There is an inverse relationship between triglyceride and HDL concentrations because triglycerides are related to increased HDL catabolism. Triglycerides are also related to cardiovascular risk factors, such as insulin resistance, obesity and diabetes mellitus (one of the major causes of coronary heart disease in women). Very high levels of triglycerides can cause acute pancreatitis, which is potentially life-threatening.

LIPID ABNORMALITIES

Hypercholesterolemia

Hypercholesterolemia affects at least one-third of the adult population in the western world. Although cholesterol is a major risk factor for coronary heart disease, it is not the only risk factor, and should be put into perspective. The majority of patients who develop coronary heart disease and have myocardial infarctions, for example, do not have raised cholesterol, and the majority of patients who have raised cholesterol do not have coronary heart disease.

There are several causes of hypercholesterolemia, including hereditary factors, overproduction of VLDL, hypothyroidism, diabetes mellitus, nephrotic syndrome, obstructive liver disease, and drugs, such as thiazides, retinoids and glucocorticoids. These factors should be taken into consideration when assessing the lipid profile of a patient.

In hereditary cholesterol disorders, genetic abnormalities of the LDL receptor result in reduced clearance and catabolism of LDL. More commonly, overproduction of VLDL leads to increased amounts of LDL, which overload the receptor clearance system. Although most patients presenting with hypercholesterolemia will fall into this category, postmenopausal women should be assessed for secondary causes, such as hypothyroidism and diabetes. Postmenopausal women are at high risk of developing these conditions, and therefore they should be excluded or identified.

Hypertriglyceridemia

Hypertriglyceridemia is most commonly seen in patients with obesity and diabetes mellitus. Patients with diabetes mellitus are also likely to be dyslipidemic in terms of HDL and LDL concentrations. Other causes of hypertriglyceridemia include alcohol, chronic renal failure and, very rarely, acute myocardial infarction. Triglyceride levels are raised by some non-selective β-blockers and by orally administered estrogens, whereas they are reduced by non-orally administered estrogens.

Hyperlipidemia

Hyperlipidemia (i.e. raised cholesterol and triglyceride levels) is seen in patients with hypothyroidism, diabetes mellitus, chronic renal disease and liver disease. Drugs inducing hyperlipidemia include thiazides, corticosteroids and retinoids.

CORONARY HEART DISEASE

Cholesterol and coronary heart disease

Cholesterol is an important factor in the development of coronary heart disease. Atheroma can be induced in animals fed a high cholesterol diet, but it is debatable whether there is a true animal model for human atheroma. The Cynomolgus macaques have a condition very similar to human atheroma, but to induce atheroma in animals takes much effort; the serum cholesterol has to be raised to at least 20 mmol/l, which is rarely seen in humans. The exception is in patients with homozygous hypercholesterolemia, who have extremely high cholesterol levels and develop coronary heart disease at a young age. They die in their teens and early 20s from coronary heart disease as a direct result of high cholesterol levels.

Coronary heart disease is more common in human populations that have high saturated fat diets and a high prevailing cholesterol level. Coronary heart disease rates are low in populations with a low cholesterol level, e.g. in Japan. The risk of coronary heart disease changes when members of the population migrate, quite possibly because of changes in diet. Raised cholesterol levels and increased risk of coronary heart disease are probably the result of both environmental and genetic factors.

Further evidence of the importance of cholesterol in coronary heart disease is that cholesterol-lowering therapies have been conclusively shown to reduce the risk of coronary heart disease. There is a definite relationship between cholesterol and coronary heart disease, but it is not a simple one because the majority of people with coronary heart disease do not have inappropriately raised cholesterol levels.

Lipoproteins and coronary heart disease

There is a relationship between the levels of LDL and the incidence of coronary heart disease. Approximately, for every 1% increase in LDL, there is a 2% increase in coronary heart disease, and, for every 1% decrease in LDL by therapy, there is a 2% decrease in coronary heart disease. Interestingly, LDL levels appear to be less important in the development of coronary heart disease in women compared with men. The levels of HDL and triglycerides are thought to be more important in women.

Many observational studies have been conducted to assess the roles of lipoproteins and other lipids in coronary heart disease. Extrapolation of results from these studies to give statements such as 'HDL cholesterol is an important independent risk factor for coronary heart disease' is scientifically unsound. HDL cannot be an independent risk factor because it is dependent on the other lipids.

The relative benefits of changing HDL levels compared with changing triglyceride levels in the development of coronary heart disease are not yet known. This is a key point because estrogens and progestogens often have the unusual effect of causing both HDL and triglyceride levels to be moved in the same direction (i.e. both increased or both decreased), so they do not change both parameters in a beneficial direction (or only rarely). This causes a dilemma; is it better for the patient to have decreased triglycerides at the expense of decreased HDL, or increased HDL with concomitant increased triglycerides? Unfortunately, the answer is not known.

Triglycerides and coronary heart disease

Triglycerides are also an important factor in the development of coronary heart disease. As discussed earlier, fasting triglyceride levels are related to lipid metabolism. They are positively associated with LDL levels[10] and negatively associated with LDL particle size[1], so the higher the triglyceride level, the smaller and denser the LDL. They are also negatively related to HDL$_2$ subfraction[10].

High triglyceride levels are also related to the following cardiovascular risk factors: increased insulin, increased non-esterified fatty acids, increased uric acid, which may reflect abnormalities of the glycolytic pathways, increased factor VII and increased plasminogen activator inhibitor (PAI)-1 (i.e. the hemostatic factors that are linked to atherogenesis), and abnormalities of vascular function (high triglyceride levels are significantly related to increased E-selectin, a cell adhesion molecule, and increased angiotensin-converting enzyme activity[2]). Clearly, endogenous triglycerides are linked with many risk factors for coronary heart disease.

INSULIN RESISTANCE SYNDROME

Triglycerides are also a marker of the insulin resistance syndrome. Several different metabolic abnormalities, such as dyslipidemia and hypertension, are linked with insulin resistance in the development of coronary heart disease (Figure 3).

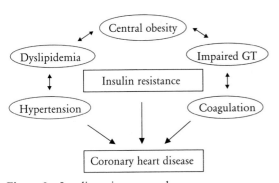

Figure 3 Insulin resistance syndrome

Lipids and insulin resistance

Insulin resistance is associated with low HDL and HDL$_2$ subfraction, increased triglycerides, small dense LDL and non-esterified fatty acid flux, and increased central adiposity, which is the fat distribution associated with increased risk of coronary heart disease.

Glucose and insulin resistance

Patients with insulin resistance will also have impaired glucose tolerance and increased insulin response to a glucose challenge (this alone is a concern). These patients will also have increased proportions of certain insulin propeptides, which have been shown to be linked with increased risk of coronary heart disease[11]. Interestingly, it has recently been shown that patients with insulin resistance have increased levels of leptin[12].

Coagulation and insulin resistance

The insulin resistance syndrome is also linked with other coronary heart disease risk factors, including increased factor VII, decreased tissue plasminogen activator and increased PAI-1.

THE MENOPAUSE

The menopause is an important coronary heart disease risk factor unique to women. The menopause is associated with increased coronary heart disease risk (this is independent of age, which is one of the most important factors affecting lipids and coronary heart disease risk) and adverse metabolic changes. Considerable data have been published on these adverse changes in different metabolic systems[13,14]. The data for lipids are discussed below (Figure 4)[10].

Lipids and menopause

We divided over 500 healthy non-obese pre- and postmenopausal women (aged 18–70 years) according to their menopausal status. Fasting serum lipids and lipoproteins were measured and standardized for age, body mass index, and gravidity, and lifestyle factors, including smoking,

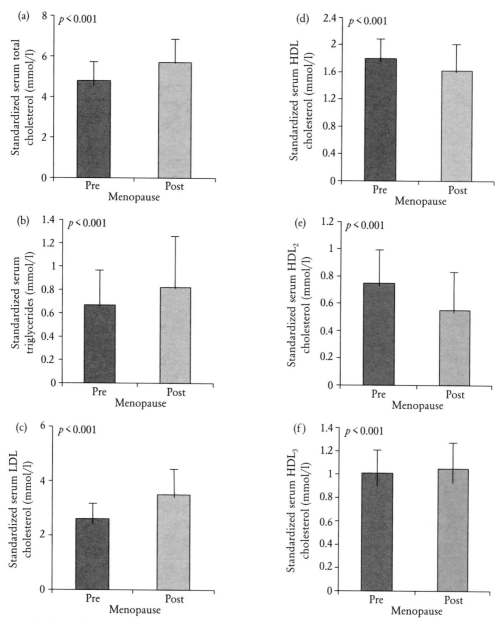

Figure 4 Lipids and menopause. (a) Total cholesterol; (b) triglycerides; (c) LDL cholesterol; (d) HDL cholesterol; (e) HDL$_2$ cholesterol; (f) HDL$_3$ cholesterol. Data are standardized for age, body mass index, gravidity, smoking, alcohol and exercise. Reproduced from reference 10 with permission from Elsevier Science

alcohol and exercise, and any differences were attributed to the difference in menopausal status[10].

The study showed that postmenopausal women have a statistically significantly higher level of total cholesterol, triglycerides and LDL (which explains the higher total cholesterol) compared with pre-menopausal women (all $p < 0.001$) (Figure 4). Postmenopausal women may also have higher levels of small dense LDL and lipoprotein(a).

Postmenopausal women have significantly lower HDL levels compared with premenopausal women ($p < 0.001$) (Figure 4). Although statistically significant, this difference is only small in terms of serum levels, and it masks a larger difference in the HDL subfractions. There is a large difference in serum HDL_2 levels between premenopausal and postmenopausal women (lower in postmenopausal women) and a small difference in serum HDL_3 levels (higher in postmenopausal women), but both differences are statistically significant ($p < 0.001$).

CONCLUSION

Lipids are essential for life, but abnormalities in lipid metabolism can lead to health problems. The role of lipids in coronary heart disease, which is potentially life-threatening, has been overstated in the past, but care must be taken not to understate this role. A significant proportion of the population in the western world has a lipid disorder which increases coronary heart disease risk, such as hyperlipidemia or dyslipidemia.

The menopause has a major effect on several metabolic risk factors for coronary heart disease, including lipid metabolism. HRT has a significant beneficial effect on lipid metabolism; however, this is only a small part of its overall benefit to the arterial system.

References

1. Austin MA. Triglyceride, small, dense low-density lipoprotein, and the atherogenic lipoprotein phenotype. *Curr Atheroscler Rep* 2000;2:200-7
2. Stevenson JC, Proudler AJ. Unpublished data, 2001
3. Austin MA, Breslow JL, Hennekens CH, *et al.* Low density lipoprotein subclass patterns and risk of myocardial infarction. *J Am Med Assoc* 1988;26: 1917-21
4. Williams KJ, Tabas I. The response-to-retention hypothesis of early atherogenesis. *Arterioscler Thromb Vasc Biol* 1995;15:551-61
5. Crook D, Howell R, Sidhu M, Edmonds DK, Stevenson JC. Elevated serum lipoprotein(a) levels in young women with endometriosis. *Metabolism* 1997;46:735-9
6. Cobbaert C, Mulder P, Lindemans J, *et al.* Serum LP(a) levels in African aboriginal Pygmies and Bantus, compared with Caucasian and Asian population samples. *J Clin Epidemiol* 1997;50:1045-53
7. Rubin EM, Krauss R, Spangler E, *et al.* Inhibition of early atherogenesis in transgenic mice by human apolipoprotein A-I. *Nature* 1991;353:265-7
8. Mahrabian M, Qiao J-H, Hyman R, *et al.* Influence of the apoA-II gene locus on HDL levels and fatty streak development in mice. *Arterioscler Thromb* 1993;13:1-10
9. Warden CH, Hedrick CC, Qiao J-H, *et al.* Atherosclerosis in transgenic mice overexpressing apolipoprotein AII. *Science* 1993;261:469-71
10. Stevenson JC, Crook D, Godsland IF. Influence of age and menopause on serum lipids and lipoproteins in healthy women. *Atherosclerosis* 1993;98: 83-90
11. Båvenholm P, Proudler AJ, Tornvall P, *et al.* Insulin, intact and split proinsulin and coronary artery disease in young men. *Circulation* 1995;92: 1422-9
12. Leyva F, Godsland IF, Ghatei M, *et al.* Hyperleptinemia as a component of a metabolic syndrome of cardiovascular risk. *Arterioscler Thromb Vasc Biol* 1998;18:928-33
13. Stevenson JC. Metabolic effects of the menopause and oestrogen replacement. In Barlow DH, ed. *Baillière's Clinical Obstetrics and Gynaecology. The Menopause: Key Issues.* London: Ballière Tindall, 1996:449-67
14. Spencer CP, Godsland IF, Stevenson JC. Is there a menopausal metabolic syndrome? *Gynecol Endocrinol* 1997;11:341-55

Diabetes, obesity and cardiovascular disease 4

E. Friday

WORLD-WIDE BURDEN OF DIABETES MELLITUS

Diabetes mellitus is a major cause of morbidity and mortality throughout the world. The World Health Organization has estimated that the world-wide burden of diabetes mellitus will more than double from 140 million to 300 million by the year 2026, with the largest increase predicted in developing countries[1]. The American Diabetes Association estimates that there are 15.7 million people affected with diabetes mellitus in the United States, although only two-thirds of these people, or approximately 10.3 million people, have actually been diagnosed with diabetes[2]. The remaining one-third remains undiagnosed and untreated. Unfortunately, the prevalence of diabetes is increasing rapidly in many countries[3,4]. Those that are diagnosed frequently receive inadequate treatment of hyperglycemia as well as risk factors for co-morbid conditions associated with diabetes mellitus. Diabetes is the leading cause of blindness in adults aged 20–74 years, as well as the leading cause of end-stage renal disease[2,5]. Diabetes-related neuropathies and peripheral vascular diseases are the most frequent causes of amputation. People with diabetes are two to four times more likely to suffer from heart disease or stroke and 75% of deaths in diabetic patients can be attributed to cardiovascular diseases. The American Diabetes Association estimates that 5–10% of people living with diabetes have type 1 diabetes, 90–95% have type 2 diabetes and 2–5% have gestational diabetes[2].

OBESITY AND DIABETES RISK

The prevalence of obesity is increasing rapidly in many industrialized countries[6]. In the United States (US), the number of overweight and obese men and women has risen dramatically since 1960; 54% of adults over the age of 20 are overweight (body mass index ≥ 25) and 22% are obese[7]. This alarming increase is also present in youth; 25% of US children are overweight or obese. Obesity is clearly a risk factor for type 2 diabetes[8]. It is clear that obesity will fuel a future explosion in the incidence of type 2 diabetes throughout the world. We desperately need to incorporate preventive measures such as routine exercise and calorie restriction into our lives to combat the threat of type 2 diabetes. Furthermore, modest weight loss through lifestyle modification has been shown to reduce blood glucose levels in overweight people without diabetes, and weight loss reduces blood glucose in some patients with type 2 diabetes[9].

CARDIOVASCULAR DISEASE IN DIABETIC WOMEN

Cardiovascular diseases, especially coronary heart disease and cerebrovascular disease, are the leading causes of death in women and claim more women's lives than all forms of cancer[10]. While several risk factors contribute to the development of atherosclerosis, diabetes is devastating for women. The Nurses' Health Study revealed that diabetic women have a five-fold higher risk of coronary heart disease than non-diabetic women[11,12]. Furthermore, diabetes negates the protective cardiovascular effect that women usually enjoy[13,14]; women without diabetes tend to develop cardiovascular disease approximately 10 years later than men on average[10]. Diabetic patients represent approximately one-third of all patients with cardiovascular disease in many studies[15,16]. However, when the patients are broken down by gender, approximately 25–30% of men with known atherosclerosis have diabetes, but the percentage for women is higher, with approximately 36–46% of female cardiovascular patients having known diabetes[15-17].

CARDIOVASCULAR DISEASE MORTALITY IN DIABETIC MEN AND WOMEN

Multiple studies have demonstrated an increase in cardiovascular mortality in diabetic patients[11,18,19]. Increases in short-term mortality (28–60 days after myocardial infarction), as well as 1–5-year mortality after infarction have been demonstrated in diabetic subjects compared to non-diabetic subjects[19,20]. While there have been significant reductions in age-adjusted heart disease mortality in non-diabetic men (-21%, $p < 0.001$) and women (-12.6%, $p = 0.04$) between 1971 and 1984 in the United States, heart disease mortality/1000 diabetic person-years has trended upward in diabetic women ($+15.2\%$, non-significant)[18]. Thus, diabetic patients, particularly diabetic women, continue to experience high rates of cardiovascular mortality.

DIABETES AND MYOCARDIAL INFARCTION

Among middle-aged diabetic patients, myocardial infarction rates are typically twice those of the non-diabetic population in men and three times higher in women[19]. Diabetic patients admitted with a heart attack are older[20,21], more likely to be female and more likely to have a prior history of myocardial infarction or ischemic heart disease than non-diabetic patients[21]. Diabetic women and men admitted with myocardial infarction have more frequent rates of hypertension, tachycardia, acute arrhythmias and cardiogenic shock than non-diabetic men and women[19,20], despite no increase in infarction size compared to non-diabetic patients[19]. Furthermore, congestive heart failure and cardiogenic shock appear to be more common and severe than would be predicted from infarction size in diabetic patients[22]. One recent study showed that diabetic women, but not diabetic men, had longer delays in time to hospitalization following angina symptoms, and higher rates of cardiac arrest and death following myocardial infarction compared to non-diabetic patients[20]. Diabetic women were also less likely to receive thrombolysis, coronary angiography, or exercise stress testing than non-diabetic women[20]. Cardiac ischemia or angina may have been asymptomatic or atypical in these diabetic women, thus delaying the diagnosis of myocardial infarction and effectively reducing the early use of thrombolytic agents. In another study, both diabetic women and men were significantly less likely to be treated with streptokinase, β-blockers and aspirin following an acute myocardial infarction than were non-diabetic women and men[21]. They were also significantly less likely to receive β-blockers at the time of discharge, despite the fact that treatment with β-blockers has been shown to significantly reduce the relative risk of 5-year mortality in diabetic subjects[20]. Research has also shown that several cardiovascular pharmaceutical interventions, including thrombolytic drugs, β-blockers and antiplatelet medications, have been shown to have similar efficacy in reducing cardiovascular mortality in diabetic and non-diabetic subjects following myocardial infarction[20]. Therefore, aggressive medical management should be included in the management of diabetic patients following a myocardial infarction whenever possible.

In-hospital mortality rates following myocardial infarction are 1.5–2 times higher in diabetic patients than non-diabetic patients[22]. Diabetic women have a particularly poor prognosis; mortality rates are nearly twofold higher than those of men[22]. Decreases in short-term (< 60 days) and long-term survival after myocardial infarction have been demonstrated in diabetic patients compared to non-diabetic patients[19].

CONGESTIVE HEART FAILURE

Diabetes mellitus is a significant risk factor for congestive heart failure[19,22]. In the participants age 45–74 years in the Framingham study, rates of congestive heart failure were twofold higher in diabetic men and fivefold higher in diabetic women compared to non-diabetic women[19,23]. Likely contributors to the development of congestive heart failure in diabetic patients include myocardial infarction or ischemia, cardiomyopathy, atrial fibrillation, long-standing hypertension with diastolic dysfunction, renal insufficiency, microvascular disease and possibly cardiac muscle insulin resistance[22].

CARDIAC RISK FACTORS IN DIABETIC PATIENTS

Hyperglycemia

While poor glucose control has been associated with an increased risk of cardiovascular disease in several large epidemiological studies, there is little evidence to suggest a causal link between hyperglycemia and atherosclerosis[24]. In European women with type 1 diabetes, those subjects with known cardiovascular disease had significantly lower concentrations of hemoglobin A1c (6.21 vs 6.88%, $p < 0.05$) than diabetic women without known cardiovascular disease[25]. While there is clear evidence that good glucose control can limit the development of microvascular complications such as nephropathy, neuropathy and retinopathy, it is widely accepted that other risk factors largely contribute to the burden of macrovascular atherosclerosis in diabetic patients.

Hyperinsulinemia

High plasma insulin concentrations are clearly associated with hypertension, insulin resistance, obesity, dyslipidemia and type 2 diabetes mellitus. Populations with endogenous hyperinsulinemia appear to be at increased risk for cardiovascular diseases[26]. However, insulin resistance is associated with a number of other cardiovascular risk factors, including hypertension, reduced levels of high density lipoprotein (HDL) cholesterol, hypertriglyceridemia, increased numbers of small dense low-density lipoprotein (LDL) particles, and increased levels of plasminogen activator inhibitor-1. Insulin resistance has been correlated with increasing carotid intimal medial wall thickness after adjusting for smoking, lipid levels, hypertension, medications, diabetes and gender in the Insulin Resistance Atherosclerosis Study (IRAS)[26,27]. Therefore, it is unclear if insulin itself is atherogenic or if it is a surrogate marker for something else that increases cardiovascular risk. The UK Prospective Diabetes Study (UKPDS) showed similar rates of cardiovascular disease in insulin-treated patients compared to diabetic subjects initially randomized to oral diabetic agents[28]. Furthermore, the Diabetes and Insulin-Glucose Infusion in Acute Myocardial Infarction (DIGAMI) Study showed reduced cardiovascular mortality at 1 year and 3.4 years following an acute myocardial infarction in patients receiving initial insulin infusions followed by multiple injections of insulin for at least 3 months, to achieve improved glucose control, compared to a group receiving usual care[29]. Therefore, the limited research data currently available suggest that exogenous insulin treatment does not increase the risk of cardiovascular disease in patients with diabetes.

Dyslipidemia

Patients with well-controlled type 1 diabetes frequently have a normal lipid pattern and frequently have elevated HDL cholesterol levels when compared to non-diabetic populations[30]. Hypertriglyceridemia, however, may be present in patients with poorly controlled type 1 diabetes or some other genetic risk for hypertriglyceridemia. Dyslipidemia with elevations in very low density lipoprotein (VLDL) cholesterol and triglyceride as well as reduced HDL cholesterol is common in type 2 diabetes[30-32]. Hypertriglyceridemia is a risk factor for cardiovascular disease in diabetic subjects and may play an even more important role in diabetic women than men. A recently published article has demonstrated a significant reduction in long-term survival and cardiac event-free survival in diabetic women, following coronary artery bypass grafting with triglyceride concentrations in the highest quartile (> 3.12 mmol/l or 276 mg/dl) compared to women with triglyceride concentrations < 3.12 mmol/l[33]. Hypertriglyceridemia levels in the highest quartile had no effect on long-term survival in diabetic men but non-significantly increased cardiac events (relative risk 1.28, confidence interval 0.99–1.66). Low density lipoprotein cholesterol levels are usually normal or slightly elevated in patients with type 2 diabetes, but the LDL particles may be smaller and denser in diabetic patients, especially if triglyceride concentrations are elevated. These small, dense LDL particles are more readily oxidized in the vessel wall and likely to contribute to the early atherosclerotic lesion. Treatment of hypercholesterolemia with statins to lower levels of LDL cholesterol in subsets of diabetic patients with known coronary artery disease has been shown to significantly reduce cardiac events in the Scandinavian Simvastatin Survival Study (4S)[34,35] and the Cholesterol and Recurrent Events (CARE) study[36]. Gemfibrozil treatment in the Helsinki Heart Study and the Veterans Administration HDL Intervention Trial (VA-HIT) produced a statistically non-significant reduction in coronary heart disease events or death in diabetic subgroups[37,38]. There are several on-going lipid-lowering trials that specifically address lipid risk factor modification in patients with diabetes mellitus. The American Diabetes Association currently recommends that LDL cholesterol be reduced to less than 100 mg/dl in all patients with diabetes mellitus[30], although there are no outcome studies to date that demonstrate a cardiovascular benefit with LDL cholesterol < 100 mg/dl for primary prevention in patients with diabetes mellitus.

Lipoprotein oxidation

Multiple studies have reported enhanced oxidation of plasma lipoproteins in diabetic patients and animals[39,40]. Oxidized LDL is taken up more readily by endothelial macrophages and may represent one of the early steps in the pathological development of atherosclerotic plaque in diabetic patients. One unpublished study has demonstrated reductions in the susceptibility of LDL lipoproteins to copper-induced oxidation[41] in women with type 2 diabetes treated with estrogen, although another published study demonstrated no change in LDL oxidation in estrogen-treated diabetic women[42].

Hypertension

Hypertension is frequently present in diabetic patients. In diabetic women with type 1 diabetes, hypertension, microalbuminuria (albumin excretion rate 20–200 µg/min) and macroalbuminuria (albumin excretion > 200 µg/min) were significantly more common in women with known cardiovascular disease[25]. The UKPDS has clearly shown that blood pressure control with captopril or atenolol reduces the incidence of diabetes-related deaths (combined myocardial infarction, sudden death, stroke, peripheral vascular disease or renal failure deaths), strokes and microvascular complications[43,44]. At the end of the 9-year study, 29% of the patients assigned to the relatively modest tight control group (< 150/85 mmHg) required three or more blood pressure medications to achieve an average blood pressure of 144/82 mmHg. Many, but not all, blood pressure treatment trials in diabetic subjects have demonstrated additional benefits of angiotensin converting enzyme inhibitors for the reduction of myocardial infarction and cardiovascular events in diabetic patients[45]. The Hypertension Diabetes Executive Committees Working Group of the National Kidney Foundation has recently recommended that blood pressure be lowered to less than 130/80 mmHg in diabetic individuals to reduce the risk of cardiovascular disease and renal failure, even though most patients will need treatment with two or more blood pressure medications to achieve this blood pressure goal[46].

Proteinuria and microalbuminuria

Proteinuria and microalbuminuria have been highly associated with cardiovascular disease, renal disease and retinopathy[47]. Patients with microalbuminuria have been shown to have a higher incidence of silent myocardial ischemia, as measured by exercise stress test, along with a reduced total exercise time and workload[48]. Diabetic patients with proteinuria have been shown to have a significant reduction in cardiovascular event-free survival over an average of 20.2 months following percutaneous coronary revascularization, compared to diabetic patients without proteinuria determined by routine urinalysis[16]. Furthermore, diabetic patients with the largest degree of proteinuria had the worst event-free survival rate (50%), whereas diabetic patients without proteinuria had an improved event-free survival (75%) that was similar to non-diabetic patients. In the Wisconsin Epidemiologic Study of Diabetic Retinopathy, the cardiovascular mortality rate increased significantly from 36.9/1000 person-years in the normo-albuminuric group to 85.5/1000 person-years in diabetic subjects with microalbuminuria (0.03–0.29 g/l) and 123/1000 person-years in subjects with gross proteinuria (≥ 0.3 g/l)[47].

Coagulation and fibrinolysis

Elevated levels of fibrinogen and increased platelet adhesiveness are frequently present in patients with diabetes[19,22] and have been associated with an increased risk of atherosclerosis in epidemiological studies. High fibrinogen concentrations have been associated with vascular conditions such as coronary heart disease, stroke and carotid atherosclerosis[19]. Plasminogen activator inhibitor (PAI-1) levels also appear to be elevated in diabetic individuals[19]. High PAI-1 levels are associated with impaired fibrinolysis and thus may contribute to impaired clot lysis in diabetic subjects.

OBESITY AND CARDIOVASCULAR RISK

The prevalence of obesity is rapidly increasing in the United States and many other industrialized nations[49]. Excess weight is independently associated with an increased risk of coronary heart disease in men and women[49]. Obesity, particularly central abdominal obesity, is associated with a number of risk factors for cardiovascular disease, including hypertension, dyslipidemia and endogenous hyperinsulinemia[7,50]. Modest weight loss of 5–10% of body weight has been associated with improvements in blood pressure, glucose and cholesterol concentrations. Given the overwhelming burden of cardiovascular disease throughout the world, lifestyle modification and obesity prevention will be important in the primary prevention of cardiovascular disease. More research is clearly needed to improve our efforts to prevent obesity and develop obesity treatment strategies.

ESTROGEN REPLACEMENT THERAPY IN POSTMENOPAUSAL DIABETIC WOMEN

Estrogen replacement therapy has been shown to improve blood lipoproteins and apolipoproteins[51,52], enhance vascular relaxation[53], and reduce the incidence of cardiovascular disease in several epidemiological studies[54,55]. However, the majority of these findings were demonstrated in Caucasian, healthy, postmenopausal women.

Because of concerns about the safety of estrogen replacement therapy in diabetic women, they were excluded from early prospective trials of estrogen replacement therapy[56].

There are now a few small, short-term, human studies that have demonstrated improved glucose metabolism in postmenopausal diabetic women treated with 17β-estradiol[57,58] or conjugated equine estrogen[59,60]. Treatment with 2 mg/day of oral 17β-estradiol for 60–68 days significantly improved blood glucose control when compared to placebo treatment in 25 hyperandrogenic women with non-insulin-dependent diabetes mellitus in a blinded, cross-over study by Andersson and colleagues[57]. Brussaard and co-workers also demonstrated improvements in hemoglobin A1c during a 6-week, dual-arm, placebo-controlled trial of 2 mg micronized 17β-estradiol per day ($n = 20$) vs placebo ($n = 20$) in postmenopausal diabetic women with non-insulin-dependent diabetes mellitus[58]. A randomized, prospective, but non-placebo-control trial by Samaras and colleagues with 2 months of conjugated equine estrogen 0.625 mg/day followed by 4 months of conjugated equine estrogen/medroxyprogesterone acetate 0.625 mg/5 mg in a small group of diabetic women ($n = 14$) showed that hormone replacement significantly improved hemoglobin A1c, and reduced the waist-to-hip ratio and central fat mass compared to 6 months of control observation[60]. We have also demonstrated that conjugated equine estrogen 0.625 mg/day for 8 weeks significantly reduced fasting and postprandial glucose as well as glycated hemoglobin in a placebo-controlled, randomized, cross-over design in 25 postmenopausal women with type 2 diabetes[59].

Several prospective studies of estrogen replacement in diabetic women thus far have demonstrated significant reductions in LDL cholesterol and significant elevations in HDL cholesterol[57-59]. Brussard and colleagues have also shown that 17β-estradiol also increases HDL_2 cholesterol and apolipoprotein A-1 as well as reducing apolipoprotein B in diabetic women[58]. Conjugated equine estrogen has been shown to raise fasting triglyceride by 12%; however, incremental postprandial triglyceride concentrations throughout the day were significantly improved during estrogen treatment, which may negate any increase in fasting triglyceride[59]. In contrast, there were no statistically significant triglyceride elevations detected during 17β-estradiol therapy in the diabetic women[57,58]. Another unpublished report demonstrated improvements in endothelial vasodilatation in diabetic women treated with estrogen, but diabetic women were still found to have less endothelium-dependent vasodilatation than non-diabetic women treated with estrogen[61]. Thus, estrogen replacement in diabetic women produces fairly similar lipid and lipoprotein changes to those observed in non-diabetic women, but other cardiovascular risk factors may not be fully normalized with estrogen/hormone treatment in women with type 2 diabetes.

Several case–control and prospective epidemiological studies have shown that postmenopausal women treated with estrogen or estrogen plus progesterone have a lower incidence of cardiovascular disease than women not receiving estrogen[54,55]. Limited epidemiological data are available in diabetic women, but one article suggests that the risk of myocardial infarction in postmenopausal diabetic women is only reduced in current estrogen users, with a cumulative duration of use greater than 6 years[62]. Furthermore, the Heart and Estrogen/progestin Replacement Study (HERS), which included 18–19% women with diabetes mellitus and coronary artery disease in the study population, showed a worsening in cardiovascular events in the first year of study but cardiovascular benefits in women taking conjugated equine estrogen plus medroxyprogesterone after 4 and 5 years of use[63]. More recently, however, Herrington and colleagues have reported that neither conjugated equine estrogen 0.625 mg/day nor conjugated equine estrogen 0.625 mg plus medroxyprogesterone acetate 2.5 mg/day for a mean duration of 3.2 years reduced the progression of coronary atherosclerosis in women with at least one coronary artery stenosis greater than 30%, as measured by quantitative angiography[64]. Diabetic women (total diabetic subjects in all treatment arms, $n = 69$), however, appeared to have more severe progression of atherosclerosis during treatment with conjugated equine estrogen plus medroxyprogesterone acetate than with conjugated equine estrogen alone, although this comparison was not analyzed for statistical significance in the original publication. Therefore, it is difficult to determine at this time if estrogen therapy will actually reduce the incidence of clinically significant cardiovascular disease in diabetic women. The results from additional prospective, randomized, clinical trials will be necessary to determine if estrogen and/or hormone replacement therapy benefits women at high risk for cardiovascular disease.

THERAPIES TO REDUCE THE RISK OF CARDIOVASCULAR DISEASE IN DIABETIC PATIENTS

Several therapies have been recommended to reduce the risk of symptomatic cardiovascular disease in diabetic women and men[65]. Exercise has been associated with a reduced number of cardiovascular events in diabetic women[66,67]. Hypertension treatment has also been shown to reduce the incidence of cardiovascular events in diabetic subjects[43,44]. Aspirin use has been shown to significantly reduce the number of cardiovascular events in diabetic subjects in several prospective randomized trials[68,69]. The American Diabetes Association recommends the use of aspirin 81–325 mg/day in men and women with known atherosclerosis. Aspirin use should also be considered for primary prevention of cardiovascular disease in diabetic patients over the age of 30 years with multiple risk factors. In diabetic patients with known cardiovascular disease, lipid-lowering therapy has clearly been shown in prospective randomized trials to reduce the number of secondary cardiovascular events[31,34–36]. Improved glucose regulation has been clearly shown to inhibit microvascular disease; however, the effects of glucose control on macrovascular disease is less clear. Metformin has been shown to reduce the number of diabetes-related clinical endpoints, diabetes-related deaths and all-cause mortality[70]. Ongoing trials are examining the role of other glucose regulating agents, insulin sensitizers and lipid-lowering agents in the prevention of atherosclerosis and cardiovascular events.

ACKNOWLEDGEMENTS

Dr Friday currently receives funding from the American Heart Association, Southeast Affiliate and the Department of Health and Human Services, Office of Women's Health.

References

1. Diabetes. World Health Organization web site. Available at http://www.who.int/ncd/dia/indexhtm. Accessed March 19, 2001

2. Diabetes Facts and Figures. American Diabetes Association web site. Available at http://www.diabetes.org/ada/facts.asp#toll. Accessed March 19, 2001

3. Mokdad AH, Ford ES, Bowman BA, Nelson DE, Engelgau MM, Vinicor R, Marks JS. Diabetes trends in the US: 1990-1998. *Diabetes Care* 2000;23:1278-83

4. Harris MI, Flegal KM, Cowie CC, Eberhardt MS, Goldstein DE, Little RR, Wiedmeyer H, Byrd-Holt DD. Prevalence of diabetes, impaired fasting glucose, and impaired glucose tolerance in US adults. *Diabetes Care* 1998;21:136-44

5. American Diabetes Association. Diabetic retinopathy. *Diabetes Care* 2001;24:S73-6

6. Hill JO, Peters JC. Environmental contributions to the obesity epidemic. *Science* 1998;280:1371-4

7. Expert Panel on the Identification, Evaluation and Treatment of Overweight and Obesity in Adults. Executive summary of the clinical guidelines on the identification, evaluation and treatment of overweight and obesity in adults. *Arch Intern Med.* 1998;158:1855-67

8. American Diabetes Association. Report of the expert committee on the diagnosis and classification of diabetes mellitus. *Diabetes Care* 2001;24:S5-S20

9. American Diabetes Association. Nutrition recommendations and principles for people with diabetes mellitus. *Diabetes Care* 2001;24:S44-7

10. Mosca L, Manson JE, Sutherlane SE, Langer RD, Manolio T, Barrett-Connor E. Cardiovascular disease in women. *Circulation* 1997;96:2468-82

11. Bierman EL. Atherogenesis in diabetes. *Arterioscler Thromb* 1992;12:647-56

12. Manson JE, Colditz GA, Stampfer MJ, Willett WC, Krolewski AS, Rosner B, Arky RA, Speizer FE, Hennekens CH. A prospective study of maturity-onset diabetes and risk of coronary heart disease and stroke in women. *Arch Intern Med* 1991;151:1141-7

13. Sowers JR. Diabetes mellitus and cardiovascular disease in women. *Arch Intern Med* 1998;158:617-21

14. Barrett-Connor EL, Cohn BA, Wingard DL, Edelstein SL. Why is diabetes mellitus a stronger risk factor for fatal ischemic heart disease in women than in men? *J Am Med Assoc* 1991;265:627-31

15. Mehta RH, Ruane TJ, McCargar PA, Eagle KE, Stalhandske EJ. The treatment of elderly diabetic patients with acute myocardial infarction: insight from Michigan's Cooperative Cardiovascular Project. *Arch Intern Med* 2000;160:1301-6

16. Marso SP, Ellis SG, Tuzcu EM, Whitlow PL, Franco I, Raymond RE, Topol EJ. The importance of proteinuria as a determinant of mortality following percutaneous coronary revascularization in diabetics. *J Am Coll Cardiol* 1999;33:1269-77

17. Kjaergaard SC, Hansen JJ, Fog L, Bulow I, Christensen PD. In-hospital outcome for diabetic patients with acute myocardial infarction in the thrombolytic era. *Scand Cardiovasc J* 1999;33:166-70

18. Gu K, Cowie CC, Harris MI. Diabetes and decline in heart disease mortality in US adults. *J Am Med Assoc* 1999;281:1291-7

19. Wilson PWF. Diabetes mellitus and coronary heart disease. *Am J Kidney Dis* 1998;32:S89-100

20. Löwel H, Koenig W, Engel S, Hörmann A, Keil U. The impact of diabetes mellitus on survival after myocardial infarction: can it be modified by drug treatment? *Diabetologia* 2000;43:218-26

21. Lim LL-Y, Tesfay GM, Heller RF. Management of patients with diabetes after heart attack: a population-based study of 1982 patients from a heart disease register. *Aust NZ J Med* 1998;28:334-42

22. Aronson D, Rayfield EJ, Chesebro JH. Mechanisms determining course and outcome of diabetic patients who have had acute myocardial infarction. *Ann Intern Med* 1997;126:296-306

23. Kannel WB, Hjortland MC, Castelli WP. Role of diabetes in congestive heart failure. The Framingham Study. *Am J Cardiol* 1974;34:29-34

24. Barrett-Connor E. Does hyperglycemia really cause coronary heart disease? *Diabetes Care* 1997;20:1620-3

25. Orchard TJ, Stevens LK, Forrest KY-Z, Fuller JH. Cardiovascular disease in insulin dependent diabetes mellitus: similar rates but different risk factors in the US compared with Europe. *Int J Epidemiol* 1998;27:976-83

26. Hsueh WA, Law RE. Cardiovascular risk continuum: implications of insulin resistance and diabetes. *Am J Med* 1998;105(1A):4-14S

27. Howard G, O'Leary DH, Zaccaro D, *et al.* Insulin sensitivity and atherosclerosis. *Circulation* 1996;93:1809-17

28. UK Prospective Diabetes Study Group. The incidence of myocardial infarction in white, South Asian, and Afro-Caribbean patients with type 2 diabetes (UK Prospective Diabetes Study 32). *Diabetes Care* 1998;21:1271-7

29. Malmberg K, Norhammer A, Wedel H, Rydén L. Glycometabolic state at admission: important risk marker of mortality in conventionally treated patients with diabetes mellitus and acute myocardial infarction. Long-term results from the Diabetes and Insulin-Glucose Infusion in Acute

Myocardial Infarction (DIGAMI) Study. *Circulation* 1999;99:2626–32

30. American Diabetes Association. Management of dyslipidemia in adults with diabetes. *Diabetes Care* 2001;24:S58–61

31. Haffner SM. Management of dyslipidemia in adults with diabetes (Technical Review). *Diabetes Care* 1998;21:160–78

32. Howard BV, Cowan LD, Go O, Welty TK, Robbins DC, Lee ET. Adverse effects of diabetes on multiple cardiovascular disease risk factors in women. *Diabetes Care* 1998;21:1258–65

33. Sprecher DL, Pearce GL, Park EM, Pashkow FJ, Hoogwerf BJ. Preoperative triglycerides predict post-coronary artery bypass graft survival in diabetic patients. *Diabetes Care* 2000;23:1648–53

34. Pyörälä K, Pedersen TR, Kjekshus J, *et al*. Cholesterol lowering with simvastatin improves prognosis of diabetic patients with coronary heart disease: a subgroup analysis of the Scandinavian Simvastatin Survival Study (4S). *Diabetes Care* 1997;20:614–20

35. Haffner SM, Alexander CM, Cook TJ, Bocuzzi SJ, Musliner TA, Pedersen TR, Kjekshus J, Pyörälä K. Reduced coronary events in simvastatin-treated patients with coronary heart disease and diabetes or impaired fasting glucose levels. *Arch Intern Med* 1999;159:2661–7

36. Goldberg RB, Mellies MJ, Sacks FM, Moye LA, Howard BV, Howard WJ, Davis BR, Cole TG, Pfeffer MA, Braunwald E. Cardiovascular events and their reduction with pravastatin in diabetic and glucose-intolerant myocardial infarction survivors with average cholesterol levels: subgroup analyses in the cholesterol and recurrent events (CARE) trial. The Care Investigators. *Circulation* 1998;98: 2513–19

37. Koskinen P, Mänttäri M, Manninen V, Huttunen JK, Heinonen OP, Frick MH. Coronary heart disease incidence in NIDDM patients in the Helsinki Heart Study. *Diabetes Care* 1992;15:820–5

38. Rubins HB, Robins SJ, Collins D, Fye CL, Anderson JW, Elam MB, Faas FH, Linares E, Schaefer EJ, Schectman G, Wilt TJ, Wittes J. Gemfibrozil for the secondary prevention of coronary heart disease in men with low levels of high-density lipoprotein cholesterol. Veterans Affairs High-Density Lipoprotein Cholesterol Intervention Trial Study Group. *N Engl J Med* 1999;341:410–18

39. Tan KC, Ai VH, Chow WS, Chau MT, Leong L, Lam KS. Influence of low density lipoprotein (LDL) subfraction profile and LDL oxidation on endothelium-dependent and independent vasodilation in patients with type 2 diabetes. *J Clin Endocrinol Metab* 1999;84:3212–16

40. Chisolm GM, Irwin KC, Penn MS. Lipoprotein oxidation and lipoprotein-induced cell injury in diabetes. *Diabetes* 1992;41 (Suppl 2):61–5

41. Friday KE, Morel DW. Estrogen replacement therapy inhibits lipoprotein oxidation in post-

menopausal diabetic women. *Diabetes* 1999;48 (Suppl 1):A253

42. Brussard HE, Gevers Leuven JA, Kluft C, Krans HMJ, van Duyvenvoorde W, Buytenhek R, van der Laarse A, Princen HMG. Effect of 17β-estradiol on plasma lipids and LDL oxidation in postmenopausal women with type II diabetes mellitus. *Arterioscler Thromb Vasc Biol* 1997;17:324–30

43. UK Prospective Diabetes Study Group. Tight blood pressure control and risk of macrovascular and microvascular complications in type 2 diabetes (UKPDS 30). *Br Med J* 1998;317:703–13

44. UK Prospective Diabetes Study Group. Efficacy of atenolol and captopril in reducing risk of both macrovascular and microvascular complications in type 2 diabetes (UKPDS 39). *Br Med J* 1998;317: 713–20

45. Pahor M, Psaty BM, Alderman MH, Applegate WB, Williamson JD, Furberg CD. Therapeutic benefits of ACE inhibitors and other antihypertensive drugs in patients with type 2 diabetes. *Diabetes Care* 2000;23:888–92

46. Bakris GL, Williams M, Dworkin L, Elliott WJ, Epstein M, Toto R, Tuttle K, Douglas J, Hsueh W, Sowers J. Preserving renal function in adults with hypertension and diabetes: a consensus approach. *Am J Kidney Dis* 2000;36:646–60

47. Valmadrid CT, Klein R, Moss SE, Klein BE. The risk of cardiovascular disease mortality associated with microalbuminuria and gross proteinuria in persons with older-onset diabetes mellitus. *Arch Intern Med* 2000;160:1093–100

48. Rutter MK, McComb JM, Brady S, Marshall SM. Silent myocardial ischemia and microalbuminuria in asymptomatic subjects with non-insulin-dependent diabetes mellitus. *Am J Cardiol* 1999;83: 27–31

49. Tsang TS, Barnes ME, Gersh BJ, Hayes SN. Risks of coronary heart disease in women: current understanding and evolving concepts. *Mayo Clin Proc* 2000;75:1289–303

50. Eckel RH, Krauss RM. American Heart Association call to action: obesity as a major risk factor for coronary heart disease. *Circulation*. 1998;97:2099–100

51. Walsh BW, Schiff I, Rosner B, Greenberg L, Ravnikar V, Sacks FM. Effects of postmenopausal estrogen replacement on the concentrations and metabolism of plasma lipoproteins. *N Engl J Med* 1991;325:1196–204

52. Writing Group for the PEPI Trial. Effects of estrogen or estrogen/progestin regimens on heart disease risk factors in postmenopausal women. *J Am Med Assoc* 1995;273:199–208

53. Gilligan DM, Bada DM, Panza JA, Quyyumi AA, Cannon RO. Acute vascular effects of estrogen in postmenopausal women. *Circulation* 1994;90: 786–91

54. Stampfer MJ, Colditz GA, Willett WC, Manson JE, Rosner B, Speizer FE, Hennekens CH.

Postmenopausal estrogen therapy and cardio-vascular disease: ten-year follow-up from the Nurses' Health Study. *N Engl J Med* 1991;325:756-62

55. Grodstein F, Stampfer MJ, Manson JE, Colditz GA, Willett WC, Rosner B, *et al.* Postmenopausal estrogen and progestin use and the risk of cardiovascular disease. *N Engl J Med* 1996;335:453-61

56. Friday KE. Estrogen replacement therapy for postmenopausal women with diabetes. *Diabetes Spectrum* 1997;10:230-4

57. Andersson B, Mattsson L, Hahn L, Mårin P, Lapidus L, Holm G, *et al.* Estrogen replacement therapy decreases hyperandrogenicity and improves glucose homeostasis and plasma lipids in postmenopausal women with non-insulin-dependent diabetes mellitus. *J Clin Endocrinol Metab* 1997;82:638-43

58. Brussaard HE, Gevers Leuven JA, Frölich M, Kluft C, Krans HMJ. Short-term oestrogen replacement therapy improves insulin resistance, lipids and fibrinolysis in postmenopausal women with NIDDM. *Diabetologia* 1997;40:843-9

59. Friday KE, Dong C, Fontenot RU. Conjugated equine estrogen improves glycemic control and blood lipoproteins in postmenopausal women with type 2 diabetes. *J Clin Endocrinol Metab* 2001;86:48-52

60. Samaras K, Hayward CS, Sullivan D, Kelly RP, Campbell LV. Effects of postmenopausal hormone replacement therapy on central abdominal fat, glycemic control, lipid metabolism and vascular factors in type 2 diabetes: a prospective study. *Diabetes Care* 1999;22:1401-8

61. Yeo JK, Kim KS, Bae JH, Lee HW, Won KC. The effect of estrogen supplementation on the endothelium dependent vasodilation in postmenopausal women with type 2 diabetes mellitus. *Diabetes* 1999;48 (Suppl 1):A372

62. Kaplan RC, Heckbert SR, Weiss NS, Wahl PW, Smith LN, Newton KM, Psaty BM. Postmenopausal estrogens and risk of myocardial infarction in diabetic women. *Diabetes Care* 1998;21:1117-21

63. Hulley S, Grady D, Bush T, Furberg C, Herrington D, Riggs B, Vittinghoff E. Randomized trial of estrogen plus progestin for secondary prevention of coronary heart disease in postmenopausal women. *J Am Med Assoc* 1998;280:605-13

64. Herrington DM, Revoussin DM, Brosnihan KB, Sharp PC, Shumaker SA, Snyder TE, Furberg CD, Kowalchuk GJ, Stuckey TD, Rogers WJ, Givens DH, Waters D. Effects of estrogen replacement on the progression of coronary artery atherosclerosis. *N Engl J Med* 2000;343:522-9

65. American Diabetes Association. Standards of medical care for patients with diabetes mellitus. *Diabetes Care* 2001;24 (Suppl 1):S33-43

66. Walker KZ, Piers LS, Putt RS, Jones JA, O'Dea K. Effects of regular walking on cardiovascular risk factors and body composition in normoglycemic women and women with type 2 diabetes. *Diabetes Care* 1999;22:555-61

67. Hu FB, Stampfer MJ, Solomon C, Liu S, Colditz A, Speizer FE, Willett WC, Manson JE. Physical activity and risk for cardiovascular events in diabetic women. *Ann Intern Med* 2001;134:96-105

68. American Diabetes Association. Aspirin therapy in diabetes. *Diabetes Care* 2001;24 (Suppl 1):S62-8

69. Harpaz D, Gottlieb S, Graff E, Boyko V, Kishon Y, Behar S. Effects of aspirin treatment on survival in non-insulin-dependent diabetic patients with coronary artery disease. *Am J Med* 1998;105:494-9

70. UK Prospective Diabetes Study (UKPDS) Group. Effect of intensive blood-glucose control with metformin on complications in overweight patients with type 2 diabetes (UKPDS34). *Lancet* 1998;352:854-65

Endothelial function in hypertension: role of gender

A. Virdis, L. Ghiadoni, I. Sudano, S. Buralli, G. Salvetti, S. Taddei and A. Salvetti

5

INTRODUCTION

There is an important gender difference in the incidence of cardiovascular morbidity and mortality, with premenopausal women being at lower risk than males. This finding suggests that sex hormones could be important factors for modulating cardiovascular disease[1]. Among the various direct and indirect mechanisms through which sex hormones can influence both cardiovascular function and structure, their effect on endothelial function may be important. The reasons for this will be discussed below.

ENDOTHELIAL FUNCTION

Endothelial cells play an important local regulatory role by secreting substances that control both vascular tone and structure[2]. The endothelium produces several relaxing factors including nitric oxide (NO), prostacyclin and an as yet unidentified hyperpolarizing relaxing factor (EDHF)[2]. The best characterized, and probably the most important, relaxing factor is NO[3], which is derived from transformation of the amino acid L-arginine into citrulline by the activity of NO synthase (NOS)[4], a constitutive enzyme present in endothelial cells. NO is produced and released under the influence of agonists, such as acetylcholine, bradykinin, substance P, serotonin and others acting on specific endothelial receptors, and by mechanical forces, such as shear stress[2]. Endothelial cells can also induce relaxation by causing hyperpolarization[5]. This possibility has been identified by the finding that in some experimental conditions endothelium-dependent relaxation cannot be abolished by NO synthase antagonists, thereby ruling out NO as responsible for this activity[5]. Moreover, recent data seem to indicate that in humans with impaired NO availability, such as

hypertensive patients[6] or normal subjects treated with *N*-monomethyl-L-arginine (L-NMMA)[7], a competitive antagonist of NOS, endothelium-dependent vasodilation is accounted for by the activation of a relaxing pathway involving hyperpolarization[7].

In certain conditions endothelial cells can evoke contractions. Experimental evidence indicates that in aging, menopause and pathological conditions such as hypertension, diabetes mellitus, atherosclerosis, vasospasm and reperfusion injury, activation of endothelial cells can lead to the production and release of contracting factors including cyclooxygenase-derived endothelium-dependent contracting factors (EDCFs), represented mainly by prostanoids (thromboxane A_2 and prostaglandin H_2)[8] and oxygen free radicals[9], which counteract the relaxing activity of NO. Moreover, oxygen free radicals can also impair endothelial function by causing NO breakdown[10]. It is of relevance that the concept of endothelial dysfunction is related above all to the parallel activation of the NO and EDCF pathways. Even in the presence of preserved NO production, EDCFs can impair NO availability or biological effects. Thus in some experimental conditions, EDCF pathway blockade can lead to complete restoration of the L-arginine–NO pathway.

ENDOTHELIAL DYSFUNCTION IN HUMAN HYPERTENSION

Evidence

Endothelial function is usually assessed in humans by studies on vascular reactivity performed in different vascular beds. The classical approach is to evaluate changes in flow or in diameter of large arteries in response to locally-infused endothelial agonists or to mechanical stimuli, as compared with those induced by endothelium-independent stimuli. Moreover, it is possible to evaluate the mechanism(s) underlying endothelial function, such as activation of the L-arginine–NO pathway through local infusion of L-arginine, NO availability through the inhibitory effect of L-NMMA, and the role of oxidative stress by evaluating the effect of vitamin C, a scavenger of oxygen free radicals[11].

In essential hypertensive patients, impaired endothelium-dependent vasodilation has been clearly documented in various vascular beds including the forearm, the skin and the subcutaneous and renal microcirculation, as well as in large arteries such as the brachial and epicardial arteries[12].

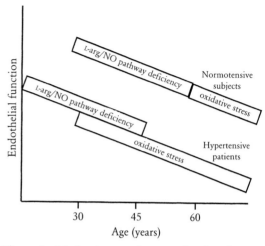

Figure 1 Mechanism causing age-related endothelial dysfunction in normotensive subjects and hypertensive patients. For further explanations see text. L-Arg, L-arginine; NO, nitric oxide

Mechanisms causing endothelial dysfunction

At least in the forearm circulation, the main mechanism causing endothelial dysfunction seems to be an impairment of NO availability, since vasodilation caused by acetylcholine and bradykinin, two endothelial agonists, is not reduced by simultaneous infusion of L-NMMA[6,13,14]. This alteration seems to be related to the production of EDCFs, induced by activation of the cyclooxygenase pathway[15] and mainly represented by oxygen free radicals, as shown by the fact that intrabrachial infusion of the scavenger vitamin C increases endothelium-dependent vasodilation and restores the inhibiting effect of L-NMMA[6]. However, mechanisms causing endothelial dysfunction are clearly influenced by aging, which is in itself an important mechanism determining endothelial dysfunction both in normotensive subjects[16,17] and in hypertensive patients[17]. In normotensive subjects, age-related decline in endothelial function starts after the age of 30 years and is caused by an L-arginine–NO pathway alteration until the age of 60 years, when the effect of EDCFs – possibly oxidative stress – starts to be relevant[18] (Figure 1). In essential hypertension the mechanisms involved in endothelial dysfunction are likewise age-related, but characterized by earlier onset, since alteration of the L-arginine–NO pathway can be observed

from the age of 18 years, and EDCF production can appear after the age of 30 years[18] (Figure 1). It is therefore conceivable that essential hypertension merely causes earlier onset of the endothelial dysfunction which is characteristic of aging.

Clinical significance of endothelial dysfunction

Available data indicate that endothelial dysfunction linked to essential hypertension is not related to hemodynamic load attributable to blood pressure increase[19], a finding which suggests that impaired endothelium-dependent relaxation may not play a role in causing and/or maintaining high blood pressure values. Endothelial dysfunction is now viewed as an important mechanism promoting atherosclerosis and thrombosis, a hypothesis which is substantiated by several observations. NO and EDCFs not only exert opposite effects on vascular tone but also inhibit and activate, respectively, those mechanisms such as platelet aggregation, vascular smooth muscle cell migration and proliferation, adhesion molecule expression and monocyte adhesion, which are known to play an important role in the genesis of atherothrombosis[2]. Endothelial dysfunction is detectable in the presence of the great majority of other cardiovascular risk factors, such as aging, post-menopause, hypercholesterolemia, diabetes mellitus, smoking and hyperhomocysteinemia, and in the presence of coronary atherosclerosis. It is further increased by the association of two or more cardiovascular risk factors[12].

In essential hypertensive patients, impaired forearm endothelial-dependent vasodilation is correlated with intima–media thickening of carotid arteries, an index of atherosclerotic vascular damage[20]. In epicardial arteries of normotensive subjects, endothelial dysfunction correlates with the extent of atherosclerotic wall thickening detected by intravascular echography[21]. Finally, in epicardial arteries of heart transplant patients, endothelial dysfunction predicts the development of allograft arteriosclerosis[22].

Four recent prospective studies have evaluated the incidence of cardiovascular events according to baseline endothelial function, evaluated in the coronary circulation of patients with mild or absent coronary atherosclerosis but with more than one cardiovascular risk factor including hypertension in about 40–50% of patients[23-25], and in the brachial artery in patients with chest pain (angina in 60% and coronary artery stenosis greater than 30%)[26]. Overall, these studies indicate that in a mean follow-up of 2-10 years, cardiovascular events such as cardiac death, myocardial infarction, unstable angina, PTC, CABC and, in one study, congestive heart failure, stroke and peripheral revascularization, were significantly increased in patients with reduced endothelial function.

In conclusion, the available data indicate that endothelial dysfunction may be an important mechanism causing atherothrombosis, thus increasing the occurrence of cardiovascular events.

GENDER AND ENDOTHELIAL DYSFUNCTION

As already mentioned, aging is associated with a progressive decline in endothelial function both in normotensive subjects[16,17] and hypertensive patients[17,18]. However, in normally menstruating normotensive women, no endothelial dysfunction has been observed, and age-related impairment in endothelial-dependent vasodilation is evident only after the menopause[16,27]. In premenopausal hypertensive women, aging is associated with endothelial dysfunction although the deterioration of endothelial-dependent vasodilation is less marked than that in men[27]. In contrast, after the menopause, the age-related endothelial dysfunction in hypertensive women is similar to that observed in men[27]. Age-related impairment of endothelial function therefore occurs only after the menopause in normotensive women and mainly after the menopause in hypertensive women.

This finding suggests that sex hormones are involved in the modulation of endothelial function, and it is therefore rational to evaluate whether estrogen protects endothelial function in women and whether testosterone impairs it in men.

Estrogen and endothelial function

In normotensive women, endogenous estrogens improve endothelial function. This effect seems to be mediated both by activation of the L-arginine–NO pathway and by inhibition of oxidative stress[28,29]. We therefore examined the mechanism(s) involved in control of endothelial function in the forearm microcirculation of normotensive and hypertensive premenopausal women and age-matched normotensive and hypertensive men. The L-arginine–NO pathway was evaluated by observing the effect of local L-arginine infusion on acetylcholine-induced vasodilation. NO availability was inferred from the inhibitory effect of local infusion of L-NMMA on endothelium-dependent vasodilation. Oxidative stress was studied through the effect of local infusion of vitamin C on endothelium-dependent vasodilation. Data obtained so far indicate that endothelium-dependent vasodilation, which is significantly greater in normotensive women as compared with normotensive men, is characterized by reduced NO availability in men, in whom L-arginine increases endothelium-dependent vasodilation to a greater extent than in women. Vitamin C did not change endothelium-dependent vasodilation in either gender. Taken together, these data suggest that in normotensive women endogenous estrogen protects endothelial function through preservation of the L-arginine–NO pathway (Figure 2).

In hypertensive premenopausal women, endothelium-dependent vasodilation was significantly greater that in age-matched men. In addition, local L-NMMA infusion reduced endothelium-dependent vasodilation in women but not in men, a finding which indicates that NO availability is present only in premenopausal women. L-Arginine infusion restored endothelium-dependent vasodilation in premenopausal women but not in men, while local infusion of vitamin C improved endothelium-dependent vasodilation only in men. Taken together, these data indicate that endogenous estrogen also pro-

tects endothelial function in hypertensive premenopausal women, an effect which seems to be due to activation of the L-arginine–NO pathway and above all to inhibition of oxidative stress (Figure 3).

Endogenous androgen and endothelial function

Experimental data concerning vascular actions of testosterone are contradictory. It has been reported that 2-week treatment with this hormone enhances the vasoconstrictor response of pig coronary

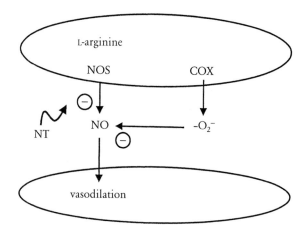

Figure 2 The protective effect of endogenous estrogen on endothelial function in normotensive premenopausal women seems to be due to the activation of the L-arginine–nitric oxide (NO) pathway. NOS, nitric oxide synthase; COX, cycloxygenase; NT, normotensive patients

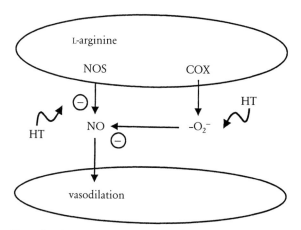

Figure 3 The protective effect of endogenous estrogen on endothelial function in hypertensive premenopausal women seems to be due to the activation of the L-arginine–nitric oxide (NO) pathway and above all to the inhibition of oxidative stress. NOS, nitric oxide synthase; COX, cycloxygenase; HT, hypertensive patients

arteries, an effect which is reduced by endothelial denudation[30], and that *in vitro* testosterone impairs endothelial dysfunction associated with hypercholesterolemia and environmental tobacco smoke exposure in the male rabbit aorta[31]. On the other hand, it has been reported that *in vitro* testosterone causes endothelium-independent relaxation in rabbit coronary arteries and aorta[32], while *in vivo* intracoronary infusion of testosterone induces vasodilation in canine coronary conductance and resistance arteries, an effect which is partially mediated by endothelium-derived NO[33]. In humans, data on the possible effect of testosterone on endothelial function are scarce and conflicting. For example, while intracoronary infusion of testosterone, which causes local vasodilation, did not change epicardial and microcirculatory coronary responses to acetylcholine in patients with coronary heart disease[34], acute intravenous infusion of testosterone improved flow-mediated dilation in the brachial artery of similar patients[35]. However, this latter finding does not prove that testosterone improves endothelial function, since in this study endothelium-independent vasodilation caused by nitroglycerine was not assessed[35]. In contrast, it has been reported that in androgen-deprived aged men with prostatic carcinoma, endothelium-dependent, but not endothelium-independent, vasodilation in the brachial artery is significantly higher than in controls[36]. The latter controlled study suggests that physiological levels of testosterone could impair endothelial function in men.

CONCLUSIONS

The endothelium is an important paracrine-autocrine organ which exerts a crucial role in the modulation of vascular tone and structure. A normally functioning endothelium is characterized by the production and availability of NO, which causes local vasodilation and counteracts processes leading to atherothrombosis. A dysfunctioning endothelium, on the other hand, is characterized by reduced or absent NO availability owing to impairment of the L-arginine–NO pathway and above all to production of EDCFs, represented mainly by oxygen free radicals. This leads to impairment of local vasodilation and to activation of those processes that cause atherothrombosis. Endothelial dysfunction is therefore associated with structural alterations in carotid and coronary arteries and with a greater incidence of cardiovascular events. Aging is an important condition determining endothelial dysfunction both in normotensive subjects and in hypertensive patients, and hypertension seems to induce earlier onset of those mechanisms which cause age-related endothelial dysfunction. Available data indicate that premenopausal normotensive women are protected against the deleterious effect of aging on endothelial function and that age-related impairment of endothelial function is attenuated in premenopausal hypertensive women. This protective effect on endothelial function seems to be mediated by endogenous estrogen, which preserves NO availability by activating the L-arginine–NO pathway in normotensive women, and also by inhibiting oxidative stress in hypertensive women. It is tempting to hypothesize that the protective effect of endogenous estrogen on endothelial function could be a plausible mechanism contributing to the lower cardiovascular risk of premenopausal women.

Finally, whether endogenous androgen can impair endothelial function is still an unresolved issue, since data concerning the effect of testosterone on endothelial function are few and contradictory.

References

1. Gerhard M, Ganz P. How do we explain the clinical benefits of estrogen? From bedside to bench. *Circulation* 1995;92:5–8

2. Luscher TF, Vanhoutte PM. *The Endothelium: Modulator of Cardiovascular Function*. Boca Raton: CRC Press, 1990

3. Palmer RMJ, Ferrige AG, Moncada S. Nitric oxide release accounts for the biological activity of endothelium-derived relaxing factor. *Nature* 1987;327:424-526

4. Bredt DS, Hwang PM, Glatt CE, *et al.* Cloned and expressed nitric oxide synthase structurally resembles cytochrome P-450 reductase. *Nature* 1991;351:714

5. Cohen RA, Vanhoutte PM. Endothelium-dependent hyperpolarization – beyond nitric oxide and cyclic GMP. *Circulation* 1995;92:3337-49

6. Taddei S, Virdis A, Ghiadoni L, *et al.* Vitamin C improves endothelium-dependent vasodilation by restoring nitric oxide activity in essential hypertension. *Circulation* 1998;97:2222-9

7. Taddei S, Ghiadoni L, Virdis A, *et al.* Vasodilation to bradykinin is mediated by an ouabain-sensitive pathway as a compensatory mechanism for impaired NO availability in essential hypertensive patients. *Circulation* 1999;100:1400-5

8. Altiere RJ, Kiritsy-Roy JA, Catravas JD. Acetylcholine-induced contractions in isolated rabbit pulmonary arteries: role of thromboxane A_2. *J Pharmacol Exp Ther* 1986;236:535-41

9. Katusic ZS, Vanhoutte PM. Superoxide anion is an endothelium-derived contracting factor. *Am J Physiol* 1989;257:H33-H37

10. Gryglewski RJ, Palmer RMJ, Moncada S. Superoxide anion is involved in the breakdown of endothelium-derived vascular relaxing factor. *Nature* 1986;320:454-6

11. Bendich A, Machlin IJ, Scandurra O, *et al.* The antioxidant role of vitamin C. *Adv Free Radic Biol Med* 1986;2:419-44

12. Taddei S, Virdis A, Ghiadoni L, *et al.* Endothelial dysfunction in hypertension: fact or fancy? *J Cardiovasc Pharmacol* 1998;32(Suppl 3):S41-47

13. Taddei S, Virdis A, Ghiadoni L, *et al.* Cyclooxygenase inhibition restores nitric oxide activity in essential hypertension. *Hypertension* 1997;29:274-9

14. Panza JA, Garcia CE, Kilcoyne CM, *et al.* Impaired endothelium-dependent vasodilation in patients with essential hypertension: evidence that nitric oxide abnormality is not localized to a single signal transduction pathway. *Circulation* 1995;91:1732-8

15. Taddei S, Virdis A, Mattei P, *et al.* Vasodilation to acetylcholine in primary and secondary forms of human hypertension. *Hypertension* 1993;21:929-33

16. Celermajer DS, Sorensen KE, Spiegelhalter DJ, *et al.* Aging is associated with endothelial dysfunction in healthy men years before the age-related decline in women. *J Am Coll Cardiol* 1994;24:471-6

17. Taddei S, Virdis A, Mattei P, *et al.* Aging and endothelial function in normotensive subjects and essential hypertensive patients. *Circulation* 1995;91:1981-7

18. Taddei S, Virdis A, Mattei P, Ghiadoni L, Basile Fasolo C, Sudano I, Salvetti A. Hypertension causes premature aging of endothelial function in humans. *Hypertension* 1997;29:736-43

19. Panza JA, Quyyumi AA, Callahan TS, Epstein SE. Effect of antihypertensive treatment on endothelium-dependent vascular relaxation in patients with essential hypertension. *J Am Coll Cardiol* 1993;21:1145-51

20. Ghiadoni L, Taddei S, Virdis A, *et al.* Endothelial function and common carotid wall thickening in essential hypertensive patients. *Hypertension* 1998;32:25-32

21. Zeiher AM, Schächinger V, Hohnloser ST, *et al.* Coronary atherosclerotic wall thickening and vascular reactivity in humans. *Circulation* 1994;89:2525-32

22. Davis SF, Yeung AC, Meredith IT, *et al.* Early endothelial dysfunction predicts the development of transplant coronary artery disease at 1 year post-transplant. *Circulation* 1996;93:457-62

23. Suwaidi JA, Hamasaki S, Higano ST, *et al.* Long-term follow-up of patients with mild coronary artery disease and endothelial dysfunction. *Circulation* 2000;101:948-54

24. Schächinger V, Britten MB, Zeiher AM. Prognostic impact of coronary vasodilator dysfunction on adverse long-term outcome of coronary heart disease. *Circulation* 2000;101:1899-1906

25. Murakami T, Mizuno S, Kaku B. Clinical morbidities in subjects with Doppler-evaluated endothelial dysfunction of coronary artery. *J Am Coll Cardiol* 1998;31(Suppl A):abstr 1165-64

26. Neunteufl T, Heher S, Katzenschlager R, *et al.* Late prognostic value of flow-mediated dilation in the brachial artery of patients with chest pain. *Am J Cardiol* 2000;86:207-10

27. Taddei S, Virdis A, Ghiadoni L, *et al.* Menopause is associated with endothelial dysfunction in women. *Hypertension* 1996;28:576-82

28. Virdis A, Ghiadoni L, Pinto S, *et al.* Mechanisms responsible for endothelial dysfunction associated with acute estrogen deprivation in normotensive women. *Circulation* 2000;101:2258-63

29. Virdis A, Ghiadoni L, Sudano I, *et al.* Estrogen and endothelial function. In Paoletti R, *et al.*, eds. *Women's Health and Menopause.* Amsterdam: Kluwer Academic Publishers, 1999:89-98

30. Farhat MY, Wolfe R, Vargas R, *et al.* Effect of testosterone treatment on vasoconstrictor response of left anterior descending coronary artery in male and female pigs. *J Cardiovasc Pharmacol* 1995;25:495-500

31. Hutchinson SJ, Sudhir K, Chou TM, *et al.* Testosterone worsens endothelial dysfunction associated with hypercholesterolemia and enviromental tobacco smoke exposure in male rabbit aorta. *J Am Coll Cardiol* 1997;29:800-7

32. Yue P, Chatterjee K, Beale C, *et al.* Testosterone relaxes rabbit coronary arteries and aorta. *Circulation* 1995;91:1154-60

33. Chou TM, Sudhir K, Hutchinson SJ, *et al.* Testosterone induces dilation of canine coronary artery conductance and resistance arteries *in vivo. Circulation* 1996;94:2614–19

34. Webb CM, McNeill JG, Hayward CS, *et al.* Effects of testosterone on coronary vasomotor regulation in men with coronary heart disease. *Circulation* 1999;100:1690–6

35. Ong PJL, Patrizi G, Chong WCF, *et al.* Testosterone enhances flow-mediated brachial artery reactivity in men with coronary artery disease. *Am J Cardiol* 2000;85:269–72

36. Herman SM, Robinson JTC, McCredie RJ, *et al.* Androgen deprivation is associated with enhanced endothelium-dependent dilation in adult men. *Arterioscler Thromb Vasc Biol* 1997;17:2004–9

Venous thromboembolism and hormone replacement therapy

6

P. M. Mannucci

Clinical manifestations of venous thromboembolism range from superficial thrombophlebitis, which is a benign condition with no long-term adverse effects or risks of major complications, to pulmonary embolism, which is life-threatening[1]. More frequent and of intermediate severity is deep vein thrombosis, which may not only cause pulmonary embolism but carries a risk of post-phlebitic syndrome, a disabling condition affecting many people who have experienced deep vein thrombosis.

Population-based studies of the annual incidence of venous thromboembolism in three different geographical locations have provided similar results, respectively, 1 per 1000 inhabitants in the USA[2] and 1.6–1.8 per 1000 in Sweden[3,4]. An important aspect of the epidemiology of venous thromboembolism in the context of the assessment of the absolute risks associated with oral contraceptives and hormone replacement therapy is that annual incidence increases dramatically with age, from 1 per 100 000 in childhood to 1 per 10 000 in adults of an age appropriate for use of the pill, and up to 1 per 100 in elderly people[2-5]. Postmenopausal women have an intermediate rate of annual incidence of venous thromboembolism of between 1 per 1000 and 1 per 5000, and this rate increases with age[2].

PATHOPHYSIOLOGY OF VENOUS THROMBOEMBOLISM

The first example of deep vein thrombosis of the legs did not appear in the literature until the thirteenth century, when it was described in a young man in France[6]. Such sources as the Bible, Galen and Hippocrates are silent on deep vein thrombosis, which may reflect the fact that symptoms of unilateral leg swelling and inflammation were perhaps confused with those of other pathological conditions. The first significant study on the pathophysiology of venous thromboembolism was made in the mid-nineteenth century by the German pathologist Rudolf Virchow, whose work still remains the basis of our current understanding of the disease[7]. He defined three essential factors for the onset of venous thromboembolism, still termed 'Virchow's triad', namely, damage to the vessel wall, the slowing of blood flow (stasis) and increased blood coagulability.

Modern studies have confirmed that damage to the endothelium of the vessel wall is an etiological factor in deep vein thrombosis, but it is not as important as in arterial thrombosis[1]. Stasis is undoubtedly an important factor in deep vein thrombosis, as evidenced by the fact that prevention of reduced blood flow is an important strategy in the prevention of this condition. Methods for preventing venous thromboembolism in patients undergoing major surgery, for example, include the use of graduated compression stockings[8], and the use of stockings which can be intermittently inflated during the operation and postoperatively[9]. Although the inflatable devices are not widely used in clinical practice, as they are rather cumbersome and inconvenient to deploy, they have been shown to be effective, indicating the importance of venous stasis as a precipitating cause of venous thromboembolism[8,9].

Increased blood coagulability is now recognized as probably the most significant part of the Virchow's triad in the pathogenesis of venous thromboembolism, whereas it probably has a less important role in arterial thromboembolism. Hypercoagulability has been defined in slightly different ways by different authors. In 1980, Wessler[10] defined it in terms of 'a perturbed but partially contained system in which intravascular coagulation is occurring but has not yet progressed to actual thrombus deposition'. More recently, Bauer and Rosenberg[11] offered a more biochemical definition of hypercoagulability, which they termed 'the prethrombotic state', which 'can be defined as an imbalance between the procoagulant and natural anticoagulant mechanisms that eventually leads to the development of overt thrombotic phenomena...'. The key point to note in this definition of hypercoagulability is that not only is there no clinical evidence of thrombosis, but that the coagulation cascade is activated, a state that can now be demonstrated by means of sensitive biochemical tests (prothrombin fragment 1 + 2, thrombin–antithrombin complex and others)[11].

The hypercoagulable state has now been recognized as a feature of a wide variety of acquired clinical conditions (Table 1). Most notable in the present context is the use of oral contraceptives, which are known to increase the risks of venous thromboembolism four- to six-fold, especially with third-generation products[12-15], though such risks need to be balanced against the inherent hypercoagulability and associated risks of pregnancy and the puerperium (Table 1). Also, as considered in more detail below, there is now evidence that hormone replacement therapy carries an increased

Table 1 Acquired and heritable conditions associated with hypercoagulability and an increased risk of venous thromboembolism

Acquired conditions	Heritable conditions
Pregnancy and puerperium	Deficiencies of naturally occurring anticoagulants (antithrombin, protein C, protein S)
Oral contraceptive use	Factor V Leiden, Arg506Gln
Hormone replacement therapy	Prothrombin G20210A mutation
Surgery and trauma	Some dysfibrinogenemias
Prolonged bed rest	Resistance to activated protein C in the absence of factor V Leiden*
Malignancy	Moderate hyperhomocysteinemia*
Cardiac failure	Elevation of fibrinogen*
Antiphospholipid syndrome	Elevation of factor VIII*
	Elevation of factor IX*
	Elevation of factor XI*

*The exclusively genetic basis of these risk factors of venous thromboembolism has not been confirmed

risk for venous thrombosis and pulmonary embolism[16].

INHERITED HYPERCOAGULABLE STATES

One of the most important findings on hypercoagulability in recent years has been that certain conditions associated with it, and therefore with increased risks of venous thromboembolism, can be inherited (Table 1)[1]. A minority of the inheritable risk factors can be explained in terms of a genetically determined deficiency or decreased function of proteins involved in the regulation of coagulation enzymes (antithrombin, protein C, protein S), leading to a procoagulant imbalance and hence to hypercoagulability. However, in the general population, a deficiency of the naturally occurring anticoagulants is very rare (less than 1% combined) (Table 2)[1]. On the other hand, the gain of function factor V mutation Arg506Gln and the prothrombin mutation G20210A exhibit polymorphic frequencies in the general population and are substantially more prevalent in people with venous thromboembolism (Table 2)[1]. However, these mutations are equally prevalent in centenarians[17] as in the general population, demonstrating that, although they are pointers for venous thromboembolism, they have little or no effect on mortality. Nonetheless, these mutations are associated with increased risks of venous thromboembolism (Table 2) and, in particular, are much more likely to be found in unexplained than consecutive cases of venous thromboembolism (Table 2), as well as in selected cases characterized by thrombosis in adolescence and in the young (less than 40–50 years)[18,19].

Other risk factors related to the hemostasis system have been identified recently, although it is not yet fully established whether they are risk factors for venous thromboembolism, nor whether they are genetically determined[1]. These putative risk factors are the acquired resistance to the anticoagulant action of activated protein C, moderate hyperhomocysteinemia and elevations of plasma levels of factor VIII, factor IX, factor XI and fibrinogen (which is not only a risk factor for arterial thrombosis but also for venous thromboembolism) (Table 1).

Table 2 Approximate prevalence of inherited thrombophilic abnormalities in the female healthy population and female patients with venous thromboembolism (VTE)

Abnormality	Healthy population (%)	VTE patients (%)
Antithrombin deficiency	0.2	1.1
Protein C deficiency	0.2	2.7
Protein S deficiency	0.3	1.3
Factor V Leiden	3–5	20/50*
Prothrombin G20210A mutation	1–3	6/20*

*Consecutive/unexplained VTE cases

Inherited risk factors are particularly important in venous thromboembolism when they are combined with other risk factors. For example, in healthy women of an age appropriate for the use of oral contraceptives, but who do not use them, the annual incidence of venous thromboembolism is 1 per 10 000[2]. In women who take oral contraceptives, but do not have mutant factor V, the annual risk of venous thromboembolism rises to 4 per 10 000 women (perhaps as high as 6 per 10 000 with third-generation pills). The presence of mutant factor V in women who are not taking oral contraceptives increases the risk to 8 per 10 000, whilst in those using oral contraceptives the risk increases multiplicatively to 32 per 10 000, so that the annual incidence of venous thromboembolism becomes as high as 1 per 300[20]. Despite these increases of risk of venous thromboembolism with mutant factor V Leiden, it has been calculated that two million women contemplating oral contraceptive use would have to be screened in order to prevent a single case of fatal pulmonary embolism or 100 cases of deep vein thrombosis[21]. Clearly, such screening would be regarded as not being cost-effective. Corresponding figures have not apparently been calculated for the screening of older women before starting hormone replacement therapy.

HYPERCOAGULABILITY AND HORMONE REPLACEMENT THERAPY

There are some data that suggest that hypercoagulability occurs prevalently in women who take hormone replacement therapy. One relatively small placebo-controlled study of women taking conjugated estrogens at conventional doses (0.625 and 1.25 mg/day) has, for example, demonstrated increased levels of prothrombin fragment 1 + 2, and hence, by definition, the presence of hypercoagulability[22]. Such effects, which can be predicted to increase risks of venous thromboembolism, are observed whether estrogens are given by mouth or transdermally[23]. Estrogen delivered by either route were also shown to have converse effects that would be expected to decrease the risk of venous thromboembolism, namely, a reduction in fibrinogen, which is a well-established risk factor for venous thromboembolism[22]. It seems, therefore, as with lipid metabolism, that no single measurement can be used as an indicator of hypercoagulability in such a complex system as hemostasis, and it is necessary to balance positive and negative effects of different parameters.

Several studies have compared hemostatic changes induced by estrogen-only replacement therapy and progestogen/estrogen replacement therapy, which is now the preferred treatment for women with an intact uterus. Two large prospective studies, namely, the Postmenopausal Estrogen and Progestogen Intervention (PEPI) trial using the progestogen medroxyprogesterone acetate[24], and the Medical Research Council (MRC) trial using norgestrel[25], have both shown that fibrinogen is equally reduced by estrogen-only replacement therapy and combined hormone replacement therapy (Table 3). However, only the MRC trial showed any effects on factor VII, a putative risk factor for thrombosis, especially arterial thrombosis. In this study, factor VII was increased with estrogen-only replacement therapy, but not with combined hormone replacement therapy, suggesting that the progestogen component of the latter mitigates the effects of estrogen. The complexity of the processes affected by estrogen-only replacement therapy and combined hormone replacement therapy is also apparent in lipid changes (Table 3), which were similar in both studies, with the exception of trends in triglycerides.

Comparative effects of estrogen-only and combined hormone replacement therapy on hemostasis have also been studied in the large cross-sectional Atherosclerosis Research In Communities (ARIC) study[26]. This showed no significant difference in their effects on fibrinogen, which decreased with both estrogen-only and combined hormone replacement therapy, nor on the anticoagulant protein antithrombin, which decreased slightly in both. With estrogen-only replacement therapy, there was an increase in factor VII, a result which confirms the findings from the prospective studies. Also, in the cross-sectional study, protein C was increased only with estrogen replacement therapy, a change which can be interpreted as protective for venous thromboembolism, since protein C is a potent inhibitor of blood coagulation (Table 3).

Overall, the results of the prospective and cross-sectional studies suggest that the progestogen component of combined hormone replacement therapy appears to attenuate, but not abolish, the procoagulant imbalance associated with estrogen-only preparations.

RISK OF VENOUS THROMBOEMBOLISM IN USERS OF HORMONE REPLACEMENT THERAPY

All the evidence for possible links between the use of hormone replacement therapy and venous thromboembolism is based on epidemiological data. Early studies suggested no increased risks of venous thromboembolism in hormone replacement therapy users, although more recent studies taken together have suggested an approximately two-fold increased risk for current users[27-34] (Table 4). Most of these investigations used case-control or cohort studies, without randomization or placebo controls[27-32,34]. A meta-analysis of these accumulated data suggests that an increased risk of venous thromboembolism with hormone replacement therapy use is likely, but indicates that there remains an element of uncertainty[16]. This has now been addressed in two randomized, controlled, double-blind clinical trials, namely the Heart and Estrogen/progestin Replacement Study (HERS)[35] and the Estrogen in Venous Thromboembolism Trial (EVTET)[36].

In the HERS trial, 2763 postmenopausal women with coronary heart disease, but without a

Table 3 Effects of combined progestogen/estrogen hormone replacement therapy (HRT) and estrogen-only replacement therapy (ERT) on lipids and hemostatic factors in prospective and cross-sectional studies

Parameter	Effect of ERT	Effect of combined HRT
PEPI and MRC trials (prospective)		
Cholesterol		
total	—	↓
HDL	↑	↓
LDL	↓	↓
Triglycerides	↑	↑*
Factor VII	↑†	—
Fibrinogen	↓	↓
ARIC study (cross-sectional)		
Fibrinogen	↓	↓
Antithrombin	↓	↓
Protein C	↑	—
Factor VII	↑	—

PEPI trial, Postmenopausal Estrogen and Progestogen Intervention trial[24]; MRC trial, Medical Research Council trial[25]; ARIC study, Atherosclerosis Research in Communities study[26]; HDL, high-density lipoprotein; LDL, low-density lipoprotein; *effect shown in PEPI trial only; †effect shown in MRC trial only

Table 4 Risk ratios for venous thromboembolism associated with hormone replacement therapy

Study	Estrogen route	Risk ratio (95% CI)
Case-control studies		
Boston CDSP[27]	oral	2.3 (0.5–8.6)
Pettiti et al.[28]	oral	0.7 (0.2–2.5)*
Devor et al.[29]	oral	0.8 (0.3–2.1)
Daly et al.[30]	oral	4.6 (2.1–10)
	transdermal	2.0 (0.5–7.6)
Daly et al.[31]	oral	2.3 (0.6–8.1)
Jick et al.[32]	oral	3.6 (1.6–7.8)
Perez-Gutthann et al.[34]	oral	2.1 (1.3–3.6)
	transdermal	2.1 (0.9–4.6)
Prospective study		
Grodstein et al.[33]	oral	2.1 (1.2–3.8)

CI, confidence interval; *90% confidence interval; CDSP, Collaborative Drug Surveillance Program

history of venous thromboembolism, were randomized to daily hormone replacement therapy with 0.625 mg conjugated estrogens plus 2.5 mg medroxyprogesterone acetate or placebo[35]. They were followed up for an average of 4.1 years. There were 34 venous thromboembolic events in the hormone replacement therapy group compared to 13 in the placebo group, with a relative risk of 2.7 (95% confidence interval 1.4–5.0), and a *p*-value for the difference of 0.003. The cumulative incidence of venous thromboembolism increased in both groups, due to the effects of increasing age. Further analysis showed that in users of hormone replacement therapy venous thromboembolism was most strongly associated with fractures of the lower extremity (Table 5). Other factors found to be linked with venous thromboembolism in the HERS trial, all of which are known from other evidence to be risk factors for the disease, were cancer, recent surgery, and hospitalization for medical reasons. In the context of hospitalization, it should be noted that risks of venous thromboembolism in medical patients confined to bed for long periods can be reduced substantially with the use of low molecular-weight heparin. HERS also demonstrated that venous thromboembolism was 50% less frequent in women taking aspirin (or a statin), suggesting that it may be possible to reduce deep vein thrombosis by using simple, inexpensive drugs with relatively few side-effects.

The EVTET study was completely different from HERS, as it was carried out in high-risk women with a history of venous thromboembolism, who were randomized to hormone replacement therapy or placebo[36]. The results showed a relatively rapid increase with time in the proportion of women suffering from venous thromboembolism episodes under hormone replacement therapy, compared with little change in the placebo group. Such a marked difference in the incidence of recurrent venous thromboembolism caused the trial to be terminated prematurely. The clearcut implication of the EVTET study, incomplete as it was, is that women with a previous episode of venous thromboembolism should not be prescribed hormone replacement therapy unless there are strong overriding reasons, in which case the possibility of giving at the same time drugs to prevent venous thromboembolism should be considered.

CONCLUSIONS

Despite considerable efforts to elucidate the links between hormone replacement therapy and venous thromboembolism, there is still uncertainty in this field. There is little doubt that hormone replacement therapy leads to a clinically relevant increased risk of venous thromboembolism in postmenopausal women. The estimated risk seems higher in the first year of treatment. There is no clear evidence for a dose-response relationship with estrogens or for differences between estrogen-only and combined hormone replacement therapy. Since most of the studies have been carried out in women using oral hormone replacement therapy, no conclusion is possible at the moment on the risk of venous thromboembolism related to transdermal preparations. It would be interesting to determine the role of the thrombophilic inherited gain of function mutations in the risk of thrombosis, a subject which was not addressed in HERS; unlike women starting oral contraceptive intake, it is possible that these older women should be screened for this mutation and the resultant hypercoagulability before commencing hormone replacement therapy, but the case cannot at present be made with absolute clarity. On the whole, in women with no risk factors for venous thromboembolism, the excess risk of venous thromboembolism with hormone replacement therapy use appears to be small in relation to the well-established potential benefits. However, women with a history of a previous episode of venous thromboembolism should not be prescribed hormone replacement therapy.

Table 5 Determinants of venous thromboembolism in the Heart and Estrogen/progestin Replacement Study (HERS)[35]

Determinant	Relative risk (95% CI)
Lower extremity fracture	18.1 (5.4–60.4)
Cancer	3.9 (1.6–9.4)
Recent surgery (within 90 days)	4.9 (2.4–9.8)
Non-surgical hospitalization	5.7 (3.0–10.8)
Aspirin treatment	0.5 (0.2–0.8)
Statin treatment	0.5 (0.2–0.9)

CI, confidence interval

References

1. Rosendaal FR. Venous thrombosis: a multicausal disease. *Lancet* 1999;353:1167-73
2. Anderson FA, Wheeler HB, Goldberg RJ, *et al.* A population-based perspective of the hospital incidence and case-fatality rates of deep vein thrombosis and pulmonary embolism. *Arch Intern Med* 1991;151:933-8
3. Nordström M, Lindblad B, Bergqvist D, Kjellstrom T. A prospective study of the incidence of deep vein thrombosis within a defined urban population. *J Intern Med* 1992;232:155-60
4. Hansson PO, Welin L, Tibblin G, Eriksson H. Deep vein thrombosis and pulmonary embolism in the general population. 'The Study of Men Born in 1913'. *Arch Intern Med* 1997;157:1665-70
5. Rosendaal FR. Thrombosis in the young: epidemiology and risk factors; a focus on venous thrombosis. *Thromb Haemost* 1997;78:1-6
6. Dexter L, Folch-Pi W. Venous thrombosis. An account of the first documented case. *J Am Med Assoc* 1974;228:195-6
7. Virchow R. Phlogose und Thrombose in Gefässystem. In *Gesammelte Abhandlungen zur Wissenschaftlichen Medizin*. Frankfurt: Staatsdruckerei, 1856
8. Agu O, Hamilton G, Baker D. Graduated compression stockings in the prevention of venous thromboembolism. *Br J Surg* 1999;86:992-1004
9. Turpie AG, Hirsh J, Julian D, Johnson J. Prevention of deep vein thrombosis in potential neurosurgical patients. A randomized trial comparing graduated compression stockings alone or graduated compression stockings plus intermittent pneumatic compression with control. *Arch Intern Med* 1989:149:679-81
10. Wessler S. Thrombosis and sex hormones: a perplexing liaison. *J Lab Clin Med* 1980;96:757-61
11. Bauer KA, Rosenberg RD. The pathophysiology of the prethrombotic state in humans: insights gained from studies using markers of hemostatic system activation. *Blood* 1987;70:343-50
12. Vessey M, Mant D, Smith A, Yeates D. Oral contraceptives and venous thromboembolism: findings in a large prospective study. *Br Med J (Clin Res Edn)* 1986;292:526
13. Venous thromboembolic disease and combined oral contraceptives: results of an international multicentre case-control study. Word Health Organization Collaborative Study of Cardiovascular Disease and Steroid Hormone Contraception. *Lancet* 1995;346:1575-82
14. Gerstman BB, Piper JM, Tomita DK, Ferguson WJ, Stadel BV, Lundin FE. Oral contraceptive estrogen dose and the risk of deep venous thromboembolic disease. *Am J Epidemiol* 1991;133:32-7
15. Carr B, Ory H. Estrogen and progestin components of oral contraceptives: relationship to vascular disease. *Contraception* 1997;55:267-72
16. Oger E, Scarabin PY. Assessment of risk for venous thromboembolism among users of hormone replacement therapy. *Drugs Aging* 1999;14:55-61
17. Mari D, Mannucci PM, Duca F, Bertolini S, Franceschi C. Mutant factor V (Arg506Gln) in healthy centenarians. *Lancet* 1996;347:1044
18. Lane DA, Mannucci PM, Bauer KA, *et al.* Inherited thrombophilia: part 1. *Thromb Haemost* 1996;76:651-62
19. Lane DA, Mannucci PM, Bauer KA, *et al.* Inherited thrombophilia: part 2. *Thromb Haemost* 1996;76:824-34
20. Vandenbroucke JP, Koster T, Briet E, Reitsma PH, Bertina RM, Rosendaal FR. Increased risk of venous thrombosis in oral-contraceptive users who are carriers of factor V Leiden mutation. *Lancet* 1994;344:1453-7
21. Vandenbroucke JP, van der Meer FJ, Helmerhorst FM, Rosendaal FR. Factor V Leiden: should we screen oral contraceptive users and pregnant women? *Br Med J* 1996;313:1127-30
22. Caine YG, Bauer KA, Barzegar S, *et al.* Coagulation activation following estrogen administration to post-menopausal women. *Thromb Haemost* 1992;68:392-5
23. Scarabin PY, Alhenc-Gelas M, Plu-Bureau G, Taisne P, Agher R, Aiach M. Effects of oral and transdermal estrogen/progesterone regimens on blood coagulation and fibrinolysis in postmenopausal women. A randomized controlled trial. *Arterioscler Thromb Vasc Biol* 1997;17:3071-8
24. The Writing Group for the PEPI Trial. Effect of estrogen or estrogen/progestin regimens on heart disease risk factors in post-menopausal women. The Post-menopausal Estrogen/Progestin Interventions (PEPI) Trial. *J Am Med Assoc* 1995;273:199-208
25. Medical Research Council's General Practice Research Framework. Randomised comparison of oestrogen versus oestrogen plus progestogen hormone replacement therapy in women with hysterectomy. *Br Med J* 1996;312:473-8
26. Nabulsi AA, Folsom AR, White A, *et al.* Association of hormone-replacement therapy with various cardiovascular risk factors in postmenopausal women. (The Atherosclerosis Risk in Communities Study Investigators). *N Engl J Med* 1993;328:1069-75
27. Boston Collaborative Drug Surveillance Program, Boston University Medical Center. Surgically confirmed gallbladder disease, venous thromboembolism and breast tumors in relation to

postmenopausal estrogen therapy. *N Engl J Med* 1974;290:15–19

28. Petitti DB, Wingerd J, Pellegrin F, Ramcharan S. Risk of vascular disease in women. Smoking, oral contraceptives, noncontraceptive estrogens, and other factors. *J Am Med Assoc* 1979;242:1150–4

29. Devor M, Barrett-Connor E, Renvall M, Feigal D, Ramsdell J. Estrogen replacement therapy and the risk of venous thrombosis. *Am J Med* 1992;92: 275–82

30. Daly E, Vessey MP, Painter R, Hawkins MM. Case-control study of venous thromboembolism risk in users of hormone replacement therapy. *Lancet* 1996;348:1027

31. Daly E, Vessey MP, Hawkins MM, Carson JL, Gough P, Marsh S. Risk of venous thromboembolism in users of hormone replacement therapy. *Lancet* 1996;348:977–80

32. Jick H, Derby LE, Wald Myers MW, Vasilakis C, Newton KM. Risk of hospital admission for idiopathic venous thromboembolism among users of post-menopausal oestrogens. *Lancet* 1996;348: 981–3

33. Grodstein F, Stampfer MJ, Goldhaber SZ, *et al.* Prospective study of exogenous hormones and risk of pulmonary embolism in women. *Lancet* 1996; 348:983–7

34. Perez Gutthann S, Garcia Rodriguez LA, Castellsague J, Duque Oliart A. Hormone replacement therapy and risk of venous thromboembolism: population-based case-control study. *Br Med J* 1997;314:796–800

35. Grady D, Wenger NK, Herrington D, *et al.* Postmenopausal hormone therapy increases risk for venous thromboembolism disease. *Ann Intern Med* 2000;132:689–96

36. Hoibraaten E, Ovigstad E, Arnesen H, Larsen S, Wickstrom E, Sandset PM. Increased risk of recurrent venous thromboembolism during hormone replacement therapy – results of the randomized, double-blind, placebo-controlled Estrogen in Venous Thromboembolism Trial (EVTET). *Thromb Haemost* 2000;84:961–7

Acute coronary syndromes in women

7

G. M. C. Rosano, C. Vitale, D. Onorati and M. Fini

INTRODUCTION

The group of acute ischemic syndromes includes the clinical syndromes of unstable angina and myocardial infarction with or without ST segment elevation. Women admitted to hospital with acute ischemic syndromes have different clinical presentations and outcomes from men (Figure 1)[1]. Women present more frequently than men with unstable angina and less frequently with acute myocardial infarction. Among patients presenting with acute ischemic syndromes, previous angina is more frequent in women while previous myocardial infarction is more frequent in men. While the lower incidence of previous myocardial infarction in women presenting with acute ischemic syndromes may be the result of a lower female survival rate after a first myocardial infarction, the differences in prior angina may relate to gender differences in anginal mechanisms and perception of

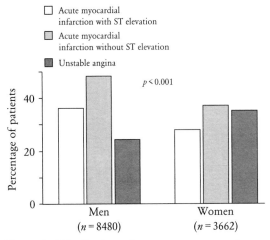

Figure 1 Distribution of acute coronary syndromes by gender. Women have a greater incidence of unstable angina, while men more frequently present with acute myocardial infarction with or without ST segment elevation. Adapted from reference 1

pain or in the distribution of risk factors between sexes.

CLINICAL PRESENTATION

Chest pain is the commonest symptom of acute ischemic syndromes in both men and women. Women, however, are more likely than men to present with dyspnea, fatigue, nausea and abdominal pain. The presence of these symptoms may contribute to the higher rate of undiagnosed myocardial infarctions and the longer time to make a diagnosis and therefore to initiate specific therapy in women than in men.

Women presenting with acute ischemic syndromes are usually older and have a higher prevalence of risk factors for coronary artery disease, such as smoking, arterial hypertension and diabetes, compared with their male counterparts, even when similar age groups are compared. In women, therefore, the cluster of risk factors may unfavorably affect prognosis and incidence of complications during hospitalization. Furthermore, not only do women have a higher prevalence of risk factors, but the weight of these risk factors is higher than in men. Indeed, ranking risk factors by their ability to predict coronary events after age adjustment, diabetes ranks seventh in females but only 21st in males, and cigarette smoking ranks fourth in women but seventh in men. Studies have shown that diabetes confers a 3–7-fold elevation in the risk of coronary events in women, compared to a 2–3-fold increase in men[2]. The risk associated with smoking is higher in women than in men, independently of age and other risk factors.

An important factor differing between men and women with acute ischemic syndromes is the delay in seeking and receiving care when chest pain is experienced. Women with acute ischemic syndromes tend to present later at hospital than men, and this delay in seeking care leads to a longer delay in the women receiving appropriate treatment. In the GUSTO I study[3], women had a significantly longer delay in presentation at hospital compared with men; this increase in delay was about half an hour and was comparable to delays reported by other studies. The delay between symptom onset and treatment influences the response to therapy, especially to thrombolysis and primary percutaneous transluminal coronary angioplasty (PTCA).

OUTCOME OF ACUTE ISCHEMIC SYNDROMES

Outcomes in patients presenting with acute ischemic syndromes vary according to the clinical syndrome, although most of the differences in prognosis, especially in cases of acute myocardial infarction, are related to the longer delay in women in seeking and receiving care (Figure 2)[1].

Among patients with unstable angina, women tend to have less extensive disease and the frequent finding of normal coronary arteries, which translates to a better outcome than in men. Indeed, the adjusted odds ratio for a major cardiac event in the 30 days after hospitalization is 0.65, compared with men. When presenting with an acute myocardial infarction without ST segment elevation, men and women have the same prognosis. This seems to be related to the fact that although women in this group have less extensive coronary

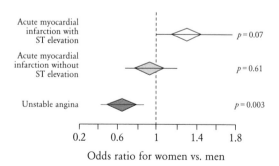

Figure 2 Adjusted 30-day risk of death or infarction in men and women admitted with acute ischemic syndromes. Women have a better prognosis when admitted with the diagnosis of unstable angina but have a worse fate when presenting with acute myocardial infarction with ST segment elevation. Adapted from reference 1

artery disease they are older and have more comorbidity. Furthermore, in this group of patients, more time is spent in making the diagnosis, abolishing or reducing the male/female time difference in receiving thrombolysis. When presenting with acute myocardial infarction and ST segment elevation, women have a significantly worse outcome than men. A major problem in evaluating the fate of men and women presenting with acute myocardial infarction is the presence of comorbidities and the age difference between sexes. Women present later with acute myocardial infarction because in them the disease appears later in life than in men, and therefore, in our view, the adjustment for age when comparing prognosis of acute myocardial infarction between sexes is not justified. Some authors have suggested that female gender is not an independent predictor of prognosis in patients with acute ischemic syndromes after adjustment for age and comorbidities. Advanced age *per se*, however, cannot explain the gender-related difference in outcome as recently shown by Vaccarino and colleagues[4], who demonstrated that among patients of 50 years of age or less, mortality was more than twice as high in women as in men, and that the difference decreased with age and was no longer significant after the age of 74 years.

The different mortality rate in women presenting with acute myocardial infarction does not seem to be dependent upon a different response to thrombolysis. Indeed, a meta-analysis conducted by the Fibrinolytic Therapy Trialists[5] showed that women had a 60% greater 35-day mortality rate than men, independently of whether or not thrombolytic therapy was used. The ISIS-3 study[6] showed a significantly higher 35-day mortality rate and a higher probability of cardiac rupture, reinfarction and cardiogenic shock in women with acute myocardial infarction receiving thrombolysis than in men. These data were confirmed by a large thrombolytic therapy trial; GUSTO I showed that women have a nearly two-fold higher 30-day relative risk of death compared with men before adjusting for age and comorbidities, and a relative risk of 1.15 after adjustment[3]. In this study, women had higher 30-day rates of shock, congestive heart failure and reinfarction than men (Figure 3). The GUSTO I sub-study confirmed the more recurrent ischemia and a higher 30-day mortality rate in women than in men, despite similar 7-day left ventricular ejection fraction and extent of coronary atherosclerosis and presence of collateral circulation at coronary angiography[7]. This substudy also showed that global left ventricular ejection fraction after 90 min of thrombolysis and the degree of reperfusion (thrombolysis in myocardial infarction (TIMI) grade of flow III) were similar in men and women, suggesting that there is no gender difference in the response to thrombolysis (Figure 4)[7].

TREATMENT OF ACUTE ISCHEMIC SYNDROMES IN MEN AND WOMEN

The therapeutic options for the treatment of unstable angina and acute myocardial infarction are similar in men and women, but it seems that men

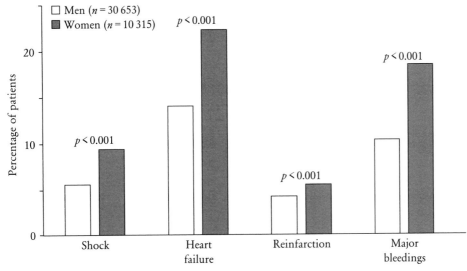

Figure 3 In-hospital complications in men and women in the GUSTO I study. Women have a nearly two-fold higher 30-day relative risk of death compared with men before adjusting for age and comorbidities, and a relative risk of 1.15 after adjustment. In this study, women had higher 30-day rates of shock, congestive heart failure and reinfarction than men. Adapted from reference 3

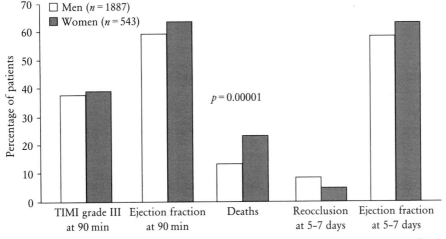

Figure 4 Effect of thrombolysis on vessel patency, left ventricular ejection fraction and mortality in men and women in the GUSTO I study. Despite similar effectiveness of thrombolysis on vessel patency and left ventricular function, women have a higher mortality rate. Adapted from reference 7. TIMI, thrombolysis in myocardial infarction

and women may have different responses to different therapeutic approaches, and that despite an equivalent response to therapy, women receive effective treatments less frequently than men.

The question of whether women respond differently from men to thrombolysis has been addressed by the GUSTO I angiographic sub-study in which patency rates and left ventricular function were assessed at 90 min and 5–7 days after thrombolysis (Figure 4)[7]. Patency and reocclusion rates as well as global left ventricular function were similar in men and women. However, in this study more women than men died before the 5–7-day angiogram (23% vs. 11%, $p < 0.00001$). It is therefore possible that this excess mortality in the first few days of hospitalization after thrombolysis reflected either thrombolysis failure (reocclusion) or side-effects (hemorrhage, cardiac rupture). A randomized comparison of male/female outcome after either thrombolysis or primary angioplasty has been carried out by the PAMI investigators[8]. The study, which included 395 patients, showed that among patients randomized to thrombolysis, women had a higher mortality rate compared with men, but that the outcome among patients randomized to primary PTCA was similar in the two sexes. The study showed that in women the choice of treatment significantly influenced prognosis, and therefore that in women with acute myocardial infarction, primary PTCA, where available, is superior to thrombolysis. A partial explanation of these results is the higher incidence of intracranial hemorrhage in women receiving thrombolysis, which in this study was particularly elevated (5.3% women vs. 0.7% men, $p = 0.037$). Other studies using weight-adjusted administration of recombinant tissue plasminogen activator failed to show this increased incidence of intracranial hemorrhage in women.

The FRISC 2 study[9] has recently evaluated the effects of two different therapeutic strategies in men and women admitted with unstable angina and has shown that an early aggressive strategy with coronary angiography and PTCA is preferable in men, while women seem to benefit more from a conservative therapeutic approach with a delayed invasive assessment (Figure 5)[9,10]. Thrombolysis and primary PTCA therefore seem to have a similar effectiveness in men and women,

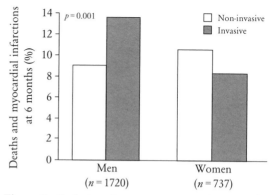

Figure 5 Early invasive versus conservative strategies in men and women admitted with unstable angina. An early aggressive strategy with coronary angiography and PTCA is preferable in men, while women seem to benefit more from a conservative therapeutic approach with a delayed invasive assessment. Adapted from reference 9

but different therapeutic strategies confer better prognoses in the two sexes according to clinical presentation[11-14]. Women presenting with acute myocardial infarction seem to benefit more from primary angioplasty, while women presenting with unstable angina benefit more from standard therapy and an initially conservative approach. Despite evidence of a similar efficacy of standard therapies in men and women, several studies have shown an underutilization of thrombolysis, aspirin, beta-blockers, heparin and revascularization procedures in women compared with men[15-24]. This evidence, together with the longer time spent in diagnosis and giving care, may explain the worse outcome after hospitalization of women with an acute myocardial infarction compared with men.

CONCLUSION

Acute ischemic syndromes have different incidences in men and women. Women more frequently have unstable angina, while men tend to present more frequently with acute myocardial infarction. Treatment strategies in women yield different results according to clinical presentation. Women presenting with an acute myocardial infarction benefit more from primary PTCA, while women presenting with unstable angina benefit more from standard therapy and a delayed invasive approach.

Compared with men, women have a higher early mortality rate when presenting with an acute myocardial infarction. This higher mortality rate is not explained by advanced age, comorbidities or extent of coronary artery disease. Possible explanations are the higher prevalence of underlying risk factors, and the greater incidence of recurrent ischemia, reinfarction, cardiac rupture and stroke (when weight-adjusted rates of thrombolysis are given) in women compared with men. However, important additional factors which play a major role in determining the worse outcome in women are the longer time delay in presentation at hospital, the longer delay in receiving care and therapy, and the underutilization of effective therapy compared with male counterparts. These factors are related to social and cultural prejudices which suggest that angina is not important in women. An effort should be made to alert women and doctors so that earlier and better treatment of women presenting with chest pain in the emergency room can be achieved.

References

1. Hochman JS, Tamis EJ, Thompson TD, *et al.* for the Global Use of Strategies to Open Occluded Coronary Arteries in Acute Coronary Syndromes IIb Investigators. Sex, clinical presentation and outcome in patients with acute ischemic syndromes. *N Engl J Med* 1999;341:226–32

2. Malmberg K, Yusuf S, Gerstein HC, Brown J, Zhao F, *et al.* Impact of diabetes on long-term prognosis in patients with unstable angina and non-Q-wave myocardial infarction: results of the OASIS (Organization to Assess Strategies for Ischemic Syndromes) Registry. *Circulation* 2000;102:1014–19

3. Weaver WD, White HD, Wilcox RG, *et al.* for the GUSTO I Investigators. Comparison of characteristics and outcomes among women and men with acute myocardial infarction treated with thrombolytic therapy. *J Am Med Assoc* 1996;275:777–82

4. Vaccarino V, Parsons L, Every NR, *et al.* Sex-based differences in early mortality after myocardial infarction. *N Engl J Med* 1999;341:217–25

5. Fibrinolytic Therapy Trialists Collaborative Group. Indications for fibrinolytic therapy in suspected acute myocardial infarction: collaborative review of early mortality and major morbidity results from all randomized trials of more than 1000 patients. *Lancet* 1994;343:311–22

6. Malacrida R, Genon M, Maggioni AP, *et al.* for the Third International Study of Infarct Survival Collaborative Group. A comparison of early outcome of acute myocardial infarction in women and men. *N Engl J Med* 1998;338:8–14

7. Woodfield SL, Lundergan CF, Reiner JS, *et al.* Gender and acute myocardial infarction: is there a different response to thrombolysis? *J Am Coll Cardiol* 1997;29:35–42

8. Stone GW, Grines CL, Browne KF, *et al.* Predictors of in-hospital and 6-month outcome after acute myocardial infarction in the reperfusion era: the Primary Angioplasty in Myocardial Infarction (PAMI) Trial. *J Am Coll Cardiol* 1995;25:370–7

9. FRISC Investigators. Long-term low-molecular-mass heparin in unstable coronary-artery disease: FRISC II prospective randomised multicentre study. FRagmin and Fast Revascularisation during Instability in coronary artery disease. *Lancet* 1999;354:701–7

10. Adams PC, Skinner JS, Cohen M, McBride R, Fuster V. Acute coronary syndromes in the United States and United Kingdom: a comparison of approaches. The Antithrombotic Therapy in Acute Coronary Syndromes Research Group. *Clin Cardiol* 1998;21:348–52

11. Alexander KP, Peterson ED, Granger CB, *et al.* Potential impact of evidence-based medicine in acute coronary syndromes: insights from GUSTO-IIb. Global Use of Strategies to Open Occluded Arteries in Acute Coronary Syndromes trial. *J Am Coll Cardiol* 1998;32:2023–30

12. Al-Khalili F, Svane B, Wamala SP, Orth-Gomer K, Ryden L, Schenck-Gustafsson K. Clinical importance of risk factors and exercise testing for prediction of significant coronary artery stenosis in women recovering from unstable coronary artery disease: the Stockholm Female Coronary Risk Study. *Am Heart J* 2000;139:971–8

13. Goldschmidt-Clermont PJ, Schulman SP, Bray PF, Chandra NC, Grigoryev D, *et al.* Refining the treatment of women with unstable angina – a randomized, double-blind, comparative safety and efficacy evaluation of integrelin versus aspirin in the

management of unstable angina. *Clin Cardiol* 1996; 19:869–74

14. Hochman JS, McCabe CH, Stone PH, *et al*. Outcome and profile of women and men presenting with acute coronary syndromes: a report of TIMI IIIB. *J Am Coll Cardiol* 1997;30:141–8

15. Johanson P, Abrahamsson P, Rosengren A, Dellborg M. Time trends in thrombolytics: women are catching up. *Scand Cardiovasc J* 1999;33:39–43

16. Lincoff AM, Califf RM, Ellis SG, Sigmon KN, Lee KL, Leimberger JD, Topol EJ. Thrombolytic therapy for women with myocardial infarction: is there a gender gap? Thrombolysis and Angioplasty in Myocardial Infarction Study Group. *J Am Coll Cardiol* 1993;22:1780–7

17. Matsui K, Polanczyk CA, Gaspoz JM, Theres H, Kleber FX, *et al*. Management of patients with acute myocardial infarction at five academic medical centers: clinical characteristics, resource utilization, and outcome. *J Invest Med* 1999;47:134–40

18. Mohler ER III, Ryan T, Segar DS, Sawada SG, Sonel AF, *et al*. Clinical utility of troponin T levels and echocardiography in the emergency department. *Am Heart J* 1998;135:253–60

19. Naunheim KS, Fiore AC, Arango DC, Pennington DG, Barner HB, *et al*. Coronary artery bypass grafting for unstable angina pectoris: risk analysis. *Ann Thorac Surg* 1989;47:569–74

20. Ornato JP. Chest pain emergency centers: improving acute myocardial infarction care. *Clin Cardiol* 1999;22(Suppl 8):IV3–9

21. Puletti M, Sunseri L, Curione M, Erba SM, Borgia C. Acute myocardial infarction: sex-related differences in prognosis. *Am Heart J* 1984;108:63–6

22. Stone GW, Grines CL, Browne KF, *et al*. Comparison of in-hospital outcome in men versus women treated by either thrombolytic therapy or primary coronary angioplasty for acute myocardial infarction. *Am J Cardiol* 1995;75:987–92

23. Toss H, Wallentin L, Siegbahn A. Influences of sex and smoking habits on anticoagulant activity in low-molecular-weight heparin treatment of unstable coronary artery disease. *Am Heart J* 1999;137:72–8

24. Wexler LF. Studies of acute coronary syndromes in women – lessons for everyone. *N Engl J Med* 1999; 341:275–6

Estrogen receptor-β and women's health   8

M. Warner, G. Cheng, L. Wang, Z. Weihua, S. Saji and J.-Å. Gustafsson

ESTROGEN RECEPTOR-β

Endocrinologists often ask how it is possible that estrogen receptor-β (ERβ) remained undetected for 30 years after the discovery of estrogen receptor-α (ERα)[1]. The answer is that for a long time estrogen was regarded solely as a hormone responsible for female reproductive function, and its major target organ was seen as the uterus. Indeed, the mature uterus is a rich source of ERα with little ERβ. We now know that estrogen has multiple functions in many extrauterine tissues in the body, both male and female, and that in many of these tissues there is no detectable ERα. ERβ was cloned from a rat prostate cDNA library in 1995[2]. It belongs to the same nuclear receptor family as do all other steroid hormone receptors and it binds to estradiol with an affinity similar to that of ERα.

DISTRIBUTION OF ERβ IN THE BODY

ERβ is widely distributed throughout the body; in females the highest expression is in the granulosa cells in the ovary and in males in the prostate epithelium[2,3]. However, ERβ is also present in the cardiovascular system, bone, brain, colon, urinary bladder, mammary gland, lung and immune system[4]. Surprisingly, in the immature uterus, ERα and ERβ are expressed at similar levels[5], and ERβ but not ERα is highly expressed in the myometrium during pregnancy where it is thought to have a role in prevention of premature labor[6].

ERβ IN DISEASES OF THE OVARY

Mice in which the ERβ gene has been inactivated (BERKO mice)[7] have revealed previously unsuspected functions for ERβ in the ovary, and these novel functions may lead to new insights into human diseases such as ovarian cancer, polycystic ovarian disease, early ovarian failure and infertility.

The abundance of an estrogen receptor in cells which synthesize estrogen was at first puzzling. Studies with BERKO mice have shown that ERβ does, in fact, play an extremely important role in follicular maturation, and without it ovulation very rarely occurs. BERKO mice have normal levels of estradiol and luteinizing hormone (LH) and a very reduced capacity to ovulate[8]. Ovulation can be stimulated by human chorionic gonadotropin (hCG), but very few ova are produced. Occasionally, BERKO mice do get pregnant and deliver their litters. The litter size is small (approximately four pups per litter).

Mice in which the ERα gene is inactivated (ERKO) also have ovarian abnormalities and are infertile, but the abnormalities can be completely reversed by normalizing the plasma concentration of LH, indicating regulation at the level of the hypothalamic–pituitary axis[9]. The major defect in BERKO ovaries, i.e. failure to ovulate, is reversed by the antiandrogen, flutamide. Since there are large numbers of healthy primary, preantral and antral follicles in BERKO ovaries, it is apparent that there is excessive recruitment of primordial follicles into the growing pool. In 2-year-old BERKO ovaries there is almost complete absence of follicles, compared with the wild-type ovaries in which a multitude of follicles still remain at this age. This early ovarian failure is supportive evidence that more primordial follicles enter the growth pool early in these animals.

In addition to the increase in follicular atresia, there is also a marked disorganization of the germinal epithelium of the BERKO ovary. Since this is the site of development of most human ovarian cancers, a role for ERβ in regulation of the growth of this layer would suggest novel approaches for understanding and perhaps for treatment of ovarian cancer.

The etiology of ovarian cancer is poorly understood. A high life-time number of ovulatory cycles and excessive gonadotropin and androgen stimulation of the ovary are risk factors, and protective factors include multiparity and use of oral contraceptives. Since ovulation is a cytokine-regulated process in the ovarian epithelium it has been suggested that cytokines and chemokines play a role in the etiology of ovarian cancer[10].

We have found that one of the major defects in the BERKO ovary is failure of down-regulation of the androgen receptor in follicles as they mature from the early antral stage. Persistence of an androgenic environment leads to follicular atresia and is one characteristic of polycystic ovarian disease. A role for the androgen receptor in follicular atresia in BERKO mice is evident from the reversal of the BERKO ovarian phenotype by treatment with flutamide. In addition to follicular atresia, overexpression of androgen receptor leads to excessive recruitment of primordial follicles into the growth pool. We speculate that a selective ovarian ERβ agonist would down-regulate ovarian androgen receptor and lead to less recruitment of primordial follicles. Such an agonist would, therefore, have two advantages. It would extend the reproductive life of a female by maintaining a large reserve of primordial follicles, and in addition, since there would be no ovulation, there would be a decreased risk of ovarian cancer.

ALZHEIMER'S DISEASE

Evidence suggests multiple roles for estrogen in the brain. It influences development, plasticity and survival of neurons, with consequences for age-related neuronal degenerative diseases. Estrogen is thought to enhance cognitive functions by modulating the production of acetylcholine in basal forebrain neurons. ERα is the predominant receptor subtype in the basal forebrain cholinergic neurons of the adult rat brain. Estrogen receptors are also involved in mediating estradiol action on central serotonergic and dopaminergic mechanisms. Estrogen can prevent or modulate insults to dopaminergic neurons and is thought, therefore, to alter the natural history of disease processes

affecting the dopaminergic circuitry in the brain, including Parkinson's disease[11,12].

Epidemiological studies suggest that estrogen replacement therapy decreases the likelihood of developing Alzheimer's disease[13-15]. Despite all of the laboratory data and trends from human epidemiological studies, the usefulness of estrogen in protection against age-related degenerative diseases in women is still an unresolved issue[15-17]. Recent studies show that replacement of estrogen in older women has no effect on incidence or progression of Alzheimer's disease. This result probably means that estrogen replacement is of no value in prevention of neurodegeneration if it is administered too late. The beneficial effects of estradiol must lie in its capacity to prevent or slow the progression of neurodegeneration.

MORPHOLOGICAL CHANGES IN BERKO MOUSE BRAINS

No morphological changes have been reported in mice lacking ERα, but there are striking abnormalities in the brains of BERKO mice[18]. The second and third layers of the somatosensory cortex are missing and there is a severe neuronal deficit throughout the cortex. In addition, neuronal cell bodies are small and there are large vacuoles surrounding the cell nuclei. In the limbic system there is an enormous proliferation of astroglia. These data suggest that there is a role for estrogen in neuronal growth and/or migration during development of the brain. In addition, continued loss of neurons as BERKO mice age suggests a role for ERβ in preventing apoptotic death of neurons. We speculate that exposure to ERβ agonists during the developmental and postmenopausal periods is essential for maintenance of healthy neurons.

BREAST CANCER

Numerous animal studies show that estrogen can induce and promote breast cancer, and removal of the ovaries or administration of antiestrogens can oppose this[19-22]. Because ERα-containing epithelial cells in the normal breast do not proliferate[23-25], the mechanisms through which estrogen induces epithelial growth in the breast are not clear. The prevailing theory is that estrogen stimulates secretion of growth factors from breast stroma and that these factors stimulate epithelial cells to proliferate.

Studies with the rodent breast[26] show that ERβ is constitutively expressed in approximately 70% of epithelial cells, regardless of the endocrine state of the breast. ERα is highly expressed during lactation when it is co-expressed with ERβ in over 70% of epithelial cells. In the virgin, pregnant and post-lactation breast, few cells express ERα, and there are very few cells where the two receptors are co-localized. During the highest proliferative phase of the breast, i.e. pregnancy, there is very little expression of ERα and high expression of ERβ, but most of the cells which express the proliferating cell nuclear antigen contain neither receptor. These results seem to indicate that the presence of estrogen receptors in epithelial cells prevents these cells from proliferating.

We have analyzed 50 human breast biopsy samples for expression of ERα and ERβ. Expression levels and function of the two receptors were measured by sucrose density gradient centrifugation in low-salt tissue extracts (unactivated estrogen receptor) with estradiol as ligand, by Western blotting of both the low-salt tissue extracts and vanadate-extracted nuclear fractions (nuclear estrogen receptor) with antibodies specific for ERα (H222) and ERβ (LBD antibody). We found that ERβ was present in all breast samples whether they were normal or displayed benign or malignant disease. ERα was not detected in normal breast or in samples displaying medullary cancer, but was expressed at very high levels in samples displaying in situ and invasive ductal cancer. Most interestingly, we found that the ERβ variant, ERβcx, was expressed in certain breast cancers. Since this ERβ isoform is a dominant repressor of ERα[27], its presence in breast cancer might define one type of ERα-positive breast cancer which is non-responsive to antiestrogen therapy.

CONCLUSIONS

Estrogen receptor-β is widely expressed in the female body. One interesting aspect of our having become aware of this receptor is that the future of hormone replacement therapy in females looks bright. Relatively selective ligands exist and more selective ligands are being developed. The postmenopausal female may look forward in the future to replacement therapies which would permit all of the beneficial effects of estrogen (in the brain, skin and cardiovascular system) without the increased risk of estrogen-related cancers.

ACKNOWLEDGEMENTS

This work was supported by the Swedish Cancer Fund and by Karo Bio AB.

References

1. Jensen EV, Jacobsen HI. Basic guides to the mechanism of estrogen action. *Rec Prog Horm Res* 1962; 18:387–414
2. Kuiper GG, Enmark E, Pelto-Huikko M, Nilsson S, Gustafsson J-Å. Cloning of a novel receptor expressed in rat prostate and ovary. *Proc Natl Acad Sci USA* 1996; 93: 5925–30
3. Sar M, Welsch F. Differential expression of estrogen receptor-beta and estrogen receptor-alpha in the rat ovary. *Endocrinology* 1999;140:963–71
4. Gustafsson J-Å. Novel aspects of estrogen action. *J Soc Gynecol Invest* 2000;7:S8–9
5. Weihua Z, Saji S, Mäkinen S, Cheng G, Jensen EV, Warner M, Gustafsson J-Å. ERβ, a modulator of ERα in the uterus. *Proc Natl Acad Sci USA* 2000; 97:5936–41
6. Wu JJ, Geimonen E, Andersen J. Increased expression of estrogen receptor-β in human uterine smooth muscle at term. *Eur J Endocrinol* 2000; 142:92–9
7. Krege JH, Hodgin JB, Couse JF, Enmark E, Warner M, Mahler JF, Sar M, Korach KS, Gustafsson J-Å, Smithies O. Generation and reproductive phenotypes of mice lacking estrogen receptor-β. *Proc Natl Acad Sci USA* 1998;95:15667–82

8. Couse JF, Bunch DO, Lindzey J, Schomberg DW, Korach KS. Prevention of the polycystic ovarian phenotype and characterization of ovulatory capacity in the estrogen receptor-alpha knockout mouse. *Endocrinology* 1999;140:5855–65

9. Couse JF, Korach KS. Estrogen receptor null mice: what have we learned and where will they lead us? *Endocr Rev* 1999;20:358–417

10. Nash MA, Ferrandina G, Gordinier M, Loercher A, Freedman RS. The role of cytokines in both the normal and malignant ovary. *Endocr Relat Cancer* 1999;6:93–107

11. Buscher U, Chen FC, Kentenich H, Schmiady H. Cytokines in the follicular fluid of stimulated and non-stimulated human ovaries; is ovulation a suppressed inflammatory reaction? *Hum Reprod* 1999;14:162–6

12. Kompoliti K. Estrogen and movement disorders. *Clin Neuropharmacol* 1999;22:318–26

13. Nakayama S, Kuzuhara S. Apolipoprotein E phenotypes in healthy normal controls and demented subjects with Alzheimer's disease and vascular dementia in Mie Prefecture of Japan. *Psychiatr Clin Neurosci* 1999;53:643–8

14. Palacios S. Current perspectives on the benefits of HRT in menopausal women. *Maturitas* 1999;33: S1–13

15. Slooter AJ, Bronzova J, Witteman JC, Van Broeckhoven C, Hofman A, van Duijn CM. Estrogen use and early-onset Alzheimer's disease: a population-based study. *J Neurol Neurosurg Psychiatr* 1999;67:779–81

16. Luoto R, Manolio T, Meilahn E, Bhadelia R, Furberg C, Cooper L, Kraut M. Estrogen replacement therapy and MRI-demonstrated cerebral white matter changes, and brain atrophy in older women. *J Am Geriatr Soc* 2000;48:467–72

17. Solerte SB, Fioravanti M, Racchi M, Trabucchi M, Zanetti O, Govoni S. Menopause and estrogen deficiency as a risk factor in dementing illness: hypothesis on the biological basis. *Maturitas* 1999; 31:95–101

18. Wang L, Anderson S, Warner M, Gustafsson J-Å. ERβ: a receptor involved in neuroprotection. *Proc Natl Acad Sci USA* 2001;98:2792–6

19. Liao DZ, Pantazis CG, Hou X, Li SA. Promotion of estrogen-induced mammary gland carcinogenesis by androgen in the male Noble rat: probable mediation by steroid receptors. *Carcinogenesis* 1998; 19:2173–80

20. Hilakivi-Clarke L, Cho E, Onojafe I, Raygada M, Clarke R. Maternal exposure to genistein during pregnancy increases carcinogen-induced mammary tumorigenesis in female rat offspring. *Oncol Reports* 1999;6:1089–95

21. Koibuchi Y, Sugamata N, Iino Y, Yokoe T, Andoh T, Maemura M, Takei H, Horiguchi J, Matsumoto H, Morishita Y. The mechanisms of antitumor effects of luteinizing hormone-releasing hormone agonist (buserelin) in 7,12-dimethylbenz(a) anthracene-induced rat mammary cancer. *Int J Mol Med* 1999;4:145–8

22. Zeps N, Bentel JM, Papadimitriou JM, D'Antuono MF, Dawkins HJ. Estrogen receptor-negative epithelial cells in mouse mammary gland development and growth. *Differentiation* 1998;62:221–6

23. Clarke RB, Howell A, Potten CS, Anderson E. Dissociation between steroid receptor expression and cell proliferation in the human breast. *Cancer Res* 1997;57:4987–91

24. Clarke RB, Howell A, Anderson E. Estrogen sensitivity of normal human breast tissue *in vivo* and implanted into athymic nude mice: analysis of the relationship between estrogen-induced proliferation and progesterone receptor expression. *Breast Cancer Res Treat* 1997;45:121–33

25. Wiesen JF, Young P, Werb Z, Cunha GR. Signaling through the stromal epidermal growth factor receptor is necessary for mammary ductal development. *Development* 1999;126:335–44

26. Saji S, Jensen EV, Nilsson S, Rylander T, Warner M, Gustafsson J-Å. Estrogen receptors alpha and beta in the rodent mammary gland. *Proc Natl Acad Sci USA* 2000;97:337–42

27. Ogawa S, Inoue S, Watanabe T, Orimo A, Hosoi T, Ouchi Y, Muramatsu M. Molecular cloning and characterization of human estrogen receptor beta-cx, a potential inhibitor of estrogen action in human. *Nucleic Acids Res* 1998;26:3505–12

Molecular biology of selective estrogen receptor modulators

9

D. M. Lonard and B. W. O'Malley

INTRODUCTION

For more than 20 years, it has been known that 4-hydroxytamoxifen (4HT), the biologically active metabolite of tamoxifen, does not behave as a 'pure' estrogen antagonist and produces estrogenic responses in some tissues. This has led to a refinement in the terminology for 4HT and other related ligands as selective estrogen receptor modulators (SERMs), reflecting their ability to behave as estrogen agonists in some tissues while behaving as antagonists in others. In the past few years, a great deal of progress has been made in our understanding of how the estrogen receptor and other nuclear hormone receptors function, which promises to shed light on the mechanism of how SERMs elicit their tissue-specific biological responses. Perhaps the largest recent contribution to our understanding of how nuclear hormone receptors function has involved the identification of nuclear hormone receptor coactivators which promise to fill in unanswered gaps in our knowledge of how SERMs function in a tissue-selective manner. Since the first nuclear receptor coactivator was identified, steroid receptor coactivator-1 (SRC-1)[1], many others have been characterized, and their contribution to the nuclear receptor activation process is being pursued aggressively[2-4]. The realization that estradiol manifests its biological actions through two estrogen receptors, the classical estrogen receptor-α (ERα) and the more recently identified estrogen receptor-β (ERβ)[5], increases the potential complexity of SERM biological action. Although largely unappreciated to this point, it has been known for many years that SERMs influence the stability of ERα. However, recent progress in the understanding of the ubiquitin–proteasome pathway in ERα function also promises to play an

important role in defining the biological character of SERMs, and will be discussed in more detail below. Additionally, co-repressors such as N-CoR and SMRT may also influence the biological response to SERMs and will also be discussed in this chapter. Integration of the many molecular factors which impinge upon the estrogen receptor promises to lead to a better understanding of how SERMs produce tissue-specific biological responses.

Binding of an agonist ligand to the estrogen receptor sets in motion a series of events which culminates in the expression of estrogen-regulated genes (Figure 1). Like other members of the nuclear hormone receptor superfamily, ERα and ERβ are modular proteins, possessing discrete domains which carry out specific functions needed for them to function as ligand-regulated transcription factors[6]. These receptors bear an *N*-terminal transcriptional activation function (AF-1), and a centrally located DNA-binding domain (DBD). The C-terminus contains the ligand binding domain (LBD), which interacts with estradiol or SERM ligands and additionally serves as a ligand-activated transcriptional activation function (AF-2). Receptor agonists such as estradiol induce a conformational change in the LBD which allows it to interact with coactivators[4], while SERM ligands such as 4HT and raloxifene induce an alternative LBD conformation which prohibits coactivator binding to the LBD. In spite of this, different SERMs induce unique LBD conformations which may account for their tissue- and promoter-specific activities and will be discussed in more detail below.

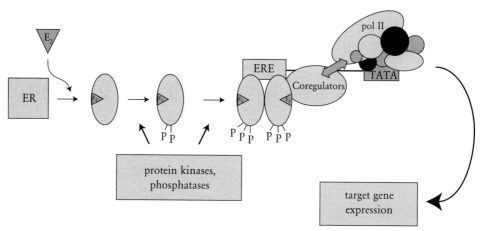

Figure 1 Model of the estrogen receptor (ER) activation process. The ligand estradiol (E_2) induces a conformational change in the receptor which sets in motion a series of events, culminating in increased transcription of estrogen-dependent genes. The E_2-bound estrogen receptor binds to its estrogen response element (ERE) and recruits coregulator proteins which serve as a physical and enzymatic bridge between the receptor and the RNA polymerase II (pol II) complex

INFLUENCE OF SERMS ON ESTROGEN RECEPTOR STRUCTURE

Crystal structural analysis of ERα and ERβ, and other nuclear hormone receptors, has revealed that their ligand binding domain consists of 12 conserved helices[7]. Helix 12, the most C-terminal of these helices, has been identified as the critical core of the AF-2 function of the receptor and plays an important role in coactivator-binding to the ligand-bound ERα[8-10]. Residues in helix 12 of the agonist-bound receptor interact with LXXLL nuclear receptor (NR) box motifs (where L is leucine and X is any amino acid) present in many coactivators such as SRC-1 and GRIP[11]. The co-crystal structure of the ERα LBD–ligand–NR box complex reveals that residues within this part of the receptor as well as within helices 3 and 5 are important for making contact with an NR box motif of GRIP1[12]. Additional crystallographic data on ERα and ERβ complexed with a variety of SERMs provide a comparative look at how these ligands produce alternative conformations in the LBD. The agonists estradiol or diethylstilbestrol (DES) induce a conformation in the receptor which forms a hydrophobic coactivator binding groove capable of interacting with the NR box of coactivators[10]. SERMs such as 4HT displace helix 12 so that it interacts with the coactivator binding groove of the receptor, excluding coactivators

from binding to the LBD. However, it should be noted that there are differences in the positioning of helix 12 in ERα when the receptor is complexed with two different SERMs, 4HT and raloxifene[10,13], which may provide a mechanism through which each of these SERMs can possess their own unique tissue-agonist/antagonist profile. Crystal structure solutions show that 4HT and raloxifene allow for the misplaced helix 12 to interact with aspartate 351 in helix 3, which has been shown to be involved in promoting the antiestrogenic activity of each of these ligands[14]. Raloxifene allows for a tighter interaction of helix 12 with aspartate 351, perhaps accounting for its more restricted agonist character.

The conformation of helix 12 of ERβ has also been shown to vary depending on which ligand it binds to. The crystal structure of ERβ bound to the phytoestrogen, genistein[15], provides an interesting example of a naturally occurring SERM ligand which causes ERβ to take on a unique conformation. In this conformation, helix 12 is in an intermediate conformation, unlike that of either the agonist or the raloxifene-bound receptor, which may yield its own unique profile of tissue-specific agonist and antagonist responses due to differing affinities and the cellular complement of co-activators. It is tempting to think that artificial SERMs such as 4HT and raloxifene mimic the alternative conformation that would normally be afforded by naturally occurring estrogens other than estradiol. Ligands such as estriol, estrone, 17α-estradiol and sulfate-conjugated estrogens may allow the receptor to take on a conformation unlike that of the estradiol-bound receptor, allowing for each ligand to produce its own distinct biological response[16].

SERM ACTION INVOLVES MECHANISMS INDEPENDENT OF AF-2

The crystal structures of the LBD of the estrogen receptor complexed with ligands does nothing, however, to reconcile the impact that the N-terminal AF-1 of ERα has on influencing the biological response to SERMs. 4HT is thought to stimulate ERα-mediated transcription through the AF-1 in certain cellular or promoter contexts[17,18] (Figure 2). Unlike 4HT, raloxifene appears to activate neither the AF-2 nor the AF-1, at least in cell and promoter contexts tested thus far. However, like 4HT, raloxifene is also an agonist in bone, resulting in an increase in bone mineral density[19,20]. This would suggest that SERMs such as raloxifene can positively stimulate gene expression through an additional mechanism other than by activation of the AF-1. Such activity may depend upon the ability of either ERα or ERβ to interact indirectly with DNA via an interaction with other transcription factors such as Sp1 and AP-1[21].

IMPACT OF ERα DEGRADATION ON SERM FUNCTION

It has been recognized for several years that SERMs can alter the stability of ERα, but the mechanism through which they influence ERα stability has received sparse attention. It has been known for over 30 years that estradiol promotes degradation of the estrogen receptor, concomitant with the activation of the receptor as a transcription factor[22], and we and others have shown that ERα is down-regulated through a proteasome-dependent mechanism[23,24]. Recent work in our laboratory has shed new light on the mechanism involved in how estradiol promotes ERα degradation[25]. Coactiva-

(a)

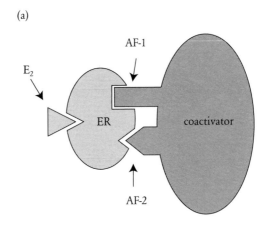

(b)

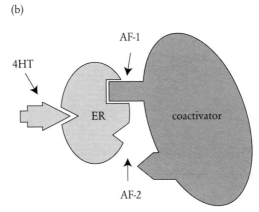

Figure 2 Selective estrogen receptor modulators (SERMs) induce an alternative conformation in the estrogen receptor (ER) which prohibits coactivator binding to the ligand-binding domain (LBD) of the receptor. (a) Estradiol (E$_2$) induces a conformation in the ER which allows for coactivators to associate with both the activation function-1 (AF-1) and the activation function-2 (AF-2). (b) A SERM such as 4-hydroxy-tamoxifen (4HT) binds in the LBD but excludes co-activator binding to the AF-2 of the receptor. In certain promoter and cell contexts, the AF-1 is activated by 4HT, allowing for this SERM to possess partial agonist activity, presumably through the interaction of co-activators with the AF-1

tor binding to the AF-2 of the estradiol-bound ERα probably contributes to the down-regulation of the receptor. Mutation of coactivator binding residues in helices 3, 5 or 12 results in altered receptor stability; in these mutants, estradiol stabilizes the receptor instead of promoting its degradation. A similar observation has been made for the retinoic acid receptor-α, where disruption of co-activator binding sites in the AF-2 of that receptor also abolishes its ligand-dependent degradation[26]. Estradiol stabilization of these coactivator binding mutants mirrors that seen for 4HT bound to the wild-type ERα, suggesting that in both of these cases, coactivator binding to the LBD is abrogated, resulting in the receptor being more stable. It is difficult, however, to explain why the compound ICI 164 384 is able to promote down-regulation of ERα, since, like 4HT, it should not pro-mote coactivator association with the receptor. Although both estradiol and ICI 164 384 promote receptor degradation, ICI 164 384 results in a much more rapid and complete down-regulation[27], and it is possible that its enhanced ability to degrade the receptor is responsible in part for its lack of agonist biological character.

As discussed above, it is likely that a coactivator or other protein that interacts with the receptor via an NR box-type mechanism is responsible for pro-moting degradation of the estradiol-bound recep-tor. This idea is bolstered by the fact that a number of coactivators and other receptor-interacting pro-teins have been identified which were previously characterized for their role in protein degradation through the ubiquitin–proteasome protein degra-dation system. Such proteins include E6-AP[28], RPF-1[29], TRIP1/SUG1[30,31] and UBC9[32,33]. The ubiquitin–proteasome system is responsible for the selective degradation of a number of short-lived transcription factors whose activity must be tightly regulated, such as NF-kB[34], STAT1[35] and fos/jun[36]. Through a series of enzymes (ubiquitin-activating, -conjugating and -ligase) the 76-amino-acid ubiquitin protein is covalently linked to proteins targeted for degradation, marking them for recognition by the 26S proteasome, a large multisubunit protease[37,38].

We have recently shown that in addition to its impact on receptor stability, the ubiquitin-proteasome protein degradation system is required for efficient transcription mediated through ERα[25]. Treatment of transiently transfected HeLa cells with the proteasome inhibitor MG132 can impair ERα-mediated transcription. MG132 can also impair progesterone receptor- and androgen receptor-mediated transcription, indi-cating that this effect is not limited to ERα. In con-trast, MG132 modestly stimulates transcription mediated via Sp1, E2F, p53 and the human glucocorticoid receptor, as well as transcription directed by the viral cytomegalovirus promoter, indicating that proteasome function is not required for transcription to proceed in general, nor for all nuclear receptors to stimulate gene expression. Proteasome function appears to be required for transcription mediated through either the AF-1 or AF-2 of ERα, as MG132 treatment is able to attenuate transcription from either domain when tethered to the GAL4 DBD. Both activation functions of steroid receptors have been shown to interact with coactivators[39,40], consistent with the possibility that MG132 is able to attenuate the transcriptional activity of either activation func-tion by interfering with the function of a common coactivator or coactivators (Figure 3).

CO-REPRESSOR INFLUENCE ON SERM BIOLOGICAL CHARACTER

Nuclear hormone receptor co-repressors also appear to play a role in determining the biological response to SERM ligands. Co-repressors such as N-CoR[41] and SMRT[42] have been identified as proteins which bind to the unliganded thyroid hormone receptor or retinoic acid receptor, respec-tively, where they actively repress transcription as part of a histone–deactylase complex[43]. In the presence of agonist ligands, the co-repressor disso-ciates from the receptor, followed by coactivator recruitment and the activation of gene transcrip-tion. Although the unliganded ERα lacks apparent repressive activity, overexpression of N-CoR is able to block the partial agonist activity of the 4HT-bound ERα[44]. This may be relevant to the phenomenon of long-term tamoxifen resistance, where estrogen-responsive breast cancers which normally respond favorably to tamoxifen therapy become resistant to, and are even promoted by, tamoxifen. Lavinsky and colleagues[45] provided evidence that this may be due to a reduction in co-repressor protein levels in breast cancer cells which have been chronically exposed to tamoxi-fen. These authors showed that MCF-7 cells implanted into nude mice which had been exposed to tamoxifen possessed lower levels of the mRNA and protein for N-CoR. They also showed that in

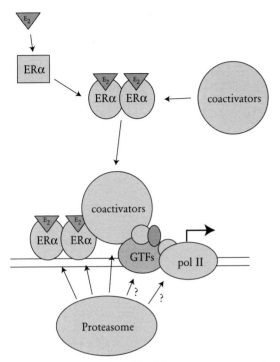

Figure 3 Role of the ubiquitin–proteasome protein degradation system in estrogen receptor-α (ERα) function. The proteasome targets the estrogen receptor (ER), coactivators and possibly general transcription factors (GTFs) and RNA polymerase II (pol II). However, the mechanism through which the proteasome contributes to ER-dependent transcription is not presently known. E_2, estradiol

cell culture, N-CoR preferentially associated with the 4HT-bound ERα, consistent with the idea that 4HT allows antagonism by promoting the association of the receptor with the co-repressor.

CONCLUSION

Our understanding of the molecular mechanisms of estrogen receptor action has been greatly expanded in the past few years. With the advent of our knowledge of coactivators and co-repressors, we are now in a better position to understand how SERMs like tamoxifen and raloxifene elicit their varied biological responses in breast, uterus, bone and other tissues. The identification of co-activators and co-repressors, and recent progress in our understanding of the effect of the ubiquitin–proteasome protein degradation system on receptor stability and function promises to provide additional critical insights into defining the mechanisms of SERM biological action. A more complete molecular picture of SERM interaction with ERα and ERβ which integrates these facts will hopefully lead to successful solutions to pressing clinical challenges in the treatment of breast cancer, such as breast cancer resistance to chronic tamoxifen therapy. In addition, such information should aid in obtaining ideal tissue-specific agonist/antagonist properties in the design of future generations of SERMs.

References

1. Oñate SA, Tsai SY, Tsai M-J, *et al.* Sequence and characterization of a coactivator for the steroid hormone receptor superfamily. *Science* 1995;270:1354-7
2. Leo C, Chen JD. The SRC family of nuclear receptor coactivators. *Gene* 2000;245:1-11
3. Westin S, Rosenfeld MG, Glass CK. Nuclear receptor coactivators. *Adv Pharmacol* 2000;47:89-112
4. McKenna NJ, Xu J, Nawaz Z, *et al.* Nuclear receptor coactivators: multiple enzymes, multiple complexes, multiple functions. *J Steroid Biochem Mol Biol* 1999;69:3-12
5. Kuiper GG, Enmark E, Pelto-Huikko M, *et al.* Cloning of a novel receptor expressed in rat prostate and ovary. *Proc Natl Acad Sci USA* 1996;93:5925-30
6. Tsai M-J, O'Malley BW. Molecular mechanisms of action of steroid/thyroid receptor superfamily members. *Annu Rev Biochem* 1994;63:451-86
7. Moras D, Gronemeyer H. The nuclear receptor ligand-binding domain: structure and function. *Curr Opin Cell Biol* 1998;10:384-91
8. Danielian PS, White R, Lees JA, *et al.* Identification of a conserved region required for hormone-dependent transcriptional activation by steroid hormone receptors. *EMBO J* 1992;11:1025-33

9. Henttu PM, Kalkhoven E, Parker MG. AF-2 activity and recruitment of steroid receptor coactivator-1 to the estrogen receptor depend on a lysine residue conserved in nuclear receptors. *Mol Cell Biol* 1997; 17:1832-9

10. Shiau AK, Barstad D, Loria PM, *et al*. The structural basis of estrogen receptor/coactivator recognition and the antagonism of this interaction by tamoxifen. *Cell* 1998;95:927-37

11. Heery DM, Kalkhoven E, Hoare S, *et al*. A signature motif in transcriptional co-activators mediates binding to nuclear receptors. *Nature* 1997;387:733-6

12. Mak HY, Hoare S, Henttu PM, *et al*. Molecular determinants of the estrogen receptor–coactivator interface. *Mol Cell Biol* 1999;19:3895-903

13. Brzozowski AM, Pike AC, Dauter Z, *et al*. Molecular basis of agonism and antagonism in the oestrogen receptor. *Nature* 1997;389:753-8

14. Levenson AS, Jordan VC. The key to the anti-estrogenic mechanism of raloxifene is amino acid 351 (aspartate) in the estrogen receptor. *Cancer Res* 1998;58:1872-5

15. Pike AC, Brzozowski AM, Hubbard RE, *et al*. Structure of the ligand-binding domain of oestrogen receptor-β in the presence of a partial agonist and a full antagonist. *EMBO J* 1999;18:4608-18

16. Gruber DM, Huber JC. Conjugated estrogens – the natural SERMs. *Gynecol Endocrinol* 1999;13:9-12

17. Metzger D, Ali S, Bornert JM, *et al*. Characterization of the amino-terminal transcriptional activation function of the human estrogen receptor in animal and yeast cells. *J Biol Chem* 1995;270:9535-42

18. Tzukerman MT, Esty A, Santiso-Mere D, *et al*. Human estrogen receptor transcriptional capacity is determined by both cellular and promoter context and mediated by two functionally distinct intramolecular regions. *Mol Endocrinol* 1994;8:21-30

19. Jordan VC, Phelps E, Lindgren JU. Effects of anti-estrogens on bone in castrated and intact female rats. *Breast Cancer Res Treat* 1987;10:31-5

20. Black LJ, Sato M, Rowley ER, *et al*. Raloxifene (LY139481 HC1) prevents bone loss and reduces serum cholesterol without causing uterine hypertrophy in ovariectomized rats. *J Clin Invest* 1994; 93:63-9

21. Gustafsson JA. Therapeutic potential of selective estrogen receptor modulators. *Curr Opin Chem Biol* 1998;2:508-11

22. Jensen EV, Suzuki T, Numata M, *et al*. Estrogen-binding substances of target tissues. *Steroids* 1969;13:417-27

23. Nawaz Z, Lonard DM, Dennis AP, *et al*. Proteasome-dependent degradation of the human estrogen receptor. *Proc Natl Acad Sci USA* 1999;96:1858-62

24. Alarid ET, Bakopoulos N, Solodin N. Proteasome-mediated proteolysis of estrogen receptor: a novel component in autologous down-regulation. *Mol Endocrinol* 1999;13:1522-34

25. Lonard DM, Nawaz Z, Smith CL, *et al*. The 26S proteasome is required for estrogen receptor-α and coactivator turnover and for efficient estrogen receptor-α transactivation. *Mol Cell* 2000;5:939-48

26. Zhu J, Gianni M, Kopf E, *et al*. Retinoic acid induces proteasome-dependent degradation of retinoic acid receptor-alpha (RARα) and oncogenic RARα fusion proteins. *Proc Natl Acad Sci USA* 1999;96:14807-12

27. Dauvois S, Danielian PS, White R, *et al*. Anti-estrogen ICI 164384 reduces cellular estrogen receptor content by increasing its turnover. *Proc Natl Acad Sci USA* 1992;89:4037-41

28. Nawaz Z, Lonard DM, Smith CL, *et al*. The Angelman syndrome-associated protein, E6-AP, is a coactivator for the nuclear hormone receptor superfamily. *Mol Cell Biol* 1999;19:1182-9

29. Imhof MO, McDonnell DP. Yeast RSP5 and its human homolog hRPF1 potentiate hormone-dependent activation of transcription by human progesterone and glucocorticoid receptors. *Proc Natl Acad Sci USA* 1999;96:1858-62

30. Lee JW, Ryan F, Swaffield JC, *et al*. Interaction of thyroid hormone receptor with a conserved transcriptional mediator. *Nature* 1995;374:91-4

31. von Baur E, Zechel C, Heery D, *et al*. Differential ligand-dependent interactions between the AF-2 activating domain of nuclear receptors and the putative transcriptional intermediary factors mSUG1 and TIF1. *EMBO J* 1996;15:110-24

32. Gottlicher M, Heck S, Coucas V, *et al*. Interaction of the Ubc9 human homologue with c-Jun and with the glucocorticoid receptor. *Steroids* 1996;61:257-62

33. Poukka H, Aarnisalo P, Karvonen U, *et al*. Ubc9 interacts with the androgen receptor and activates receptor-dependent transcription. *J Biol Chem* 1999; 274:19441-6

34. Ciechanover A, DiGiuseppe JA, Bercovich B, *et al*. Degradation of nuclear oncoproteins by the ubiquitin system *in vitro*. *Proc Natl Acad Sci USA* 1991;88:139-43

35. Palombella VJ, Rando OJ, Goldberg AL, *et al*. The ubiquitin–proteasome pathway is required for processing the NF-κB1 precursor protein and the activation of NF-κB. *Cell* 1994;78:78-85

36. Kim TK, Maniatis T. Regulation of interferon-γ-activated STAT1 by the ubiquitin–proteasome pathway. *Science* 1996;273:1717-19

37. Coux O, Tanaka K, Goldberg AL. Structure and functions of the 20S and 26S proteasomes. *Annu Rev Biochem* 1996;65:801-47

38. Baumeister W, Walz J, Zuhl F, *et al*. The proteasome: paradigm of a self-compartmentalizing protease. *Cell* 1998;92:267-80

39. Webb P, Nguyen P, Shinsako J, *et al.* Estrogen receptor activation function-1 works by binding p160 coactivator proteins. *Mol Endocrinol* 1998;12: 1605–18

40. Ma H, Hong H, Huang SM, *et al.* Multiple signal input and output domains of the 160-kilodalton nuclear receptor coactivator proteins. *Mol Cell Biol* 1999;19:6164–73

41. Horlein AJ, Naar AM, Heinzel T, *et al.* Ligand-independent repression by the thyroid hormone receptor mediated by a nuclear receptor co-repressor. *Nature* 1995;377:397–404

42. Chen JD, Evans RM. A transcriptional co-repressor that interacts with nuclear hormone receptors. *Nature* 1995;377:454–7

43. Xu L, Glass CK, Rosenfeld MG. Coactivator and corepressor complexes in nuclear receptor function. *Curr Opin Genet Dev* 1999;9:140–7

44. Smith CL, Nawaz Z, O'Malley BW. Coactivator and corepressor regulation of the agonist/antagonist activity of the mixed antiestrogen, 4-hydroxy-tamoxifen. *Mol Endocrinol* 1997;11:657–66

45. Lavinsky RM, Jepsen K, Heinzel T, *et al.* Diverse signaling pathways modulate nuclear receptor recruitment of N-CoR and SMRT complexes. *Proc Natl Acad Sci USA* 1998;95:2920–5

The estrogen receptor knock-out mouse model 10

S. Curtis Hewitt, J. F. Couse and K. S. Korach

INTRODUCTION

Estrogens, including natural, pharmacological and environmental estrogens, have numerous effects on the development and physiology of mammals. Estrogen is primarily known for its role in the development and functioning of the female reproductive system[1-4]. However, roles for estrogen in bone[5], the circulatory system[6] and the immune system have been implicated by clinical observations regarding sex differences in pathologies as well as observations following menopause or castration. The primary mechanism of estrogen action is via binding and modulation of activity of the estrogen receptor (ER), a ligand-dependent nuclear transcription factor[7-11]. The highest levels of ER are found in female reproductive tissues including the uterus, cervix, mammary glands and pituitary gland. Since other affected tissues have extremely low levels of ER, indirect effects of estrogen, for example induction of pituitary hormones that affect bone, have been proposed. The development of transgenic mouse models that lack either estrogen or ER has proven to be a valuable tool in defining the mechanisms by which estrogen exerts its effects in various systems. The aim of this chapter is to review the mouse models with disrupted estrogen signaling and describe the associated phenotypes.

Two estrogen receptors have been identified: the ERα, found primarily in the female reproductive tract, but also in other estrogen-responsive tissues; and the ERβ, a recently cloned estrogen-responsive nuclear receptor that is primarily expressed in the ovary and prostate[12-14]. Many of the roles of estrogen have been studied using castration and selective hormone replacement, but genetic disruption of one or both of the ERs is a valuable way to explore the roles and mechanisms of estrogen effects *in vivo*.

REPRODUCTIVE PHENOTYPES OF ER KNOCK-OUT MODELS

Estrogen has many roles in reproduction, and generation of the ERα and ERβ knock-out (αERKO and βERKO) mice has further illustrated its roles and mechanisms. Interestingly, both sexes of the αERKO mice are infertile, while in the βERKO mice, only the female has impaired fertility. This illustrates the importance of estrogen action through ERα in reproduction. The specific details of the impaired fertility illustrate the processes that require ERα.

The uterus and cervix

In the female αERKO mice, infertility is due in part to an underdeveloped uterus and lack of uterine growth and differentiation in response to estrogen[15,16] (Figure 1). The uteri of wild-type and βERKO mice are indistinguishable, and show the normal organization and development of the stromal, myometrial and epithelial layers (Figure 2), as well as glandular structures, meaning that ERβ is apparently not necessary for normal development of the female reproductive tract. Microscopic evaluation of uterine tissue indicates that the αERKO uterus contains all the tissue layers, but that they are immature and have a reduced number of glands (Figure 2). ERα is therefore not necessary for the initial development of the uterus, but is necessary for complete maturation and full function of the tissue. The cervical region is also identical in the wild-type and βERKO mice, with a good indication of cornification, indicating estrogen responsiveness. The cervix of the αERKO mice is again underdeveloped and is not cornified. When challenged with estrogenic compounds the uteri of wild-type and βERKO mice respond with increased weight

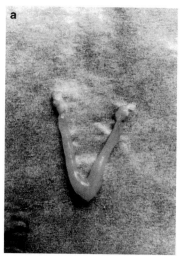
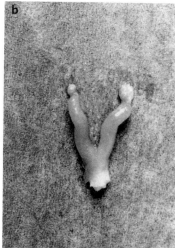
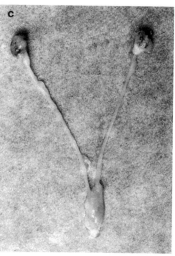

Figure 1 Gross morphology of estrogen receptor (ER) knock-out female reproductive tracts. Reproductive tracts dissected from (a) wild-type and (b) ERβ knock-out (βERKO) animals are normal, while the uterus from the ERα knock-out (αERKO) animal (c) is underdeveloped and the ovaries are enlarged and dark-colored, due to hemorrhagic cysts

and epithelial development and induction of estrogen-responsive genes[17], while the uterus of the αERKO mice is non-responsive. The uterus of the βERKO mice is fully functional, as litters are successfully carried to term and delivered.

The ovaries and ovarian hormones

The phenotypes present in both the αERKO and βERKO ovaries have been reported previously in detail[16,18,19]. The ovarian phenotypes are a major cause of infertility in the αERKO mice and sub-fertility in βERKO mice. The αERKO mice do not ovulate, while the βERKO mice are sub-fertile with reduced litter numbers and smaller litter sizes compared to wild-type littermates. Interestingly, although both ERα and ERβ are detected in the ovary, their localization differs, with ERβ in the granulosa cells and ERα in the theca and inter-stitial cells of the ovary[19]. Attempts to super-ovulate the βERKO mice results in some ovula-tion, but the number of oocytes released is five times less than in wild-type females[18]. The hall-mark phenotype of the αERKO female is the enlarged hemorrhagic cystic ovary (Figure 3), although the pre-pubertal αERKO ovary looks similar to that of wild-type littermates. This pheno-type begins to develop progressively as the animal matures and is apparently due to lack of feedback

inhibition in the pituitary, which results in chroni-cally elevated luteinizing hormone (LH)[16,20]. This indicates that ERα is responsible for mediating LH feedback inhibition in the hypothalamic-pituitary axis. The constant LH stimulation in αERKO mice results in an abnormal endocrine environment in the αERKO female, with elevated estradiol and testosterone and chronic pre-ovulatory low levels of progesterone[16,17]. The βERKO mice have ovaries that are able to func-tion, but which function sub-optimally, with the appearance of numerous unruptured follicles following super-ovulation[18]. Thus a role for ERβ in ovulation is indicated, although the mechanism is still being defined. The βERKO ovaries produce normal serum levels of estradiol, testosterone and gonadotropin[16].

The mammary glands

The mammary glands develop and function in response to ovarian hormones, most notably estro-gen and progesterone[21]. At birth, the female mammary glands are immature and consist of mainly stromal tissue, with only rudimentary epithelial duct structures confined to the nipples. In response to ovarian and pituitary hormones, the ducts grow and differentiate, eventually filling the stromal tissue with a branched tree-like structure.

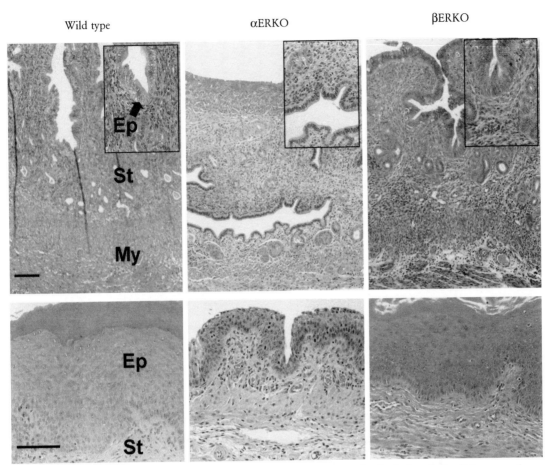

Figure 2 Uterine histology of estrogen receptor (ER) knock-out mice. Histological analysis of the uterus (upper panels) and vagina (lower panels) shows that tissue from ERβ knock-out (βERKO) mice is indistinguishable from tissue from wild-type mice, showing the normal organization of the uterine tissue into the epithelial (Ep), stromal (St) and myometrial (My) compartments. Uterine tissue from ERα knock-out (αERKO) mice is composed of all three layers, but all the layers are underdeveloped and hyperplastic. Note also that the glands are fewer in number. The vaginal tissue from the wild-type and βERKO mice is identical and is cornified, indicating response to estrogen, while tissue from the αERKO mice shows no cornification. Reproduced from reference 16, with permission

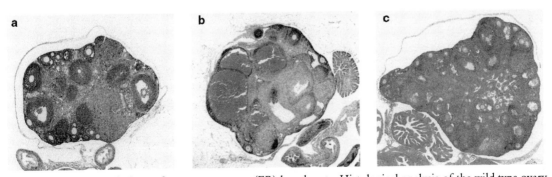

Figure 3 Ovarian pathology of estrogen receptor (ER) knock-outs. Histological analysis of the wild-type ovary (a) shows normal follicular development, with ovulation occurring. The ERα knock-out (αERKO) ovary (b) shows large cystic structures and arrested follicle development with no indication of ovulation. The ERβ knock-out (βER-KO) ovary (c) shows development of follicles, but little indication of successful ovulation

During pregnancy, lobular alveolar buds develop at the ends of these ducts. Transgenic knock-out models have been very informative in understanding the roles of estrogen and progesterone in mammary gland development. The role of progesterone is indicated by the lack of development of alveolar buds in the progesterone receptor knock-out mouse[22]. Similarly, the role of ERα is illustrated by the lack of growth of the rudimentary duct system beyond the nipple in the αERKO female[23,24] (Figure 4). The βERKO mammary gland is identical to that of wild-type littermates[16] (Figure 4) and functions normally, as βERKO mothers are able to nurse their litters. This indicates that ERβ is not needed in the mammary gland.

Progesterone action in the αERKO female

The activities of estrogen and progesterone are interdependent in the female reproductive cycle[25]. Since the progesterone receptor (PR) is regulated, in part, by estrogen, the activity of progesterone in αERKO tissues has been studied to determine whether disruption of αER signaling alters PR signaling. These observations have been reported in detail[26], but will be summarized here. PR is present at a basal level in the αERKO uterus at about 60% of the wild-type level, and its mRNA is not increased by estrogen treatment. However, this basal level of PR is sufficient to induce the mRNA of the progesterone-responsive calcitonin and amphiregulin genes. Also, the αERKO uterus can be induced to undergo a decidual reaction in response to progesterone and physical trauma. This indicates that PR is fully functional both biochemically and physiologically and is not dependent on ERα for expression or function. Interestingly, the decidual reaction is estrogen-dependent in wild-type mice, but not in αERKO mice.

The mammary gland also responds to progesterone, with development of lobular alveolar structures in the epithelium in preparation for lactation. Although the mammary epithelium of the αERKO mice is underdeveloped, it can be stimulated with progesterone to develop lobular alveolar structures, indicating that it is responsive to progesterone (Figure 5). Thus, although the PR is regulated by estrogen, the level of PR present in

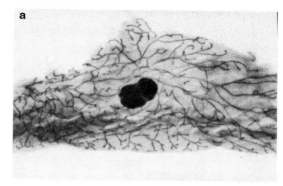

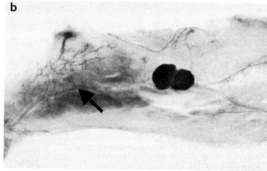

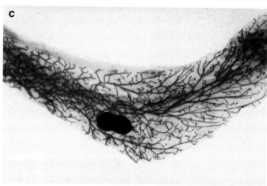

Figure 4 Mammary glands from wild-type (a) and estrogen receptor (ER) knock-out mice. The ERβ knock-out (βERKO) mice have normal mammary gland development (c). The ERα knock-out (αERKO) mice, however, have only a rudimentary underdeveloped epithelial duct (b) (arrow)

the absence of ERα is sufficient to mediate progesterone action. Although these progesterone responses have not been characterized in the βERKO mice, females can carry pregnancies to term and lactate normally, implying that the ability of the uterus and mammary glands to respond to progesterone is normal.

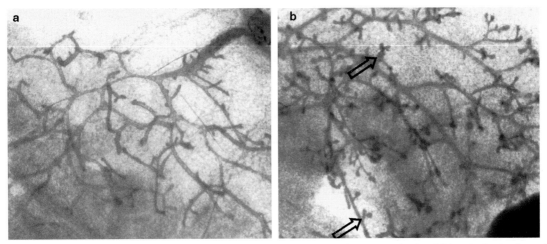

Figure 5 Mammary glands from estrogen receptor (ER)α knock-out mice, unmanipulated (a) and after 21 days of dosing with progesterone (b). Note the development of lobular-alveolar structures (arrow)

SUMMARY

The phenotypes observed in the αERKO and βERKO mice illustrate the roles of ERα and ERβ both in reproductive tissues and in more peripheral systems. Although some phenotypes are secondary results of removal of estrogen signaling (i.e. lack of negative feedback regulation of LH resulting in chronic LH stimulation of the αERKO ovary) we have learned a great deal about the role of ERα and ERβ in development and physiology. Continued evaluation and characterization of the phenotypes of classical estrogen target tissues and other organ systems should help to uncover previously unconsidered links between estrogen and other signaling pathways.

References

1. Jost A. *Recent Prog Horm Res* 1953;8:379–418
2. George FW, Wilson JD. Hormonal control of sexual development. *Vitam Horm* 1986;43:145–96
3. Wilson JD, George FW, Renfree MB. The endocrine role in mammalian sexual differentiation. *Recent Prog Horm Res* 1995;50:349–64
4. Werner MH, Huth JR, Gronenborn AM, Clore GM. Molecular determinants of mammalian sex. *Trends Biochem Sci* 1996;21:302–8
5. Turner RT, Riggs BL, Spelsberg TC. Skeletal effects of estrogen. *Endocr Rev* 1994;15:275–300
6. Farhat MY, Lavigne MC, Ramwell PW. The vascular protective effects of estrogen. *FASEB J* 1996;10:615–24
7. Evans RM. The steroid and thyroid hormone receptor superfamily. *Science* 1988;240:889–95
8. Parker MG, Arbuckle N, Dauvois S, Danielian P, White R. Structure and function of the estrogen receptor. *Ann NY Acad Sci* 1993;684:119–26
9. Tsai MJ, O'Malley BW. Molecular mechanisms of action of steroid/thyroid receptor superfamily members. *Annu Rev Biochem* 1994;63:451–86
10. Vegeto E, Wagner BL, Imhof MO, McDonnell DP. The molecular pharmacology of ovarian steroid receptors. *Vitam Horm* 1996;52:99–128
11. Chen JD, Li H. Coactivation and corepression in transcriptional regulation by steroid/nuclear hormone receptors. *Crit Rev Eukaryot Gene Expr* 1998;8:169–90
12. Kuiper GG, Enmark E, Pelto-Huikko M, Nilsson S, Gustafsson JA. Cloning of a novel receptor expressed in rat prostate and ovary. *Proc Natl Acad Sci USA* 1996;93:5925–30

13. Mosselman S, Polman J, Dijkema R. ER beta: identification and characterization of a novel human estrogen receptor. *FEBS Lett* 1996;392:49–53

14. Tremblay GB, Tremblay A, Copeland NG, *et al.* Cloning, chromosomal localization, and functional analysis of the murine estrogen receptor beta. *Mol Endocrinol* 1997;11:353–65

15. Lubahn DB, Mayer JS, Golding TS, *et al.* Alteration of reproductive function but not prenatal sexual development after insertional disruption of the mouse estrogen receptor gene. *Proc Natl Acad Sci USA* 1993;90:11162–6

16. Couse JF, Korach KS. Estrogen receptor null mice: what have we learned and where will they lead us? *Endocr Rev* 1999;20:358–417

17. Couse JF, Curtis SW, Washburn TF, *et al.* Analysis of transcription and estrogen insensitivity in the female mouse after targeted disruption of the estrogen receptor gene. *Mol Endocrinol* 1995;9:1441–54

18. Krege JH, Hodgin JB, Couse JF, *et al.* Generation and reproductive phenotypes of mice lacking estrogen receptor beta. *Proc Natl Acad Sci USA* 1998;95:15677–82

19. Schomberg DW, Couse JF, Murkhevjer A, *et al.* Targeted disruption of the estrogen receptor-alpha gene in female mice: characterization of ovarian responses and phenotype in the adult. *Endocrinology* 1999;140:2733–44

20. Couse JF, Bunch DO, Lindzey J, Schomberg DW, Korach KS. Prevention of the polycystic ovarian phenotype and characterization of ovulatory capacity in the estrogen receptor-alpha knockout mouse. *Endocrinology* 1999;140:5855–65

21. Imagawa W, Yang J, Guzman R, Nandi S. Control of mammary development. In Knobil E, Neil JD, eds. *The Physiology of Reproduction.* New York: Raven Press, 1994:1033–63

22. Lydon JP, De Mayo FJ, Funk CR, *et al.* Mice lacking progesterone receptor exhibit pleiotropic reproductive abnormalities. *Genes Dev* 1995;9:2266–78

23. Korach KS, Couse JF, Curtis SW, *et al.* Estrogen receptor gene disruption: molecular characterization and experimental and clinical phenotypes. *Recent Prog Horm Res* 1996;51:159–88

24. Bocchinfuso WP, Korach KS. Mammary gland development and tumorigenesis in estrogen receptor knockout mice. *J Mammary Gland Biol Neoplasia* 1997;2:323–34

25. Graham JD, Clarke CL. Physiological action of progesterone in target tissues. *Endocr Rev* 1997;18:502–19

26. Curtis SW, Clark J, Myers P, Korach KS. Disruption of estrogen signaling does not prevent progesterone action in the estrogen receptor or knockout mouse uterus. *Proc Natl Acad Sci USA* 1999;96:3646–51

Sex steroids in the cardiovascular system: molecular mechanisms of action

11

M. E. Mendelsohn

In the 1950s there were three world-renowned cardiologists, Professor Paul Wood in London, and Professors Paul Dudley White and Samuel Levine in Boston. Professor Wood, who was a member of, and lectured at, the Royal Society of Medicine, published a magnificent two-part article in the *British Medical Journal* in 1955 called 'An appreciation of mitral stenosis'. At just this time, Samuel A. Levine was preparing the fifth edition of his textbook *Clinical Heart Disease*, in which he gave what is believed to be the first description of a selective estrogen receptor modulator (SERM)[1]. Dr Levine was visionary, and during this time was aware of several laboratories that had shown that estrogen given to animals could inhibit the atherosclerotic process. He noted that attempts were, therefore, being made in males to try to use long-term estrogen therapy for prevention of coronary disease. He stated his hope that 'with further research, compounds might be found that would eliminate the undesirable action of such hormones and yet retain the beneficial effects'[1].

The idea that estrogen acts as a protective molecule for the cardiovascular system is, thus, a very old story. Our laboratory was fortunate to be in the right place at the right time in 1990, when we became interested in this topic just as the molecular tools to study the estrogen receptor became available[2]. Estrogen receptor (ER) α and ERβ are both expressed in human and animal cardiovascular tissues and cells in both males and females, including the endothelial cell, the smooth muscle cell and the cardiomyocyte. It is not known yet what differences in expression levels exist between different vascular beds and between the genders, nor is it clear what happens to the concentration and expression of these receptors with aging. The proteins that are recruited once these receptors bind estrogen, the coactivators discussed by Lonard and O'Malley in Chapter 9, are expressed at least in smooth muscle cells and endothelial cells, but there is far too little known to date about which coactivators are expressed in the cardiovascular system, and whether any coactivators specific for cardiovascular cells exist.

The aim in this chapter is to show how ERs are important in cardiovascular biology. This question is approached from the cell 'up', or in the reverse direction to that of clinical studies like the Heart and Estrogen/progestin Replacement Study (HERS)[3] or the Estrogen Replacement Atherosclerosis (ERA) trial[4]. We began our work simply to test the hypothesis that there are functional ERs present in the cardiovascular system and, here, an attempt has been made to provide an update as to the current state of our understanding.

Cell-specific estrogen-responsive genes are now well recognized in both smooth muscle and endothelial cells. There is now a list of 20–30 genes that are regulated in vascular tissues by estrogen[5]. The genes for the vasodilator-generating enzymes, endothelial nitric oxide synthase (eNOS), inducible NOS (iNOS), as well as for prostacyclin synthase or COX-1, are all up-regulated by estrogen in vascular cells.

One daunting problem is that there are now so many genes that are known to be estrogen-regulated in cardiovascular cells that it is difficult to choose one single gene product and implicate it as the prime actor in the cardiovascular effects of estrogen. Vasodilators were mentioned earlier and, as further examples, there are growth factors, such as vascular endothelial growth factor. It is worth mentioning that the lipoprotein effects of estrogen are due to estrogen effects on the genes that regulate production of the apolipoproteins, which are not actually in cardiovascular cells, but rather are hepatic. Thus, the lipid changes that accompany

87

hormone replacement therapy are mediated by changes in the expression of apolipoprotein production by the liver. These, of course, have cardiovascular consequences but are not direct cardiovascular effects, which are the subject of this chapter.

Beginning in 1994, the approach taken in our studies was to ask what is the role of the ER in protecting against vascular injury? To summarize, we, and others, believe that there are two general effects of estrogen in cardiovascular tissues: a rapid, vasodilatory effect that is refered to as 'non-genomic', and the longer-term effects on expression of genes regulated by the estrogen receptors that are the well-recognized manner by which

steroid hormone receptors act (Figure 1). The work discussed below focuses on these genomic (longer term) effects on gene expression. An interesting literature is evolving about the rapid effects: it is now recognized that eNOS is rapidly activated in endothelial cells exposed to estrogen in a non-transcriptional and non-genomic, but ER-dependent, fashion[6]. There is no evidence at present that this rapid effect has a physiological role. However, it is possible that there are physiological situations in which there are surges, or peaks and valleys, of estradiol when a rapid activation of eNOS might have some physiological effect. Perhaps this rapid pathway is involved in the 'hot flashes' that accompany the

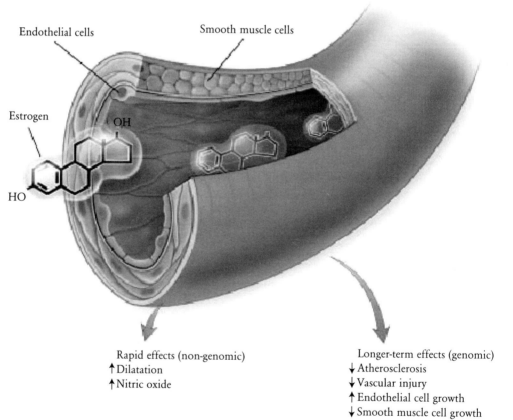

Rapid effects (non-genomic)
↑ Dilatation
↑ Nitric oxide

Longer-term effects (genomic)
↓ Atherosclerosis
↓ Vascular injury
↑ Endothelial cell growth
↓ Smooth muscle cell growth

Figure 1 Vascular endothelial and smooth muscle cells express the two known estrogen receptors. Estrogen has both rapid vasodilatory effects and longer-term actions that inhibit the response to vascular injury and prevent atherosclerosis. These effects are mediated by direct actions on vascular endothelial cells and smooth muscle cells. The rapid effects of estrogen on the blood vessel wall are believed to occur without any changes in gene expression (non-genomic effects), whereas the longer-term effects involve changes in gene expression (genomic effects) mediated by the estrogen receptors, which are ligand-activated transcription factors. Reprinted with permission from reference 5

perimenopause. Three groups are actively at work studying this question[7-9], and the subject has recently been reviewed[6] (Figure 2).

Animal models are, of course, surrogates for human physiology that have been applied in many studies for the last 50 years to study the cardiovascular effects of estrogen (reviewed in references 5 and 10). In vascular biology studies, it is important to pay attention to whether a high-cholesterol model or a normolipidemic model is being examined. The data discussed here all come from normolipidemic mouse models. The model used in our research for the past 8 years is a carotid endothelial denudation model that was first

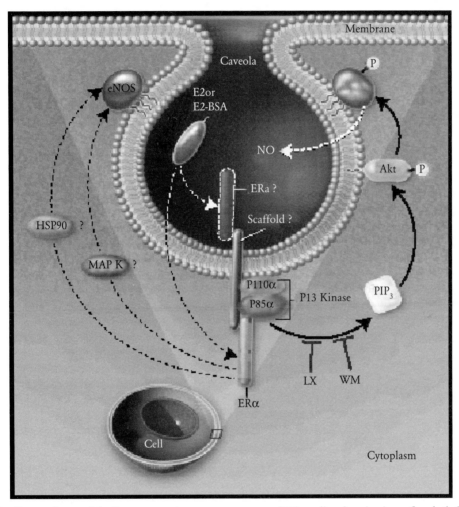

Figure 2 Composite model of non-genomic estrogen receptor (ER)-mediated activation of endothelial nitric oxide synthase (eNOS), based on published data and three recent studies[7-9]. These recent studies show immunological localization of ER to caveolae, direct interaction of ER with the p85 subunit of P13 kinase, and activation of the P13–kinase–Akt–eNOS pathway. However, many issues remain unresolved, in particular, including whether the ER hormone-binding domain is actually inside or outside the membrane, how this ER is tethered to the caveolae, and the precise primary sequence of this membrane-associated ER. The specific domains of ER that are important for the p85 interaction, as well as the identity of other potential proteins that participate in the proximal signalling events in this pathway, also remain unknown. Most importantly, compelling evidence is lacking at present that this pathway for non-genomic activation of eNOS by estrogen has a physiological or cardioprotective role. Scaffold indicates protein tethering ER to the membrane, such as a known transmembrane receptor; LY, LY294002; WT, wortmannin (P13-kinase inhibitors). Reprinted with permission from reference 6

described by Lindner and colleagues[11] and that we have modified extensively[12,13]. The model was established and the ability to inhibit the vascular injury response by estrogen in ovariectomized female mice was demonstrated in 1994–95[12]. These experiments in wild-type animals were carried out so that, if estrogen proved vasoprotective in mice as it had in other animals, it would be possible next to study the ER knock-out (ERKO) mouse that was being created at the time[14].

The mouse carotid injury model is an endothelial denudation model. When the endothelium is taken away, this removes the biochemically active protective barrier for the blood vessel that is continuously elaborating vasoprotective substances (such as nitric oxide), and the blood vessel undergoes an injury response. This is not like balloon injury models, which also cause transmural pressure and force-related breakage of vascular wall structures, nor is it like the atherosclerotic injuries that result from high lipoprotein diets in susceptible animals. The mouse carotid injury model is an endothelial denudation model in mice with normal lipid levels, with all the attendant caveats that accompany any surrogate model. First, female mice are ovariectomized and allowed 7–10 days to recover. Then the mice have pellets implanted (day −7) that release vehicle or estradiol to physiological levels, reaching a level of 0.3–0.6 nM after several days, which is maintained throughout the course of the experiment. At day 0, the mice undergo the endothelial denudation injury in which a wire is passed into the external carotid and the endothelium is denuded by three repeated passages. During the same procedure, an osmotic minipump is also implanted that releases bromodeoxy uridine (BrDU) over the subsequent 2 weeks so that any cells that proliferate may be quantitated.

There are two endpoints that are examined in the mouse carotid injury model. First, from elastin stained sections, the *medial area* can easily be quantified by computerized morphometric analyses. This is performed by two independent observers blinded to treatment group. The internal and external elastin can easily be seen, so the thickness of the vessel wall before and after an injury can be measured. This thickening is accounted for by two processes:

(1) Deposition of proteoglycans, collagen and other matrix proteins that are elaborated in response to injury;

(2) Cellular proliferation, specifically and especially smooth muscle cells in this model.

In normal C57 black 6 mice after injury there is an increase in medial area that is inhibited back to baseline by physiological levels of estradiol replacement[12]. The second endpoint is *smooth muscle cell proliferation*. Cells are stained for BrdU and then a parallel section is also stained with smooth muscle cell-specific or endothelial cell-specific antibodies which allows each poulation to be quantified. In this normolipidemic model, very few, if any, macrophages or inflammatory cells are detected in the injured area 14 days following denudation of the endothelium. Once again, we have shown in a number of studies that smooth muscle cell proliferation in response to injury is also inhibited by estradiol replacement to physiological levels.

This model was next applied to the ERαKO mouse developed in the Smithies laboratory (at the time, of course, ERβ had not yet been discovered). To our surprise, estradiol inhibited the response to injury in the ERKO mice equally well to its inhibitory effect in the wild-type littermate controls[11]. This experiment was finished in May 1996, and the exciting report of a new ER, ERβ, cloned from rat prostate was first announced at the March Keystone meeting that year[15]. Using reverse transcriptase polymerase chain reaction (RT-PCR), we were able to show that ERβ is expressed in the blood vessels of the ERαKO mice, which led to the hypothesis that ERβ was mediating the protective effects of estrogen in the ERαKO mice.

The ERβKO mouse again was developed in the Smithies laboratory, in collaboration with Jan-Ake Gustafsson and Ken Korach, and these mice were next studied using the mouse carotid injury model[16]. In this study, which required another 18 months to breed the mice, perform the study, and analyze the data, we found the identical result to the ERαKO mouse experiment. This led to only three tenable hypotheses: either there is a novel or unidentified ER, or ERα and ERβ are able functionally to complement one another *in vivo*.

In a collaboration with Jan-Ake Gustafsson and Claes Ohlsson over the last year, we have now completed a study of the ERα,β (double) KO mouse. This was a daunting breeding experiment, since only one out of 32 mice bred are predicted to be female and doubly homozygous for disruption of both the ERα and the ERβ genes. In fact, more than 820 mice were required in the breeding which allowed us to have the 26 homozygous ERα, β (double) knockout females needed to carry out the full mouse carotid injury study (wild type versus ERα,βKO mice, with vehicle control and estradiol replacement groups of 12–13 animals in all four study groups. In fact, the breeding required is quite close to the $32 \times 26 = 832$ mice predicted by simple Mendelian genetics). Some of the results of the study are discussed below, although not all the data have yet been analyzed.

The first pieces of data on the ERα,βKO mouse result include the surprising finding that the uterine weights in the ERα,βKO mice treated with estradiol were larger at the end of the experiment to a very significant degree as compared to the vehicle-treated mice. Jan-Ake Gustafsson and Claes Ohlsson have since repeated and confirmed this effect (unpublished). This finding adds a third potential explanation to the two hypotheses noted above, namely, that there is some residual and functional ERα activity in the ERαKO_Chapel Hill mice. This possibility must be considered because of the report from the Korach laboratory that described a splice variant ('E1 fragment') that is expressed and contains both DNA-binding and hormone-binding domains of ERα[17].

The results for the medial injury portion of the experiment are discussed below. For the thickening of the blood vessel endpoint (the medial area endpoint) there is no significant difference in the ERα,βKO mouse as compared to the wild-type mouse experiment. This finding was quite dramatic because it was the first time in the 7 years of studying this question that a loss of estrogen's protective effects on any endpoint was seen in any mouse. It suggests that, at least for this endpoint, ERα and ERβ are both necessary and sufficient to mediate estrogen inhibition of the medial area thickening response (which is due to gene expression of matrix proteins). We are currently analyzing the vascular smooth muscle proliferation endpoint. However, even these data demonstrate that the two known receptors together are important for this genomic protective effect of estrogen, and show further that they are able to complement each other *in vivo*. This explains the ERαKO and ERβKO experiments described earlier, i.e. when one receptor gene is disrupted, the other receptor is able to compensate.

In summary, an attempt has been made to describe our current understanding that, at least for some of the protective effects of estrogen in vascular injury, the two known estrogen receptors, ERα and ERβ, are mediating the estrogen protection, presumably by inhibiting the expression of certain genes that elaborate extracellular matrix substances and/or by increasing the expression of genes that encode proteins with a role in the breakdown of these matrix elements. These receptors are, of course, the same in all tissues, which leads to the question of how they achieve specificity for their effects in different tissues such as the blood vessel. Some of the possibilities include the types and levels of general coactivators that are expressed in many tissues, the possible existence of tissue-specific coactivators, and perhaps the expression of different splice variants of the receptors themselves. These questions are all under active investigation, but the importance of ERα and ERβ in the vascular protective effects of estrogen has now been confirmed.

References

1. Levine SA. *Clinical Heart Disease*, 5th edn. Philadelphia: W.B. Saunders Company, 1958:125

2. Walter P, Green S, Krust A, Bornert JM, Jeltsch JM, Staub A, Jensen E, Scrace G, Waterfield M, Chambon P. Cloning of the human estrogen receptor cDNA. *Proc Natl Acad Sci USA* 1985;82:7889

3. Hulley S, Grady D, Bush T, *et al.* Randomized trial of estrogen plus progestin for secondary prevention of coronary heart disease in postmenopausal women. Heart and Estrogen/progestin Replacement Study (HERS) Research Group. *J Am Med Assoc* 1998;280:605–13

4. Herrington DM, Reboussin DM, Brosnihan KB, *et al.* Effects of estrogen replacement on the progression of coronary-artery atherosclerosis. *N Engl J Med* 2000;343:522–9

5. Mendelsohn ME, Karas RH. Mechanisms of disease: the protective effects of estrogen on the cardiovascular system. *N Engl J Med* 1999;340:1801–11

6. Mendelsohn ME. Nongenomic, ER-mediated activation of endothelial nitric oxide synthase: how does it work? What does it mean? *Circ Res* 2000;87:956–60

7. Haynes MP, Sinha D, Russell KS, Collinge M, Fulton D, Morales-Ruiz M, Sessa WC, Bender JR. Membrane estrogen receptor engagement activates endothelial nitric oxide synthase via the P13–kinase-Akt pathway in human endothelial cells. *Circ Res* 2000;87:677–82

8. Simoncini T, Hafezi-Moghadam A, Brazil DP, Ley K, Chin WW, Liao JK. Interaction of oestrogen receptor with the regulatory subunit of phosphatidylinositol-3-OH kinase. *Nature* 2000;407:538–41

9. Chambliss KL, Yuhanna IS, Mineo C, Liu C, German Z, Sherman TS, Mendelsohn ME, Anderson RGW, Shaul PW. Estrogen receptor and endothelial nitric oxide synthase are organized into a functional signaling module in caveolae. *Circ Res* 2000;87:E44–52

10. Mendelsohn ME, Karas RH. Estrogen and the blood vessel wall. *Curr Opin Cardiol* 1994;9:619–26

11. Lindner V, Fingerle J, Reidy MA. Mouse model of arterial injury. *Circ Res* 1993;73:792–6

12. Sullivan TR Jr, Karas RH, Aronovitz M, Faller GT, Ziar JP, Smith JJ, O'Donnell TF Jr, Mendelsohn ME. Estrogen inhibits the response-to-injury in a mouse carotid artery model. *J Clin Invest* 1995;96:2482–8

13. Iafrati MD, Karas RH, Aronovitz M, Kim S, Sullivan TR Jr, Lubhan DB, O'Donnell TF Jr, Korach KS, Mendelsohn ME. Estrogen inhibits the vascular injury response in estrogen receptor α-deficient mice. *Nat Med* 1997;3:545–8

14. Lubahn DB, Moyer JS, Golding TS, Couse JF, Korach KS, Smithies O. Alteration of reproductive function but not prenatal sexual development after insertional disruption of the mouse estrogen receptor gene. *Proc Natl Acad Sci USA* 1993;90:11162–6

15. Kuiper GGJM, Enmark E, Pelto-Huikko M, Nilsson S, Gustafsson JÅ. Cloning of a novel estrogen receptor expressed in rat prostate and ovary. *Proc Natl Acad Sci USA* 1996;93:5925–30

16. Karas RH, Hodgin JB, Kwoun M, Krege JH, Aronovitz M, Mackey W, Gustafsson JÅ, Korach KS, Smithies O, Mendelsohn ME. Estrogen inhibits the vascular injury response in estrogen receptor β-deficient female mice. *Proc Natl Acad Sci USA* 1999;96:15133–6

17. Couse JF, Curtis SW, Washburn TF, Eddy EM, Schomberg DW, Korach KS. Disruption of the mouse oestrogen receptor gene: resulting phenotypes and experimental findings. *Biochem Soc Trans* 1995;23:929–35

Progestins and the cardiovascular system   12

R. Sitruk-Ware

INTRODUCTION

The well-recognized benefit of progestin use in hormone replacement therapy (HRT) is protection of the endometrium by opposition of the proliferative effects of estrogens. However, some of the most prescribed progestins also partially oppose the beneficial effects of estrogens. This has raised controversy about the risk/benefit ratio of combined estrogen/progestin HRT. Among the alleged risks of progestins in HRT, the risk of cardiovascular disease has been one of the most debated issues. However, given the differences between the various progestins available, and their varying pharmocologic properties, it appears to be inappropriate to claim that all progestins compromise the cardioprotective effects of estrogens.

RISK FACTORS FOR CARDIOVASCULAR DISEASE

Among the main cardiovascular risk factors recognized for both men and women, obesity, cigarette smoking, high diastolic blood pressure, hypercholesterolemia and diabetes mellitus may be preventable causes of coronary heart disease[1]. In women, estrogen deprivation following menopause may affect several of these risk factors.

Estrogen replacement therapy (ERT) has been shown to improve insulin sensitivity[2], lower diastolic blood pressure[3], increase high-density lipoprotein (HDL_2) levels[4] and stimulate the production of vasodilating factors such as nitric oxide and prostaglandin by the vessels[5]. Estrogen-induced vasodilatation occurs rapidly and this effect is referred to as a non-genomic effect[6]. Other actions of estrogens occur after several months and are dependent on changes in gene expression, and are hence referred to as genomic[6]. Progestins down-regulate the estrogen receptors and hence may interfere with some of the genomic actions of

estrogens through alterations of both the α and β isoforms of estrogen receptor.

CLASSIFICATION OF PROGESTINS

The synthetic progestins used in clinical practice are derived either from testosterone (19-nortestosterone derivatives) or from progesterone (17-OH-progesterone derivatives and 19-norprogesterone derivatives)[7].

Among the testosterone derivatives, the estrane group includes norethisterone and its metabolites, and the gonane group includes levonorgestrel and its derivatives. These derivatives, including desogestrel (also named etonogestrel), gestodene and norgestimate, have been referred to as third-generation progestins. The first-generation progestin is norethynodrel, the first progestin synthesized, and the second-generation progestins include norethisterone and levonorgestrel[7].

Several new progestins have been synthesized in the last decade. Dienogest is referred to as a hybrid progestin, being derived from the gonane group with a 17α-cyanomethyl group[8], and drospirenone derives from spirolactone[9]. The 19-nor-derivatives of progesterone are also referred to as 'pure' progestational molecules, as they bind almost exclusively to the progesterone receptor and do not interfere with the other steroid receptors[10]. This category includes progesterone, trimegestone, nomegestrol acetate and Nestorone®, as well as a new compound related to Nestorone with a methyl radical in position C18[11].

The addition of a double bond in the C6–7 position of the hydroxyprogesterone skeleton, as well as a deletion of the methyl radical in position C19, confers to nomegestrol acetate a higher progestational potency[12] than that of medroxyprogesterone acetate. In contrast, Nestorone, another

19-nor-derivative of progesterone, without a methyl radical in position C6, must be administered parenterally due to its rapid hepatic metabolism[13]. Thus very small structural changes may induce considerable differences in the effects of progestins.

Comparative progestational activities of various progestins

Progestational activity is usually tested using the McPhail Index in immature rabbits, and also the pregnancy maintenance and ovulation inhibition tests in rats. Using these *in vivo* tests, Nestorone appears to be the most potent progestin, being 10-fold more potent than levonorgestrel and 100-fold more potent than progesterone itself, when the molecules are administered subcutaneously[13]. When given orally, norethisterone, medroxyprogesterone acetate and drospirenone are more potent than progesterone, but less potent than levonorgestrel[7,9], and nomegestrol acetate is 4-fold more active than medroxyprogesterone acetate[12]. The addition to the Nestorone molecule of a methyl radical in the C18 position confers a 3–10-fold greater progestational potency using the same tests[11].

Androgenic activity of progestins

The binding affinities of the various progestins to the sex steroid receptors such as the estrogen receptor and the androgen receptor indicate considerable differences between the molecules, and these do not always correlate with the *in vivo* tests of estrogenic and androgenic potency.

Using the rat ventral prostate as a source of androgen receptor, the relative binding affinities of levonorgestrel and desogestrel are found to be 70% and 40% of that of testosterone, respectively. In contrast, Nestorone and progesterone do not show any significant binding[13]. The *in vivo* biological assay of androgenicity usually considers the effect of a given compound on the weight increase of the ventral prostate and other male sex organs in immature male rats. Using these models, levonorgestrel and 3-keto-desogestrel express androgenicity and increase the weight of ventral prostate in a dose-dependent manner, while Nestorone and progesterone do not induce such effects[13]. In similar

experiments, Bullock and Bardin[14] also showed the androgenicity of medroxyprogesterone acetate at high doses. Duc and colleagues[15] showed no effect of nomegestrol acetate, even when administered at very high doses.

Estrogenic activity of progestins

As far as the estrogenic activity of progestins is concerned, the uterine weight of ovariectomized immature female rats is significantly increased by levonorgestrel but not by Nestorone at similar doses[13]. Both compounds similarly do not bind to the estrogen receptor[13]. The 19-nor-testosterone derivatives exert some androgenic activity but only a few of them exert an estrogenic effect, and the 17-hydroxyprogesterone derivatives have varying activities. Cyproterone acetate is a potent anti-androgenic compound, while medroxyprogesterone acetate has slight androgenic activity[14] and also exerts glucocorticoid activity when given at very high doses[16]. Drospirenone, more recently synthesized in this class of compounds, is essentially an antimineralocorticoid progestin and exerts some antiandrogenic activity[9]. The 19-norprogesterone derivatives appear more specifically progestational and do not possess any androgenic, estrogenic or glucocorticoid activity[13,15]. Nomegestrol acetate has a partial anti-androgenic effect, but this is 20-fold less than that of cyproterone acetate[15].

Using the ratio between the binding affinities to the progesterone and androgen receptors as a selectivity index, Kumar and associates[13] have determined that Nestorone has the highest value of the ratio (590), followed by 3-keto-desogestrel (6) and levonorgestrel (1). When considering three 19-nortestosterone derivatives, and using the same index, 3-keto-desogestrel was considered very selective when compared to levonorgestrel and norethindrone. The 19-norprogesterone derivative Nestorone, having a high affinity for progesterone receptor but a very low affinity for androgen receptor, exhibits a very high selectivity index.

In summary, most of the progestins available to the prescriber exert a progestational effect, and all of them are able to oppose the proliferative effects of estrogens on the endometrium. However, their progestational potency varies and the dose needed to achieve the effect varies from a few micrograms to several milligrams. In addition, according to their structure and the steroid from which they are derived, the different molecules will exert other activities, some considered beneficial, and some considered to be undesirable side-effects.

PHARMACOKINETIC DIFFERENCES BETWEEN PROGESTINS

Another aspect to consider in the evaluation of the progestins is their pharmacokinetic properties and their binding to serum proteins. The measurement of radioactivity recovered in urine and faeces after oral or intravenous administration of a labelled compound indicates the absolute bioavailability of that compound and determines its absorption via the oral route. The compounds with the highest oral bioavailability are gestodene, desogestrel and cyproterone acetate[17-19].

The half-life of a compound is also determined by its binding to plasma proteins. When compared with testosterone, levonorgestrel and 3-keto-desogestrel exhibit significant but lower affinities for sex hormone binding globulin (SHBG)[13]. While both norethisterone and levonorgestrel bind to SHBG, their half-lives vary, the terminal half-life being around 7-8 h for norethisterone and up to 26 h for levonorgestrel. In contrast, cyproterone acetate has an elimination half-life of 48 h[19] and nomegestrol acetate a half-life of about 50 h[10].

Progesterone and Nestorone do not bind to SHBG and the free fraction of Nestorone is greater than that of most of the 19-nortestosterone-derived progestins. The oral bioavailability of Nestorone is only about 10%, with a shorter half-life than progestins that bind to SHBG. However, a much slower elimination rate is observed after chronic subdermal implant[20].

EFFECTS OF THE PROGESTINS ON SURROGATE MARKERS OF CARDIOVASCULAR RISK

Effects of the progestins on lipids and lipoproteins

The effects of estrogen replacement therapy (ERT) on serum lipid concentration result largely from estrogen receptor-mediated effects on the hepatic expression of apoprotein genes[6]. Most of the studies evaluating the effect of estrogens on the lipoproteins have shown a reduction of low-density lipoprotein (LDL) cholesterol levels and an increase of high-density lipoprotein (HDL) cholesterol levels by 10 to 15%[4]. Progestins with androgenic properties have been shown to oppose slightly the HDL-raising effect of estrogen[4], while natural progesterone and some 19-norprogesterone derivatives, such as nomegestrol acetate, do not affect HDL cholesterol levels[4,21].

In the Postmenopausal Estrogen/Progestin Intervention (PEPI) trial[4], 875 postmenopausal women were followed for 3 years in a randomized, double-blind, placebo-controlled trial. Five groups were evaluated. One group received placebo, one received unopposed conjugated estrogens, and three groups received combined HRT. In the combined HRT regimens, all subjects received 0.625 mg of conjugated estrogens and one of three progestin or progesterone doses: (1) medroxyprogesterone acetate, 10 mg/day, given sequentially over 12 days/month; (2) medroxyprogesterone acetate, 2.5 mg/day, given continuously; and (3) micronized progesterone, 200 mg/day for 12 days/month. All four treatment regimens induced an increase in HDL levels and a decrease in LDL levels. However, the increase in HDL cholesterol was partially reversed in the groups in which medroxyprogesterone acetate was added to oral estrogens, while oral micronized progesterone did not modify the estrogen-induced rise. The results observed for estrogen effects on LDL cholesterol were not modified by the addition of either medroxyprogesterone acetate or progesterone.

In another randomized comparative double-blind trial comparing the effects of nomegestrol acetate with those of norethisterone acetate, both given orally at a dose of 5 mg per day, the increase in HDL cholesterol observed under estradiol valerate was partially reversed by norethisterone acetate, but not by nomegestrol acetate, a 19-norprogesterone derivative[22].

The relevance of these lipid changes has been questioned. The role of HDL changes in the alleged cardiovascular protective effects of estrogens is only partial and would account for between 30% and 50% of these cardiovascular protective effects[23].

Effects of progestins on carbohydrate metabolism

Glucose intolerance and hyperinsulinemia are well-known risk factors for cardiovascular disease. Postmenopausal women have been shown to have a reduced number of peripheral insulin receptors compared with premenopausal women in the early follicular phase[24]. Insulin is a potent stimulus to endothelial cell growth and also regulates LDL receptor activity[25]. Therefore a reduction in fasting insulin levels may be important in controlling one of the mechanisms of cardiovascular disease.

Other studies using the oral glucose tolerance test (OGTT), performed before and 6 months after each treatment regimen, showed no significant changes of glucose and insulin response to the OGTT with dydrogesterone[2] or with nomegestrol acetate[26].

Godsland and colleagues[27], in an open, randomized, comparative study of 61 postmenopausal women, evaluated the effects of oral equine estrogens with sequential oral levonorgestrel (0.075 mg/day, 12 days/month), or transdermal estradiol with sequential transdermal norethisterone acetate (0.250 mg/day, 14 days/month). Using intravenous glucose tolerance tests, they found that oral therapy caused a deterioration of glucose tolerance and an overall increase in plasma insulin, most probably due to the androgenic properties of levonorgestrel. On the other hand, no change in insulin response or glucose levels occurred with the transdermal therapy. Although the progestin used also exhibited some androgenic properties on lipids, it did not affect carbohydrate metabolism when given transdermally.

In these studies of combined HRT, variations in response to oral or intravenous glucose tolerance tests were observed according to the androgenic or non-androgenic properties of the progestin used, the non-androgenic progestins having no effect on carbohydrate metabolism. However, when given transdermally this property did not induce any change.

Effects of progestins on blood pressure

Menopause by itself has no influence on high blood pressure, according to longitudinal studies[28]. Whether normotensive or hypertensive women would be at higher risk of increased blood pressure during HRT treatment has been questioned.

Drospirenone exerts a potent anti-mineralocorticoid effect and, in young women receiving oral contraceptives containing 3 mg drospirenone, a significant decrease in blood pressure was observed after 6 months of treatment[9].

DIRECT EFFECTS OF PROGESTINS ON THE VESSELS

Much attention has been directed towards the effects of sex steroids on the vessels. Although estrogens have been shown to exert beneficial effects on the vascular wall, some progestins may reverse that benefit.

The vessel wall and endothelial factors

Blood vessel walls contain smooth muscle cells and an endothelial cell lining. These structures bind estrogens with high affinity, and estrogen receptors have been identified in both types of vascular cells in women and men[29].

The presence of estrogen and progesterone binding sites in endothelial cells and in the vessel walls has been documented in animal and human arteries[30]. Estrogens have both rapid and long-term effects on the blood vessel wall. The mechanism that mediates the rapid effects of estrogens is not fully understood. These rapid effects do not appear to involve changes in gene expression. However, estrogen influences the bioavailability of endothelial-derived nitric oxide, which causes the relaxation of smooth muscle cells[6].

In postmenopausal women, the levels of vasodilator factors (nitric oxide and prostacyclin), as well as the levels of vasoconstrictive factors (endothelin-1 and thromboxane-A_2), vary under therapy. Ylikorkala and associates[5] have recently shown that women who smoke have high levels of endothelin-1. In these women, transdermal combined therapy with estradiol and norethisterone acetate was able to significantly decrease the levels of this potent vasoconstrictive agent.

Vasomotion

Major studies performed in the primate model since the early 1990s have shown that sex hormones modulate the vasomotor response of the main arteries, particularly the coronary arteries[31]. In the cynomolgus monkey, 17β-estradiol modulates the responses of the coronary arteries to acetylcholine[31,32]. Estrogen-deprived atherosclerotic monkeys were compared with animals receiving estrogen replacement therapy. The degree of coronary artery constriction following an infusion of acetylcholine was measured in both groups of animals. Paradoxical vasoconstriction occurred following acetylcholine infusion in the untreated animals, while estradiol therapy restored the normal endothelium-dependent vasodilatation. The process occurred rapidly, and vasomotion was restored to normal within 20 min of an intravenous injection of estrogens. Progesterone did not reverse the effects of estrogens. The authors concluded that estrogens preserve the normal endothelium-mediated dilation of coronary arteries, and that natural progesterone does not reverse this potential cardioprotective mechanism. However, in the same model, the addition of cyclic or continuous medroxyprogesterone acetate to estrogens inhibited acetylcholine responses by 50%[33]. In contrast, Williams and colleagues[34] reported that a non-androgenic progestin, nomegestrol acetate, did not diminish the beneficial effects of estrogens on the coronary dilator response in monkeys.

In humans, Rosano and associates[35] studied the effects of progestogens on effort-induced myocardial ischemia in female patients with coronary heart disease. They found that medroxyprogesterone acetate, but not natural progesterone, slightly reversed the beneficial effect of chronic therapy with estrogen on ST depression.

Although medroxyprogesterone acetate belongs to the pregnane group of progestins, it interacts with androgen receptors and induces synandrogenic effects[14]. These properties might explain some of its effects.

Atherosclerosis

The experiments of Adams and colleagues[36] in the female cynomolgus monkey observed no direct relationship between lipid changes and atherosclerosis. These authors examined the effects of sex hormone replacement therapy on diet-induced coronary artery atherosclerosis, expressed as the plaque area developed in the vessels of female ovariectomized monkeys. The animals received either no therapy or estradiol, or combined estradiol and progesterone, from subcutaneous implants. In parallel, the animals were fed with a highly atherogenic diet for 25 months. The plaque area was significantly decreased in both groups of animals that received steroids, although HDL and total cholesterol levels were not different from one group to the other. These results suggest that HRT has antiatherogenic effects, independent of variations in the lipid formula, and that natural progesterone does not reverse the beneficial effects of estradiol.

Other studies performed *in vitro* on vascular smooth muscle cells have shown that sex steroids, both estradiol and progesterone, inhibit their proliferation[37]. Progesterone at physiological levels inhibits DNA synthesis and proliferation in these cells in a dose-dependent manner[38].

RANDOMIZED CONTROLLED TRIALS ON HRT AND CARDIOVASCULAR DISEASE

Only double-blind, randomized, controlled trials will provide definite proof that estrogen and progesterone protect against coronary disease. Several ongoing epidemiological trials focus on primary or secondary prevention of coronary heart disease[39,40].

Primary prevention trials

The Women's Health Initiative in the USA and the Medical Research Council HRT study in Europe are designed as long-term primary prevention trials and will enrol postmenopausal women without coronary heart disease. The long-term follow-up of treatment and placebo groups will help to answer questions about the presumed protective effects of HRT, using conjugated equine estrogens and medroxyprogesterone acetate, in preventing cardiovascular and coronary heart disease[39,40].

Secondary prevention trials

In women with documented coronary heart disease, the effect of estrogens on survival was unclear before the results of the Heart and Estrogen/progestin Replacement Study (HERS) appeared[40]. The study was designed as a randomized, double-blind, placebo-controlled trial to determine whether conjugated equine estrogen plus a continuous progestagen (medroxyprogesterone acetate) is superior to placebo in preventing recurrent events in 2763 women with documented coronary heart disease.

These women have been followed up for an average of 4.1 years. The primary outcome was the occurrence of non-fatal myocardial infarction or coronary heart disease death. After 4 years of follow-up, the same number of events were recorded in both the active and the placebo groups; this finding indicates that the combined HRT regimen did not reduce the overall rate of coronary events in postmenopausal women with previous coronary heart disease. The relative hazard for a further event was 0.99 (95% confidence interval 0.8–1.2). In addition, there was no significant difference between groups in any of the secondary outcomes, despite a net decrease in LDL and an increase in HDL cholesterol levels in the hormone-treated group.

In another study, angiography was used to compare the effects of estrogens, with and without medroxyprogesterone acetate, and placebo on the vessels of women with previously documented coronary heart disease. No difference was found between the three groups in the progression of coronary atherosclerosis in women with established disease[41].

Different progestins may produce different results. Unfortunately, most of the large ongoing trials have selected the same HRT regimen for their study designs, thus preventing comparison of different regimens. Progestin consumption has varied greatly over the past two decades and varies from country to country. Also, the type of progestin mostly prescribed for HRT varies from one country to another. Therefore, the results of the epidemiological studies are difficult to compare.

The percentage of patients who received combined HRT was very low in most of the cohort studies reporting the follow-up of patients treated in the 1980s and up to the mid-1990s. Also, the type of estrogens prescribed for HRT and the doses used varied between Europe and the USA. Therefore, the hormonal balance of both estrogen and progestin varied considerably. Only randomized controlled trials of primary prevention are likely to provide an answer. However, given the magnitude and cost of these trials, very few therapeutic schedules are presently being tested. It will be very important to obtain the results of the primary prevention trials expected in 2005 and 2006. However, it will not be possible to extrapolate these results to other types of treatment.

CONCLUSION

While the benefits of progestin use in HRT, regarding endometrial protection, are well recognized, the associated risks and drawbacks have generated considerable controversy. Some progestins, with a higher androgenic potency than others, may attenuate the beneficial effects of estrogens on the lipid profile as well as vasomotion. On the other hand, other progestins devoid of androgenic properties do not exert these deleterious effects. Progesterone itself and its natural derivatives do not display androgenic properties and have a different effect on the vascular wall.

Recent results, however, suggest that in women with established coronary heart disease, HRT may not protect against further heart attacks. The epidemiological data do not show any negative effect of progestins administered with estrogens on cardiovascular morbidity or mortality. Further data are needed to compare the effects of various steroids used in clinical practice, which differ from country to country. In women without established coronary heart disease, complying with the classic contraindications of HRT and selecting progestins devoid of estrogenic, androgenic or glucocorticoid effects, can still be recommended.

References

1. Rich-Edwards JW, Mason JE, Hennekens CH, Buring JE. The primary prevention of coronary heart disease in women. *N Engl J Med* 1995;332:1758–66

2. De Cleyn K, Buytaert P, Coppens M. Carbohydrate metabolism during hormonal substitution therapy. *Maturitas* 1989;11:235–42

3. Pang SC, Greendale GA, Cedars MI, Cambone AC, Lozano K, Eggena P, Judd HL. Long-term effects of transdermal estradiol with and without medroxy-progesterone acetate. *Fertil Steril* 1993;59:76–82

4. The writing group for the PEPI trial. Effects of estrogen or estrogen/progestin regimens on heart disease risk factors in postmenopausal women: the Postmenopausal Estrogen/Progestin Interventions (PEPI) trial. *J Am Med Assoc* 1995;273:199–208

5. Ylikorkala O, Cacciatore B, Paakkari I, Tikkanen MJ, Viinikka L, Toivonen J. The long-term effects of oral and transdermal postmenopausal hormone replacement therapy on nitric oxide, endothelin-1, prostacyclin, and thromboxane. *Fertil Steril* 1998;69:883–8

6. Mendelsohn ME, Karas RH. The protective effects of estrogen on the cardiovascular system. *N Engl J Med* 1999;340:1801–11

7. Henzl MR, Edwards JA. Pharmacology of progestins: 17α-hydroxyprogesterone derivatives and progestins of the first and second generation. In Sitruk-Ware R, Mishell DR Jr, eds. *Progestins and Antiprogestins in Clinical Practice*. New York: M. Dekker Inc., 2000:101–32

8. Oettel M, Holz C. Hybrid progestins: the example of dienogest. In Sitruk-Ware R, Mishell DR Jr, eds. *Progestins and Antiprogestins in Clinical Practice*. New York: M. Dekker Inc., 2000:163–78

9. Oelkers W, Foidart JM, Dombrovicz N, Welter A, Heithecker R. Effects of a new oral contraceptive containing an antimineralocorticoid progestogen, drospirenone, on the renin–aldosterone system, body weight, blood pressure, glucose tolerance and lipid metabolism. *J Clin Endocrinol Metab* 1995;80:1816–21

10. Sitruk-Ware R, Sundaram K. Pharmacology of new progestogens: the 19-norprogesterone derivatives. In Sitruk-Ware R, Mishell DR Jr, eds. *Progestins and Antiprogestins in Clinical Practice*. New York: M. Dekker Inc., 2000:153–61

11. Tuba Z, Bardin CW, Dancsi A, *et al*. Synthesis and biological activity of a new progestogen, 16-methylene-17α-hydroxy-18-methyl-19-norpregn-4-ene-3,20-dione acetate. *Steroids* 2000;65:266–74

12. Paris J, Thevenot R, Bonnet P, Granero M. The pharmacological profile of TX 066 (17α-acetoxy-6-methyl-19-nor-4,6-pregna-diene-3,20-dione), a new oral progestative. *Drug Res* 1983;33:710–15

13. Kumar N, Koide SS, Tsong YY, Sundaram K. Nestorone®: a progestin with a unique pharmacological profile. *Steroids* 2000;65:629–36

14. Bullock LP, Bardin CW. Androgenic, synandrogenic and antiandrogenic actions of progestins. *Ann NY Acad Sci* 1977;286:321–30

15. Duc I, Botella J, Bonnet P, Fraboul F, Delansome R, Paris J. Antiandrogenic properties of nomegestrol acetate. *Arzneim Forsch/Drug Res* 1995;45:70–4

16. Hellman L, Yoshida K, Zumoff B, Levin J, Kream J, Fukushima DK. The effect of medroxy-progesterone acetate on the pituitary–adrenal axis. *J Clin Endocrinol Metab* 1976;42:912–17

17. Wilde MI, Balfour JA. Gestodene. A review of its pharmacology, efficacy and tolerability in combined contraceptive preparations. *Drugs* 1995;50:364–95

18. Shenfield GM, Griffin JM. Clinical pharmacokinetics of contraceptive steroids. An update. *Clin Pharmacokinet* 1991;20:15–37

19. Dusterberg B, Humpel M, Speck U. Terminal half-lives in plasma and bioavailability of norethisterone, levonorgestrel, cyproterone acetate and gestodene in rats, beagles and rhesus monkeys. *Contraception* 1981;24:673–83

20. Noe G, Salvatierra A, Heikinheimo O, Maturana X, Croxatto HB. Pharmacokinetics and bioavailability of ST 1435 administered by different routes. *Contraception* 1993;48:548–56

21. Conard J, Basdevant A, Thomas JL, Ochsenbein E, Denis C, Guyene TT, Degrelle H. Cardiovascular risk factors and combined estrogen–progestin replacement therapy: a placebo-controlled study with nomegestrol acetate and estradiol. *Fertil Steril* 1995;64:957–62

22. Dorangeon P, Thomas JL, Gillery P, Lumbroso M, Hazard MC. Short-term effects on lipids and lipoproteins of two progesterones used in postmenopausal replacement therapy. *Eur J Clin Res* 1992;3:187–93

23. Bush TL, Barrett-Connor E, Cowan LD, Criqui MH, Wallace RB, Suchindran CM, Tyroler HA, Rifkind BM. Cardiovascular mortality and non-contraceptive use of estrogen in women: results from the Lipid Research Clinics Program follow-up study. *Circulation* 1987;75:1102–9

24. De Pirro R, Fusco A, Bertoli A, Greco AV, Lauro R. Insulin receptors during the menstrual cycle in normal women. *J Clin Endocrinol Metab* 1978;47:1387–9

25. Chait A, Bierman EL, Albers JJ. Low-density lipoprotein receptor activity in cultured human skin fibroblasts. Mechanisms of insulin-induced stimulation. *J Clin Invest* 1979;64:1309–19

26. Dorangeon P, Thomas JL, Lumbroso M, Hazard MC, Dorangeon S. Effects of nomegestrol acetate

on carbohydrate metabolism in premenopausal women. Presented at the *XIIIth World Congress of Gynecology and Obstetrics (FIGO)*, Singapore, 1991, Abstr. No. 0636

27. Godsland IF, Gangar K, Walton C, Cust MP, Whitehead MI, Wynn V, Stevenson JC. Insulin resistance, secretion and elimination in postmenopausal women receiving oral or transdermal hormone replacement therapy. *Metabolism* 1993;42:846–53

28. Casiglia E, d'Este D, Ginocchio G, Colangeli G, Onesto C, Tramontin P, Ambrosio GB, Pessina AC. Lack of influence of menopause on blood pressure and cardiovascular risk profile: a 16-year longitudinal study concerning a cohort of 568 women. *J Hypertens* 1996;14:729–36

29. Karas RH, Patterson BL, Mendelsohn ME. Human vascular smooth muscle cells contain functional estrogen receptor. *Circulation* 1994;89:1943–50

30. Bergquist A, Bergquist D, Ferno M. Estrogen and progesterone receptors in vessels walls. *Acta Obstet Gynaecol Scand* 1993;72:10–16

31. Clarkson TB, Anthony MS, Potvin Klein K. Hormone replacement therapy and coronary artery atherosclerosis: the monkey model. *Br J Obstet Gynaecol* 1996;103(S13):53–8

32. Williams JK, Adams MR, Klopfenstein HS. Estrogen modulates responses of atherosclerotic coronary arteries. *Circulation* 1990;81:1680–7

33. Williams AK, Honore EK, Washburn SA, Clarkson TB. Effects of hormone replacement therapy on reactivity of atherosclerotic coronary arteries in cynomolgus monkeys. *J Am Coll Cardiol* 1994;24:1757–61

34. Williams JK, Cline JM, Honoré EK, Delansome R, Paris J. Coadministration of nomegestrol acetate does not diminish the beneficial effects of estradiol on coronary artery dilator responses in non-human primates. *Am J Obstet Gynecol* 1998;179:1288–94

35. Rosano GMC, Chierchia SL, Morgani GL, Gabriele M, Leonardo F, Sarrel PM, Collins P. Effect of the association of different progestogens to estradiol-17β therapy upon effort-induced myocardial ischemia in female patients with coronary artery disease. *J Am Coll Cardiol* 1997;344A:1028, abstr 167

36. Adams MR, Kaplan JR, Manuck SB, Koritnik DR, Parks JS, Wolfe MS, Clarkson TB. Inhibition of coronary artery atherosclerosis by 17-beta-estradiol in ovariectomized monkeys. Lack of an effect of added progesterone. *Arteriosclerosis* 1990;10:1051–7

37. Morey AJ, Pedram A, Razandi M, Prins BA, Hu RM, Biesiada E, Levin ER. Estrogen and progesterone inhibit vascular smooth muscle proliferation. *Endocrinology* 1997;138:3330–9

38. Lee WS, Harder JA, Yoshizumi M, Lee ME, Harbor E. Progesterone inhibits arterial smooth muscle cell proliferation. *Nat Med* 1997;3:1005–8

39. Spencer CP, Cooper AJ, Stevenson JC. Clinical trials in progress with hormone replacement therapy. *Exp Opin Invest Drugs* 1996;5:739–49

40. Hulley S, Grady D, Bush T, Furberg C, Herrington O, Riggs B, Vittinghoff E. Heart and Estrogen/Progestin Replacement Study (HERS) research group. Randomized trial of estrogen plus progestin for secondary prevention of coronary heart disease in postmenopausal women. *J Am Med Assoc* 1998;280:605–13

41. Herrington DM, Reboussin DM, Brosnihan KB, Sharp PC, Shumaker SA, Snyder TE, Furberg CD, Kowalchuk GJ, Stuckey TD, Rogers WJ, Givens DH, Waters D. Effects of estrogen replacement on the progression of coronary artery atherosclerosis. *N Engl J Med* 2000;343:522–9

Sex steroids and the cardiovascular system *in vivo*: actions in animal models

13

J. K. Williams

BRIEF REVIEW OF ANIMAL STUDIES

Studies on animal models, particularly during the last decade, have contributed extensively to our understanding of sex hormone effects on atherogenesis. A brief review of these studies is presented below.

Studies on surgically postmenopausal rabbits

Researchers have explored the effects of estrogens and progestogens on atherosclerosis progression/regression using the ovariectomized rabbit model. Atherosclerotic lesions develop in this model much as they do in humans beings, although the lipid profiles of these animals following feeding them an atherogenic diet consist primarily of beta migrating very-low-density lipoprotein (VLDL), a cholesterol ester-rich, triglyceride-poor lipoprotein. Nevertheless, this area of investigation has provided important information.

Haarbo and his group conducted studies of estrogen replacement therapy (ERT) vs. hormone replacement therapy (HRT), examining the effects of estrogen plus norethindrone acetate (NETA) or levonorgestrel in varying dosages. They found that estrogen treatment reduced aortic accumulation of cholesterol significantly, as did the combination of estrogen and progestogen treatment[1]. Alexandersen and colleagues studied the effects of diet plus estrogen alone or in combination with two progestogen regimens[2]. Eighty ovariectomized rabbits were fed a cholesterol-rich diet for 14 weeks to induce atherosclerosis. They were then divided into four groups: estrogen only, estrogen plus low-dose NETA, estrogen plus high-dose NETA, and control. Cholesterol intake was reduced to a maintenance level of 80 mg/day during the intervention period. Total serum cholesterol and ultracentrifuged lipoproteins were analyzed throughout the study. After 38 weeks, serum lipids and cholesterol content in aortic walls were measured. It was observed that NETA enhanced the antiatherogenic effects of estrogen and that this effect was only partly mediated through changes in serum lipids and lipoproteins. The enhancement of the estrogen effect may be because a portion of norethindrone is converted to ethinylestradiol[3].

The results of a particularly important study have been reported by Brehme and colleagues[4]. Using ovariectomized rabbits as models, they sought to determine if doses of hydroxyprogesterone that protected the endometrium from exogenous administered estrogen would attenuate the antiatherosclerosis effects of estradiol. Estradiol given alone was atheroprotective. The doses of hydroxyprogesterone necessary to protect the endometrium, whether given continuously or sequentially, did not attenuate the estrogen benefit (Figure 1)[4].

Studies on a rat model

Atherogenesis involves a complex sequence of events, with some components of arterial injury. The effects of estrogen and progestogens on intimal proliferation following arterial injury have been studied by Levine and colleagues. They explored the effects of estrogen (17β-estradiol) and medroxyprogesterone acetate (MPA) on the neointimal proliferative response to balloon injury of the carotid artery in intact and gonadectomized female rats. The effects of MPA on the formation of neointima, on the antiproliferative benefits of estrogen, and on the interaction between MPA and estrogen were tested[5]. Intimal proliferation in female rats was markedly reduced by estradiol

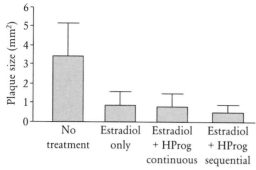

Figure 1 Atherosclerosis plaque extent of ovariectomized rabbits fed an atherogenic diet and given estradiol alone or with hydroxyprogesterone (HProg) given continuously or sequentially. Modified from Brehme *et al.*[4]

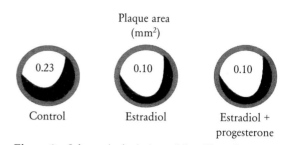

Figure 2 Schematic depiction of the effect of estrogen replacement on the extent of coronary artery atherosclerosis in surgically postmenopausal monkeys. Adapted from Adams *et al.*[6]

alone and the beneficial effect was largely abolished by the addition of MPA.

Studies in a monkey model

Direct evidence for an inhibitory effect of physiologic estrogen concentrations on progression of coronary artery atherosclerosis was found in the results of a study from our group[6]. In that study, ovariectomized monkeys were assigned randomly to one of three treatment groups:

(1) No hormone replacement;

(2) Continually administered 17β-estradiol plus cyclically administered progesterone; or

(3) Continuously administered 17β-estradiol.

Physiologic patterns of plasma estradiol and progesterone concentrations were maintained by administering the hormones in Silastic® implants. The experiment lasted 30 months. At necropsy, coronary artery atherosclerosis was reduced by about half in both hormone replacement groups (Figure 2). There was no evidence that the estradiol benefit was attenuated by progesterone.

In a subsequent 30-month study, the same researchers explored the coronary artery atherosclerosis effects of continuous oral administration of conjugated equine estrogens (CEE) alone or in combination with MPA[7]. The use of CEE alone reduced average plaque size by 72% compared with untreated controls (Figure 3). The group that received CEE plus MPA had a 28% reduction in

plaque size, suggesting some attenuation of the CEE effect. Additional trials, under somewhat different conditions, are seeking to examine further MPA effects on CEE-associated atheroprotection.

INTERPRETATION OF ANIMAL STUDIES: ARE THEY MISLEADING US?

Clearly, a new era has begun in which increasing numbers of the scientific/medical community are asking whether estrogens have any cardiovascular benefits. The doubts that have arisen are the result of two randomized prospective trials. The first, the HERS[8], recruited women who were generally beyond 65 years of age and who had definitive evidence of coronary heart disease. They were randomized into a placebo group and a group that was given a combined treatment of conjugated equine estrogens and medroxyprogesterone acetate. Initially, the treatment group showed an excess number of coronary events. By the end of the 4-year trial, no benefit could be shown in reducing coronary events by treatment with a combination of estrogens and a progestin. More recently, Herrington and his colleagues reported the results of the Estrogen Replacement Atherosclerosis (ERA) Trial[9]. In that trial, women with an average age of 65 years and with coronary heart disease demonstrated by angiography were randomized into a placebo group, a group that received CEE only, and a group that received CEE plus MPA. After treatment, coronary angiography was repeated, and no benefit could be shown for either CEE only or the combined therapy group.

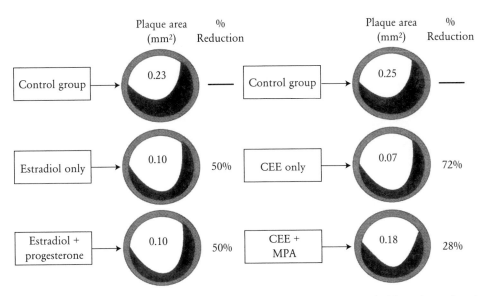

Figure 3 Effect of physiologic replacement of estradiol and progesterone compared with conjugated equine estrogen (CEE) and medroxyprogesterone acetate (MPA) on coronary atherosclerosis extent of postmenopausal cynomolgus monkeys. Modified from Adams *et al.*[7]

Given the negative findings in those two trials, we have re-examined several of our monkey experiments to gain some insight into possible explanations of the findings. In attempting to understand the incongruity between some of the observational data on human subjects, the monkey data, and the results of HERS and ERA, one must sharpen the definition of 'primary prevention'. The terms have different meanings for vascular biologists and cardiologists (Figure 4). To the vascular biologist, primary prevention of atherosclerosis means to prevent the progression of fatty streaks to atherosclerotic plaques. As cardiologists have used the term, primary prevention means to interfere with the progression of complicated plaques to coronary heart disease events.

In reconsidering several of our monkey studies, we arbitrarily divided them into three life stages (Figure 5). Life stage 1 was a situation in which the monkeys had little or no atherosclerosis before being made surgically menopausal. CEE therapy was given immediately after ovariectomy, as was the atherogenic diet. In that situation, there was an average inhibition of coronary artery atherosclerosis of about 70%[7,10].

Life stage 2 was a situation in which the animals were allowed to develop a moderate amount of atherosclerosis premenopausally, then were made surgically menopausal. CEE therapy was begun immediately and the atherogenic diet continued. In that situation, the degree of inhibition of coronary artery atherosclerosis was reduced from 70 to 50%[11]. These results could be interpreted that ERT is less effective in inhibiting progression of atherosclerosis in postmenopausal individuals with a premenopausal risk for developing atherosclerosis.

Finally, in the life stage 3 situation, the animals had low atherosclerosis risk premenopausally, were ovariectomized to make them surgically menopausal, were given an atherogenic diet, but there was a delay of 2 years (equivalent to 6 years in human life) before therapy was begun with CEE. Given that postmenopausal delay in initiating the estrogen replacement therapy, we observed no inhibition in the extensiveness of coronary artery atherosclerosis[12]. These results could be interpreted that ERT is virtually ineffective in inhibiting atherogenesis in postmenopausal individuals with more extensive atherosclerosis.

If there are lessons to be taken from the animal models about the new conundrum, they would suggest that estrogens have beneficial effects in the early stages of atherogenesis but have little or no beneficial effects in the final stages of plaque complications, instability and coronary heart disease events. In Figure 6 we have depicted this view. Key

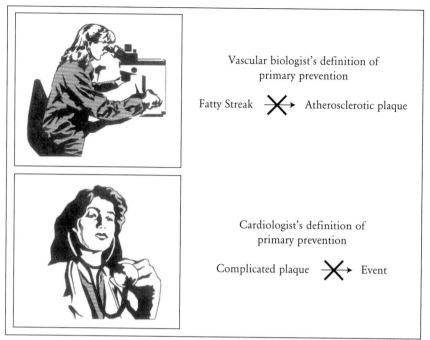

Figure 4 Comparison of 'primary prevention' as viewed by a vascular biologist in contrast to the view of cardiologist

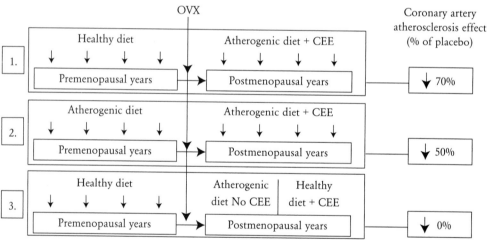

Figure 5 The relation of pre- and postmenopausal conditions to the degree of, or lack of, inhibition of coronary artery atherosclerosis

cellular events include the initiation of fatty streaks and their progression to fatty plaques and atherosclerotic plaques, the continuing recruitment of monocytes to become macrophage foam cells, low-density lipoprotein (LDL) accumulation, LDL oxidation, and smooth muscle cell proliferation. Estrogens have been shown to have favorable influences on all of those processes. On the other hand, plaque complications, plaque instability, and coronary heart disease events are influenced by neovascularization and intraplaque hemorrhage, inflammatory processes perhaps associated with C-reactive protein increases, endothelial dysfunction with the possibility of arterial spasm, and the

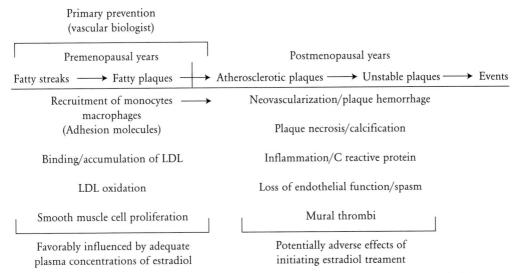

Figure 6 A mechanistic rationale for the inhibition of early events in atherogenesis by estradiol in contrast to potentially adverse effects of estradiol on late stages of plaque evolution and complication

likelihood of mural thrombi forming with any discontinuity of the endothelial surface of the plaques. There is little evidence to suggest beneficial effects of estrogen concerning those processes and, indeed, some evidence that they may be affected adversely by estrogen treatment.

CONCLUSIONS

We are left with the question: are animal models predictive of ERT or HRT effects on the atherogenesis in human beings? The answer is 'It depends'. Since almost all animal studies consist of measuring the effects of sex hormones on progression of atherosclerosis in females with no pre-existing atherosclerosis (Figure 6), they are only predictive of human studies that would measure the same endpoint. The prospective, randomized clinical studies evaluated to date include women

with pre-existing atherosclerosis, and the endpoints were either an 'event', or change in pre-existing atherosclerosis (Figure 6). Thus, it is not surprising that the animal studies were not predictive of studies in postmenopausal women with pre-existing coronary artery disease. As mentioned, the only study that was predictive of the HERS or ERA trials was one monkey study where the monkeys had extensive pre-existing atherosclerosis. Even then, the endpoint was a change in atherosclerosis extent, not the incidence or prevalence of an event.

Perhaps animal studies are more predictive of sex hormone effects on women with minimal pre-existing atherosclerosis. This raises interesting questions and possibilities of when estrogen/progestogen therapy should be initiated in women. Obviously, this is a controversial issue that will need to be addressed in the future.

References

1. Haarbo J, Leth-Espensen P, Stender S, *et al*. Estrogen monotherapy and combined estrogen–progestogen replacement therapy attenuate aortic accumulation of cholesterol in ovariectomized cholesterol-fed rabbits. *J Clin Invest* 1991;87:1274–79

2. Alexandersen P, Haabro J, Sandholdt I, *et al*. Norethindrone acetate enhances the antiatherogenic effect of 17β-estradiol: a secondary prevention study of aortic atherosclerosis in ovariectomized cholesterol-fed rabbits. *Arterioscler Thromb Vasc Biol* 1998;18:902–7

3. Kuhnz W, Heuner A, Humpel M, *et al*. *In vivo* conversion of norethisterone and norethisterone acetate to ethinyl estradiol in postmenopausal women. *Contraception* 1997;56:379–85

4. Brehme U, Bruck B, Gugel N, *et al*. Aortic plaque size and endometrial response in cholesterol-fed rabbits treated with estrogen plus continuous or sequential progestin. *Arterioscler Thromb Vasc Biol* 1999;19:1930–7

5. Levine RL, Chen S-J, Durand J, *et al*. Medroxyprogesterone attenuates estrogen-mediated inhibition of neointima formation after balloon injury of the rat carotid artery. *Circulation* 1996;94:2221–7

6. Adams MR, Kaplan JR, Manuck SB, *et al*. Inhibition of coronary artery atherosclerosis by 17-beta estradiol in ovariectomized monkeys: lack of an effect of added progesterone. *Arteriosclerosis* 1990; 10:1051–7

7. Adams MR, Register TC, Golden DL, *et al*. Medroxyprogesterone acetate antagonized inhibitory effects of conjugated equine estrogens on coronary artery atherosclerosis. *Arterioscler Thromb Vasc Biol* 1997;17:217–21

8. Hulley S, Grady D, Bush T, *et al*. Randomized trial of estrogen plus progestin for secondary prevention of coronary heart disease in postmenopausal women. *J Am Med Assoc* 1998;280:605–13

9. Herrington DM, Reboussin DM, Brosnihan KB, *et al*. Effects of estrogen replacement on the progression of coronary artery atherosclerosis. *J Am Med Assoc* 2000;343:522–9

10. Clarkson TB, Anthony MS, Jerome CP. Lack of effect of raloxifene on coronary artery atherosclerosis of postmenopausal monkeys. *J Clin Endocrinol Metab* 1998;83:721–6

11. Clarkson TB, Anthony MS, Morgan TM. Inhibition of postmenopausal atherosclerosis progression – a comparison of the effects of conjugated equine estrogens and soy phytoestrogens. *J Clin Endocrinol Metab* 2001:in press

12. Williams JK, Anthony MS, Honoré EK, *et al*. Regression of atherosclerosis in atherosclerotic monkeys. *Arterioscler Thromb Vasc Biol* 1995;15:827–36

Sex steroids and the cardiovascular system *in vivo*: actions in humans

14

P. Collins

INTRODUCTION

There have been relatively few studies conducted on the *in vivo* actions of the sex steroids, estrogen and testosterone, on the cardiovascular system. Thus, the conclusions that can be drawn about the effects of these steroids are limited, but they are believed to have beneficial vascular actions. This chapter reviews some of the data collected to date on the effects of estrogen and testosterone on vascular function. Further studies with different hormones, routes of administration and doses are required to provide definitive proof of the effects of sex steroids on the cardiovascular system.

VASORELAXANT EFFECTS OF ESTROGEN

In vitro experiments have shown that the addition of estrogen to constricted rings of coronary artery from a variety of animals results in a dose-dependent relaxation. A dose–response curve is also seen in rings of human coronary artery, and interestingly there is a sensitivity difference between the response in coronary artery from females compared with that from males, rings from females being more sensitive to the relaxing effect of estrogen than those from males (Figure 1)[1].

The dose-dependent relaxation with estrogen is independent of the endothelium; it is a direct effect of estrogen on vascular smooth muscle cells. A relaxant effect is seen at physiological concentrations of estrogen (10^{-10}–10^{-9} mol/l). At higher concentrations, estrogen may be acting as a calcium antagonist[1,2].

Estrogen inhibits the effect of constrictor agents, particularly endothelin[3] and angiotensin; it

has recently been shown that estrogen infused directly into the coronary circulation can cause a decrease in coronary sinus endothelin production[4]. Estrogen also has antioxidant effects similar to those of vitamin E and vitamin C. Estrogen may, therefore, produce a beneficial effect on the vasculature *in vivo*.

EFFECTS OF ESTROGEN ON CORONARY HEMODYNAMICS

The effects of estrogen on baseline coronary hemodynamics have been assessed by Reis and colleagues[5]. The methodology that they used (which has now been superseded) was to insert a guiding catheter into the left main stem coronary artery (which was atherosclerotic or normal) and then to insert an angioplasty guide wire. A Doppler flow probe was then placed over the guide wire to enable infusion of acetylcholine, ethinylestradiol and isosorbide dinitrate into the artery. Quantitative coronary angiography was used to calculate the blood flow from the angiographic diameter and its velocity, which was measured by a piezo-electric crystal.

The coronary artery was infused with acetylcholine, then intravenous ethinylestradiol (35 µg) and the response to acetylcholine was assessed 15 min later. The addition of ethinylestradiol to the coronary artery after acetylcholine reversed the acetylcholine effect and caused a statistically significant increase in blood flow and cross-sectional area, and a statistically significant decrease in vascular resistance (all $p < 0.01$) (Figure 2).

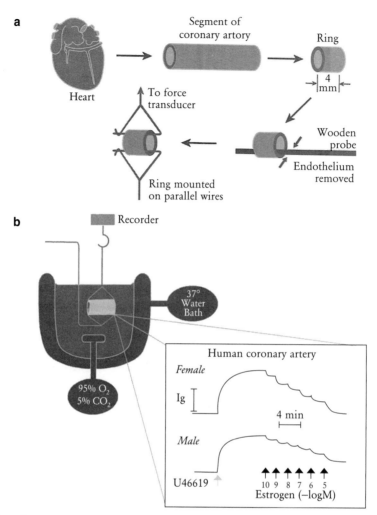

Figure 1 Effect of estrogen on human coronary artery. Estrogen was added to constricted rings of coronary artery (a). Rings from women were more sensitive than those from men (b). Adapted from reference 1

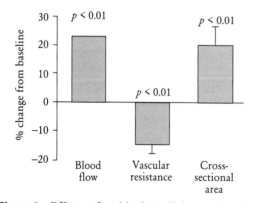

Figure 2 Effect of ethinylestradiol on baseline coronary hemodynamics. Reproduced from reference 5 with permission

DIFFERENT RESPONSES IN MALES AND FEMALES WITH CORONARY HEART DISEASE

The reversal of the acetylcholine effect in coronary arteries by estrogen was also shown by Collins and colleagues[6]. Acetylcholine (10^{-7} mol/l and 10^{-6} mol/l) was infused via a Doppler flow probe down the left anterior descending coronary artery (which was atherosclerotic) in males and females with coronary heart disease (CHD). This was followed by a 20-min infusion of estrogen down the coronary artery. The responses to acetylcholine were then assessed. The initial infusion of acetylcholine at both concentrations caused vasoconstriction of the coronary artery in males and females. This was reversed by the estrogen infusion and vasodilatation was observed.

The interesting finding in this study was the difference in response between males and females to acetylcholine after infusion of estrogen. In males, the acute response to acetylcholine after infusion of estrogen was similar to that before infusion (i.e. a similar degree of vasoconstriction occurred). In females, however, although the initial infusion of acetylcholine (pre-estrogen) caused vasoconstriction, the post-estrogen infusion of acetylcholine caused vasodilatation (the mean coronary diameter was increased by more than 5%) (Figure 3)[6].

ENDOTHELIAL CELL-SURFACE ESTROGEN RECEPTORS

The vasodilatatory effect of acetylcholine after a 20-min exposure to estrogen in females may be because of an acute estrogen receptor-dependent effect on the nitric oxide synthase (NOS) pathway. Stefano and colleagues[7] have recently shown that the addition of physiological doses of estrogen to human endothelial cells stimulates nitric oxide (NO) release via endothelial cell-surface estrogen receptors. The release of NO (as measured by an amperometric probe) occurs within 3 min after addition of estrogen; this is preceded by release of calcium (within 6 s). The reversal of the acetylcholine effect by estrogen may, therefore, be the

result of enhanced NO production from the endothelial cells in the coronary artery.

INVOLVEMENT OF THE NOS PATHWAY IN MALES AND FEMALES

The NOS pathway is likely to be switched on rapidly in females, but not in males, because females have more estrogen receptors and/or more sensitive estrogen receptors on the endothelial cell surface. Male endothelia have been shown to respond to estrogen, but the response is slower than in females. Weiner and colleagues[8] showed that the NOS pathway is not switched on until approximately 10 days after administration of estrogen to castrated male guinea pigs compared with 5 days in female guinea pigs. This may be because of differences in the number and sensitivity of arterial receptors in the male compared with the female.

The binding of estrogen to estrogen receptors on the endothelium may activate the mitogen-activated protein kinase system, which results in NO production (Figure 4).

The cell-surface estrogen receptor system is also active in neurons (causing neuroprotection), breast cancer cells (leading to cell cycle stimulation) and osteoblasts (resulting in cell proliferation and differentiation and bone conservation) (Figure 4)[9].

MEASURING THE EFFECTS OF HORMONES ON VASCULAR REACTIVITY

Brachial artery reactivity

The effects of estrogen and other hormones on vascular reactivity have been assessed using an ultrasound technique[10-12]. An ultrasound probe is placed over the brachial artery and a cuff is blown up to exclude the hand circulation for 5 min. This results in profound ischemia and metabolite release in the hand. When the cuff is released, the resistance in the hand is zero because of all the metabolites, and there is an increase in blood flow. When flow increases in the blood vessel, sheer stress activates a potassium channel on the endothelial cell surface. This leads to release of nitric

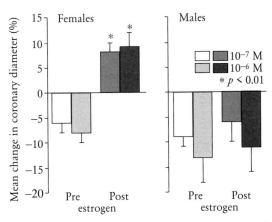

Figure 3 Differences in acute response to acetylcholine pre- and post-estrogen in females and males. Reproduced from reference 6 with permission

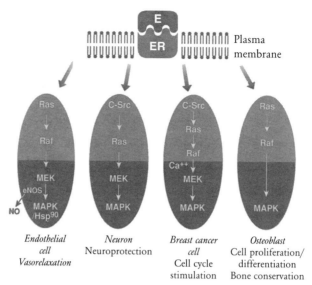

Figure 4 Effects of estrogen binding to cell-surface estrogen receptors. Reproduced from reference 9 with permission

oxide from the endothelium and vasodilatation (Figure 5). The extent of vasodilatation is measured by the ultrasound probe.

Interpreting the results

The interstudy variability in the different laboratories that use this technique needs to be known because it is uncertain whether a diameter is always being cut. This is particularly true for longitudinal studies with imaging at different time points.

EFFECTS OF ESTROGEN ON BRACHIAL ARTERY REACTIVITY

Oral estrogen

Lieberman and colleagues showed that the percentage change in diameter of the brachial artery in healthy postmenopausal women was statistically significantly greater after 1 month of oral estradiol (1 mg or 2 mg) compared with placebo ($p < 0.05$) (Figure 6)[12].

The percentage changes in diameter of the brachial artery were similar with both doses of estradiol, which indicates a ceiling in the effect of estradiol on brachial artery reactivity. Lower doses of estradiol have not yet been tested in this system, but 0.5 mg or 0.25 mg given for 1 month

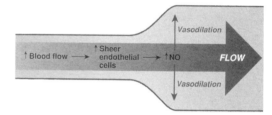

Figure 5 Endothelium-dependent   flow-mediated vasodilatation

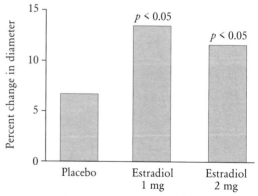

Figure 6 Effect of estrogen on brachial artery diameter. Reproduced from reference 12 with permission

may have the same enhancement effect. It is possible that the vascular effects of estradiol occur at much lower doses than the doses used for postmenopausal symptom relief. Unfortunately, there are no data yet to support or refute this hypothesis.

Transdermal estrogen and transvaginal progesterone

Gerhard and co-authors assessed the effects of transdermal estrogen (Estraderm®, Novartis) in combination with vaginally administered micronized progesterone on endothelium-dependent vasodilatation in a placebo-controlled, double-blind cross-over study[10,12]. A total of 17 postmenopausal women with mild hypercholesterolemia received two 0.1-mg Estraderm® patches twice weekly for 8 weeks, with or without 300 mg transvaginal progesterone once daily for 2 weeks, or placebo. The addition of transvaginal progesterone to the transdermal estrogen regimen did not appear to reduce the favorable estrogen effect on brachial artery reactivity (Figure 7).

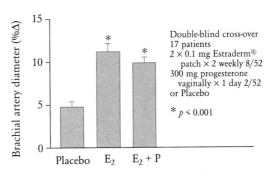

Figure 7 Endothelium-dependent vasodilatation with estrogen (E_2) and estrogen plus progesterone ($E_2 + P$). Reproduced from reference 10 with permission

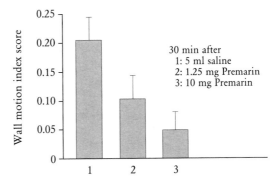

Figure 8 Effect of estrogen on myocardial ischemia (dobutamine stress echo). Reproduced from reference 14 with permission

EFFECTS OF ACUTE ESTROGEN THERAPY ON MYOCARDIAL ISCHEMIA

Exercise-induced myocardial ischemia

Estrogen affects vascular reactivity and coronary blood flow. Rosano and co-workers have shown that estrogen also has anti-ischemic effects in postmenopausal women with CHD[13]. These women were given placebo and asked to exercise until myocardial ischemia occurred (as measured by a 1-mm drop in ST segment). The mean time to ischemia was 456 s. On a different day, administration of 1 mg sublingual estrogen to the women 40 min before they exercised increased the mean time to myocardial ischemia to 579 s[13]. This increase is similar to that seen with sublingual nitrate.

Dobutamine-induced myocardial ischemia

The beneficial effects of estrogen on myocardial ischemia have also been shown by Alpaslan and colleagues[14]. They showed that short-term intravenous administration of continuous equine estrogen (Premarin®, Wyeth) at 1.25 mg or 10 mg reduced dobutamine-induced myocardial

ischemia in postmenopausal women with coronary artery disease. The wall motion index score, which is an indication of how well the heart is functioning in the presence of ischemia, was improved with both doses of estrogen compared with saline (Figure 8).

Pacing-induced myocardial ischemia

When the myocardium becomes ischemic, it produces lactic acid; therefore measurement of the pH in the coronary sinus is an extremely sensitive way of assessing myocardial ischemia. This technique was used by Rosano and co-workers in 16 postmenopausal women with CHD[15]. A pH electrode was placed directly into the coronary sinus in these women and myocardial ischemia was induced by atrial pacing. The women underwent incremental atrial pacing, starting at a rate of 100 beats/min with increments of 20 beats/min every 2 min up to

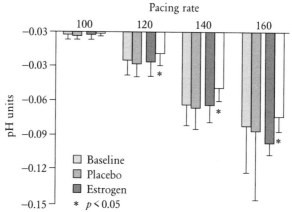

Figure 9 Effect of estrogen on myocardial ischemia. Reproduced from reference 15 with permission

160 beats/min; pacing was conducted before and 20 min after either 17β-estradiol (1 mg sublingual, nine patients) or placebo (sublingual, seven patients). The pH in the coronary sinus was continuously monitored. Estrogen statistically significantly inhibited lactic acid production into the coronary sinus at each pacing rate (all $p < 0.05$) (Figure 9).

This provides further evidence that short-term administration of sublingual estrogen could be used as an anti-ischemic agent in postmenopausal women with CHD.

EFFECTS OF CHRONIC ESTROGEN THERAPY ON MYOCARDIAL ISCHEMIA

Exercise-induced myocardial ischemia

A complex, double-blind, randomized, placebo-controlled study has been conducted by Webb and colleagues to assess whether chronic therapy with estrogen improves exercise-induced myocardial ischemia[16]. Postmenopausal women with CHD were randomized to receive either placebo patches (one patch for 4 weeks, then two patches for 4 weeks) or transdermal estrogen patches (50 μg for 4 weeks then 100 μg for 4 weeks) (phase 1) and were then crossed over to the other therapy (phase 2) (Figure 10).

The plasma concentrations of estrogen after 4 weeks of treatment with 50 μg transdermal estrogen were within the expected levels for

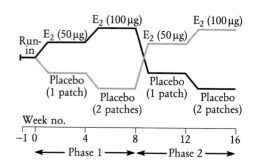

Figure 10 Cross-over design of study of Webb and colleagues[16] to assess the effect of estrogen on exercise-induced myocardial ischemia

postmenopausal women receiving this therapy. Exercise time to 1-mm ST segment depression was substantially increased after 4 weeks of estrogen therapy (50 μg) to 91 s. After 8 weeks of estrogen therapy (4 weeks 50 μg; 4 weeks 100 μg), exercise time increased to 115 s. These results indicate that chronic therapy with estrogen increases exercise time to myocardial ischemia.

LONG-TERM EFFECTS OF ESTROGEN THERAPY

Data from a variety of studies have provided strong evidence that estrogen and some progesterones affect vasculature and blood flow. Further studies are required to show whether estrogen, or estrogen combined with progesterone, has long-term beneficial effects in women with and without cardiovascular disease.

EFFECTS OF TESTOSTERONE ON THE VASCULATURE

Testosterone is structurally similar to estrogen. Although the sexual effects of these hormones are very different, they may have similar effects on the vasculature.

Rabbit coronary artery and aorta

The effects of testosterone on the vasculature were assessed in a similar way to those of estrogen using rabbit blood vessels in an organ bath (see Figure 1a). Testosterone at relatively high concentrations (0.1–10 μmol/l) caused a dose-dependent relaxation of rabbit coronary artery rings (Figure 11)[17].

Interestingly, testosterone also caused dose-dependent relaxation of the aorta from the same animals, but much higher concentrations were required (10–100 μmol/l) (Figure 11). The extent of the relaxation with testosterone is therefore dependent on the type of blood vessel; coronary arteries are much more sensitive to testosterone than the aorta.

Coronary artery in men with CHD

Men with CHD have been shown to have low levels of plasma testosterone. Webb and co-workers, therefore, conducted a study to assess the effects of testosterone on coronary blood flow in men with CHD[17]. Testosterone was infused directly into the coronary arteries of these men (all the men were hypotestosteronemic with testosterone levels below 11 nmol/l).

Testosterone was expected to have no effect or even to cause vasoconstriction, but very low concentrations of this hormone (10^{-10}–10^{-7} mol/l) caused vasodilatation and increased blood flow from approximately 35 ml/min to 40 ml/min (Figure 12).

There was no dose-dependent effect of testosterone on vasodilatation and blood flow; testosterone appeared to have an 'all or nothing' effect.

Brachial artery in men with CHD

Ong and colleagues have recently published work showing that testosterone also enhances flow-mediated brachial artery reactivity in men with

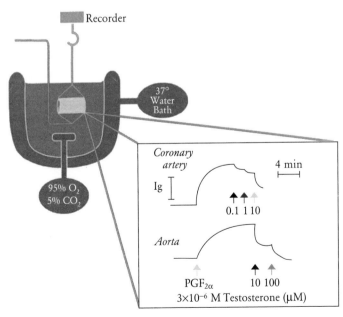

Figure 11 Effects of testosterone on rabbit vasculature. Reproduced from reference 17 with permission

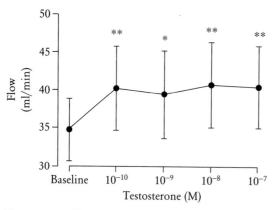

Figure 12 Effect of testosterone on coronary blood flow in men with coronary heart disease. Reproduced from reference 17 with permission

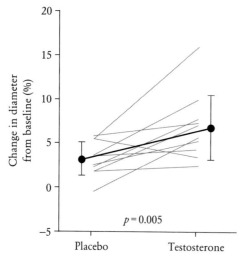

Figure 13 Effect of testosterone on brachial artery reactivity in men with coronary heart disease. Reproduced from reference 18 with permission

CHD[18]. Testosterone statistically significantly increased the change in diameter from baseline compared with placebo ($p = 0.005$) (Figure 13).

These results provide further evidence that testosterone may have beneficial effects on endothelial function in peripheral arteries.

CONCLUSION

Testosterone does not appear to be harmful to the cardiovascular system, but it is essential to select the correct dose for each patient to maximize the potential beneficial effects. If too high a dose is used, testosterone may cause harmful prothrombotic effects, particularly in patients with cardiovascular disease. It is likely that many men with coronary heart disease have low levels of plasma testosterone. This does not imply a cause and effect, but it is an interesting observation. Studies are currently being conducted to assess the potential benefits of increasing testosterone levels in men and women with coronary heart disease.

More research is required into the effects of estrogen on the cardiovascular system to define which type, route of administration and dose should be used to provide cardiovascular benefits. Other molecules are beginning to be of interest in this field; the selective estrogen receptor modulators, for example, have complicated effects on the vasculature via ion channels, the nitric oxide synthase pathway and intracellular calcium stores.

Research into the effects of sex steroids on the cardiovascular system and coronary heart disease in humans is in its infancy. Many more studies are required and there is much more to learn.

References

1. Chester AH, Jiang C, Borland JA, Yacoub MH, Collins P. Estrogen relaxes human epicardial coronary arteries through non-endothelium-dependent mechanisms. *Cor Art Dis* 1995;6:417–22

2. Collins P, Rosano GMC, Jiang C, Lindsay D, Sarrel PM, Poole-Wilson PA. Hypothesis: Cardiovascular protection by oestrogen – a calcium antagonist effect? *Lancet* 1993;341:1264–5

3. Jiang C, Sarrel PM, Poole-Wilson PA, Collins P. Acute effect of 17β-estradiol on rabbit coronary artery contractile responses to endothelin-1. *Am J Physiol* 1992;263:H271–5
4. Webb CM, Ghatei M, McNeill JG, Collins P. 17β-Estradiol decreases endothelin-1 levels in the coronary circulation of postmenopausal women with coronary artery disease. *Circulation* 2000;102: 1617–22
5. Reis SE, Gloth ST, Blumenthal RS, Resar JR, Zacur HA, Gerstenblith G, Brinker JA. Ethinyl estradiol acutely attenuates abnormal coronary vasomotor responses to acetylcholine in postmenopausal women. *Circulation* 1994;89:52–60
6. Collins P, Rosano GMC, Sarrel PM, Ulrich L, Adamopoulos S, Beale CM, McNeill J, Poole-Wilson PA. Estradiol-17β attenuates acetylcholine-induced coronary arterial constriction in women but not men with coronary heart disease. *Circulation* 1995;92:24–30
7. Stefano GB, Prevot V, Beauvillain JC, Cadet P, Fimiani C, Welters I, Fricchione GL, Breton C, Lassalle P, Salzet M, Bilfinger TV. Cell-surface estrogen receptors mediate calcium-dependent nitric oxide release in human endothelia. *Circulation* 2000;101:1594–7
8. Weiner CP, Lizasoain I, Baylis SA, Knowles RG, Charles IG, Moncada S. Induction of calcium-dependent nitric oxide synthases by sex hormones. *Proc Natl Acad Sci USA* 1994;91:5212–16
9. Collins P, Webb C. Estrogen hits the surface. *Nature Medicine* 1999;5:1130–1
10. Gerhard M, Walsh BW, Tawakol A, Haley EA, Creager SJ, Seely EW, Ganz P, Creager MA. Estradiol therapy combined with progesterone and endothelium-dependent vasodilation in postmenopausal women. *Circulation* 1998;98:1158–63
11. Lieberman EH, Gerhard MD, Uehata A, Selwyn AP, Ganz P, Yeung AC, Creager MA. Flow-induced vasodilation of the human brachial artery is impaired in patients < 40 years of age with coronary artery disease. *Am J Cardiol* 1996;78:1210–14
12. Lieberman EH, Gerhard MD, Uehata A, Walsh BW, Selwyn AP, Ganz P, Yeung AC, Creager MA. Estrogen improves endothelium-dependent, flow-mediated vasodilation in postmenopausal women. *Ann Intern Med* 1994;121:936–41
13. Rosano GMC, Sarrel PM, Poole-Wilson PA, Collins P. Beneficial effect of oestrogen on exercise-induced myocardial ischaemia in women with coronary artery disease. *Lancet* 1993;342:133–6
14. Alpaslan M, Shimokawa H, Kuroiwa-Matsumoto M, Harasawa Y, Takeshita A. Short-term estrogen administration ameliorates dobutamine-induced myocardial ischemia in postmenopausal women with coronary artery disease. *J Am Coll Cardiol* 1997;30:1466–71
15. Rosano GMC, Caixeta AM, Chierchia SL, Arie S, Lopez-Hidalgo M, Pereira WI, Leonardo F, Webb CM, Pileggi F, Collins P. Acute anti-ischemic effect of estradiol-17β in postmenopausal women with coronary artery disease. *Circulation* 1997;96: 2837–41
16. Webb CM, Rosano GMC, Collins P. Oestrogen improves exercise-induced myocardial ischaemia in women. *Lancet* 1998;351:1556–7
17. Webb CM, McNeill JG, Hayward CS, de Ziegler D, Collins P. Effects of testosterone on coronary vasomotor regulation in men with coronary artery disease. *Circulation* 1999;100:1690–6
18. Ong PJL, Patrizi G, Chong WCF, Webb CM, Hayward CS, Collins P. Testosterone enhances flow-mediated brachial artery reactivity in men with coronary artery disease. *Am J Cardiol* 2000; 85:14–17

Sex steroids and blood coagulation

15

J. Curvers, G. Tans and J. Rosing

HEMOSTASIS

Blood coagulation is an intricate process which involves many plasma proteins that participate in clot formation, down-regulation of coagulation and clot lysis (Figure 1). Coagulation is initiated when a blood vessel is damaged and tissue factor becomes exposed to the blood. Coagulation factor VII binds to tissue factor and is rapidly converted into factor VIIa. The complex formed between tissue factor and factor VIIa (TF–FVIIa) subse-

quently initiates a sequence of reactions that results in the activation of the coagulation factors IX, VIII, X and V, and prothrombin. The last coagulation factor is converted into thrombin, a protease with a key function in hemostasis, which is responsible for the conversion of fibrinogen into fibrin and thus for clot formation.

Thrombin also regulates its own formation by amplifying coagulation via activation of factor V

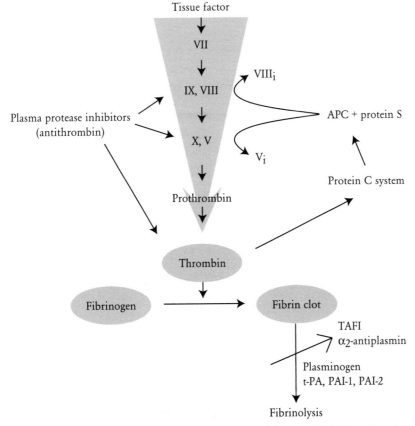

Figure 1 Simplified scheme of blood coagulation. VIII_i, inactivated factor VIII; APC, activated protein C; V_i, inactivated factor V; TAFI, thrombin activatable fibrinolysis inhibitor; t-PA, tissue type plasminogen activator; PAI, plasminogen activator inhibitor

and factor VIII and by inhibiting coagulation via activation of the protein C system. The latter pathway is activated when thrombin bound to thrombomodulin exposed at the endothelial cell surface converts the plasma protein, protein C, into activated protein C (APC). APC very effectively down-regulates coagulation by cleaving and inactivating factors Va and VIIIa in reactions in which protein S acts as cofactor.

Despite the presence of the protein C system there is a continuous slow activation of coagulation factors in the blood. Under normal conditions the activated coagulation factors are scavenged by plasma protease inhibitors (antithrombin, α_2-macroglobulin, tissue factor pathway inhibitor, α_1-antitrypsin) and traces of fibrin formed are degraded by the fibrinolytic system which comprises tissue plasminogen activator (t-PA), plasminogen and the inhibitors antiplasmin, plasminogen activator inhibitor (PAI) and thrombin activatable fibrinolysis inhibitor (TAFI). However, when the anticoagulant system, i.e. the protease inhibitors, the protein C pathway and fibrinolysis, falls short of inhibiting the ongoing coagulation, the hemostatic balance will tip over and thrombosis may occur.

VENOUS THROMBOSIS

Venous thrombosis is a common disease with an incidence of 2-4 per year per 1000 individuals[1]. The annual incidence of venous thrombosis increases with age from 1 per 100 000 during childhood to 1 per 100 in the elderly[2]. During recent years it has become clear that venous thrombosis is a multifactorial disease[3], the occurrence of which often results from an interaction between a number of hereditary and/or exogenous risk factors.

Inherited defects of anticoagulant proteins[4] (e.g. deficiencies of antithrombin, protein C or protein S), mutations in the genes of procoagulant proteins (factor V-R506Q, also called factor V Leiden[5], and prothrombin G20210A[6]) and phenotypic abnormalities (APC resistance[7,8] and high levels of factor IX[9], factor VIII[10] and factor XI[11]) predispose individuals to a higher risk of venous thrombosis. The discovery of the factor V Leiden mutation was based on the observations of Dahlbäck and colleagues[12], who reported in 1993

that in a large number of patients with deep venous thrombosis the anticoagulant protein APC was impaired in its ability to prolong the clotting of plasma. One year later it was reported that this defect, called APC resistance, was caused by a mutation in the factor V molecule (factor V-R506Q/ factor V Leiden)[5,13,14] at a predominant APC cleavage site, rendering factor V less susceptible for inactivation. This mutation, which is very common in the Caucasian population (~ 4%)[15], appears to be a major risk factor for venous thrombosis that predisposes to a seven-fold risk enhancement in heterozygotes[15,16] and an 80-fold risk increase in homozygotes[17]. However, not all APC-resistant individuals carry the factor V Leiden mutation, and later it was reported that APC resistance in the absence of the factor V Leiden mutation is an independent risk factor for venous thrombosis[7,8]. The prothrombin G20210A mutation, which was discovered in 1996[6], is a genetic variation in the 3′-untranslated region of the prothrombin gene. In heterozygous carriers this mutation is associated with elevated plasma levels of prothrombin (~ 125%) and with a three-fold increased risk of venous thrombosis[6].

Exogenous factors that increase the risk for venous thrombosis are surgery, major trauma, periods of immobilization, pregnancy, the postpartum period, and the use of oral contraceptive pills and hormone replacement therapy. The triad of Virchow (1859) represents the three factors involved in thrombosis: changes in the vessel wall, reduction in blood flow and changes in blood composition. Since the last component plays a predominant role in thrombus formation in the veins, venous thrombosis can be regarded as the clinical symptom of hypercoagulable plasma. Many investigators have therefore put effort into studying changes of hemostatic parameters in individuals at risk of venous thrombosis in an attempt to understand and explain the causes of this disease.

In numerous studies the effects of oral contraceptive use, pregnancy and hormone replacement therapy on hemostatic variables have been investigated. The parameters that have been determined can be divided into three groups: (a) plasma levels of proteins involved in coagulation, anticoagulation and fibrinolysis quantified via either an activity or an antigen assay; (b) markers of ongoing coagulation and fibrinolysis, e.g. thrombin-antithrombin (TAT) complex, prothrombin fragment 1 + 2 (F1 + 2), fibrin monomers, fibrinopeptide A, D-dimer and plasmin–antiplasmin (PAP) complexes; and (c) functional clotting tests that probe the overall activity of the coagulation and/or anticoagulation pathways, e.g. the prothrombin time (PT), the activated partial thromboplastin time (aPTT) and APC resistance tests. In the next sections of this chapter we will give an overview of the thrombotic risks and changes of hemostatic variables associated with pregnancy and the use of oral contraceptives and hormone replacement therapy.

ORAL CONTRACEPTIVES

Soon after the marketing of oral contraceptive preparations in the early 1960s it was reported that women who used oral contraceptives were exposed to an increased risk of venous thromboembolism. The incidence of venous thrombosis decreased when the estrogen dose in oral contraceptive pills was lowered to 50 μg ethinylestradiol or less[18]. In the mid-1980s, so-called third-generation oral contraceptive pills were introduced which contained, instead of levonorgestrel, lynestrenol or norethisterone, a less androgenic progestogen (desogestrel or gestodene). Although third-generation oral contraceptives were developed to reduce the risk of cardiovascular disease, it was reported in 1995 that the risk of venous thrombosis in third-generation oral contraceptive users was increased 2–3-fold compared with users of the older second-generation preparations containing levonorgestrel[19-22]. Until the present day, reports have been appearing in the literature either denying or confirming this risk difference[23-25].

The effects of oral contraceptives on the hemostatic system have been studied extensively during recent years[26-28]. In women who use oral contraceptives the plasma level of almost every protein that participates in blood coagulation changes (Table 1). The concentrations of many coagulation factors (prothrombin, factors VII, VIII, IX, X and XI) are increased. Together with the decrease of the anticoagulant proteins antithrombin and protein S, this is indicative of a net prothrombotic effect. It

Table 1 Effects of oral contraceptives on hemostatic variables

Prothrombotic effects	Antithrombotic effects
Prothrombin↑, factor VII↑, factor VIII↑, factor IX↑, factor X↑, factor XI↑, fibrinogen↑, protein S↓, antithrombin↓	protein C↑; $α_1$-antitrypsin↑, plasminogen↑, PAI-1↓

PAI-1, plasminogen activator inhibitor-1

has been argued, however, that these procoagulant changes may be counterbalanced by antithrombotic effects of the pill, such as elevated levels of protein C, $α_1$-antitrypsin and plasminogen, a decrease of plasminogen activator inhibitor-1 (PAI-1), and increased fibrinolytic activity.

Recently, a cross-over study was published[29-31] in which a direct comparison was made between a second-generation oral contraceptive (containing 30 μg ethinylestradiol and 150 μg levonorgestrel) and a third-generation oral contraceptive (containing 30 μg ethinylestradiol and 150 μg desogestrel). The trends of the changes induced by second- as well as third-generation oral contraceptives were in line with those presented in Table 1. However, there were some significant differences between the effects of the two kinds of contraceptive pills. Compared to levonorgestrel-containing oral contraceptives, the use of desogestrel-containing oral contraceptives was accompanied by significantly higher levels of factor VII, prothrombin and thrombin activatable fibrinolysis inhibitor (TAFI), and by lower levels of factor V and total and free protein S. The increased plasma levels of plasminogen, tissue plasminogen activator, D-dimer and PAP, which were observed for both oral contraceptive pills, are indicative of enhanced fibrinolytic activity. However, a clot lysis test that measures directly both the ability of plasma to lyse clots and the activity of the anti-fibrinolytic system (antiplasmin, PAI-1 and TAFI) showed that the clot lysis time was not reduced during oral contraceptive use. On the basis of these observations, Meijers and associates[31] proposed that the enhanced fibrinolytic activity during oral contraceptive use is compensated by an increased inhibition of fibrinolysis via the TAFI system.

The oral contraceptive-induced changes of the plasma levels of proteins involved in the pro-coagulant, anticoagulant and fibrinolytic pathways are moderate, and in most oral contraceptive users the values of the hemostatic parameters stay within the normal ranges. However, nowadays it is known that even relatively small increases in levels of coagulation factors are associated with an increased risk of venous thrombosis[6,9-11,32]. This suggests that the modest changes of plasma levels of coagulation factors and the differential effects on these factors of second- and third-generation oral contraceptives cannot be ignored in the discussion about the thrombotic effects of oral contraceptives.

In 1997, observations were published that are indicative of another prothrombotic effect of oral contraceptives. It was reported that the plasma of oral contraceptive users is resistant to APC and that there is a significant difference in APC resistance between users of second- and third-generation oral contraceptives[33]. There was criticism of the design of this study, but another randomized, cross-over study also established that women who use oral contraceptive pills with desogestrel are more resistant to APC than users of levonorgestrel-containing pills[34]. It is interesting to note that women in these studies who were using oral contraceptives and who were also heterozygous carriers of the factor V Leiden mutation had a degree of APC resistance that is normally observed for homozygous carriers of the factor V Leiden mutation[33]. The amplifying effects of oral contraceptive use and the factor V Leiden mutation in the APC resistance test may explain the high risk of venous thrombosis in women with the factor V Leiden mutation who use oral contraceptives[21].

PREGNANCY

It is generally accepted that there is a state of hypercoagulability during pregnancy and the puerperium. This hypercoagulable state may prevent excessive blood loss during delivery[35], but it also accounts for thrombotic complications that may occur during pregnancy. During pregnancy the incidence of venous thromboembolism is 0.3–1.0 per 1000 pregnant-woman years[36,37], of which 75% occurs antepartum[38,39]. The risk of venous throm-

bosis therefore rises during pregnancy 3–7-fold. However, with respect to the occurrence of venous thrombosis, the post-partum period can be regarded as the most dangerous period. The majority of cases of pulmonary embolism, which is the major cause of maternal death[40], occur post-partum[39]. Since the post-partum period is much shorter than the period of gestation, a 20-fold risk increase has been calculated for the puerperium[36,37,41]. Although a number of additional factors can be designated as risk factors for post-partum thrombosis (> 35 years of age, multiparity, Cesarean section, hereditary thrombophilia), it is likely that changes in the hemostatic system also contribute to the thrombotic risk in this period.

Since the 1970s, several studies have been published in which the effects of pregnancy on the hemostatic system have been described. However, most of these studies were conducted to establish changes that occur during abnormal pregnancies, e.g. pregnancies complicated by hypertension and pre-eclampsia. A detailed report on the effect of normal pregnancy on coagulation parameters was published in 1984 by Stirling and colleagues[42]. The authors showed that the plasma levels of a number of coagulation factors consistently rise during pregnancy: factor VII to 170%, factor VIII to 200% (an increase that is sustained after delivery), factor X to 130% and fibrinogen to 4.2 g/l. Prothrombin and factor V initially also increase, but after 20–30 weeks they decrease again, a phenomenon that may be due to hemodilution. The levels of the protease inhibitors α_1-antitrypsin and α_2-macroglobulin, which probably do not play an important role in the in vivo regulation of coagulation, considerably increase during pregnancy. However, the plasma level of the major physiological inhibitor antithrombin hardly changes. Furthermore, the clot lysis time decreases during pregnancy but increases enormously after delivery, indicating a vast drop in fibrinolytic capacity in the post-partum period. On the basis of these observations, Stirling and co-workers[42] concluded that the initial increase in the level of coagulation factors and fibrinogen was mediated by estradiol and that this was a mechanism to ensure integrity of the endometrium and placenta.

Many of the changes reported by Stirling and colleagues[42] were confirmed in later publications.

In addition to changes in levels of coagulation factors, these studies also provided information on the effects of pregnancy on markers of ongoing coagulation, on fibrinolytic proteins and on the protein C system. With respect to markers of coagulation, van Wersch and Ubachs[43] showed significant positive correlations between gestational age and thrombin-antithrombin (TAT) complexes and fibrin monomers. In several other studies, increased levels of TAT complexes[44-46], soluble fibrin monomers[44,47] and F1 + 2[45-48] were observed. F1 + 2 is formed when prothrombin is converted to thrombin by factor Xa, and like TAT complexes and fibrin monomers is a marker for *in vivo* thrombin formation. F1 + 2 formation increases with gestational age (correlation index 0.69), especially after 20 weeks of pregnancy[47,49,50].

With respect to fibrinolytic proteins, it has been reported that the plasma levels of plasminogen[43] and the plasminogen activator inhibitors, PAI-1 and PAI-2[43,44,47], increase with gestational age, whereas tissue plasminogen activator decreases[43,47]. Elevated levels of plasmin–antiplasmin complexes[51] and D-dimer[44,46,47] demonstrate that despite the increase of PAI-1 and PAI-2 and the decrease of t-PA, the fibrinolytic activity is enhanced during pregnancy.

Since increased plasma levels of TAT complexes, F1 + 2 and D-dimer are indicative of thrombin formation and fibrinolytic activity, it appears that in pregnant women both the coagulation and fibrinolytic systems are in activated states.

Protein S, the cofactor of APC in the anticoagulant protein C pathway, circulates in plasma in a free form and in complex with C4B binding protein. The total plasma protein S levels decrease during pregnancy to 70% of normal[52]. It has been shown that not only does total protein S decrease, but that free protein S also decreases[44,47,48,53]. Low levels of free protein S are observed at as early as 10 weeks of gestation[47], and in some cases free protein S falls to 40% of normal. This low level is sustained until after delivery (even until 8 weeks post-partum). In contrast, changes of protein C during pregnancy are much less pronounced or absent[44,53]. Since free protein S acts as a cofactor of APC in the down-regulation of coagulation, the impairment of the protein C pathway due to low levels of free protein S may contribute to the increased risk of venous thrombosis during pregnancy.

Soon after the discovery of APC resistance and the factor V Leiden mutation it was reported that pregnant women who do not carry the factor V Leiden mutation become resistant to APC[50,54-57], a phenomenon that was called 'acquired APC resistance'. Since increased resistance to APC was measured with an APC resistance assay that was based on a clotting test, and since clotting times are influenced by factor VIII and protein S levels, it is possible that increased APC resistance is due to the high levels of factor VIII and/or the low levels of protein S during pregnancy. Although a number of studies suggested that the changes in APC resistance correlated with the changes in factor VIII[48,55,56] and protein S[48], Kjellberg and co-workers[47] did not find such correlations. This indicates that other plasma components may also contribute to APC resistance.

Although significant, the extent of APC resistance determined with classical APC resistance assays is in general less pronounced than that of carriers of the factor V Leiden mutation. In 1997 we described an APC resistance test that is based on measurement of the effect of APC on thrombin formation in full plasma[58]. We found that this assay is strongly affected by pregnancy and in a preliminary report we have shown that APC resistance determined with this test increases with gestational age[59]. Using a similar assay, Sugimura and associates[60] reported an enormous increase in APC resistance in one woman who developed thrombosis during delivery, demonstrating that APC resistance which has developed during pregnancy may contribute to the risk for venous thrombosis.

HORMONE REPLACEMENT THERAPY

Although early epidemiological studies did not show that hormone replacement therapy (HRT) is associated with an increased risk for venous thromboembolism[61-63], it has been established in recent case–control studies that, compared with non-users, current users of hormone replacement therapy have a three-fold higher risk of venous thromboembolism[64,65].

With respect to the effect of HRT on hemostatic variables, there are many conflicting reports. This is probably caused by the fact that the changes of coagulation parameters during HRT are less pronounced than those occurring during oral contraceptive use or pregnancy. Also, the amount and source of estrogen, the route of administration (oral or transdermal) and the absence or presence of opposing progestogens may determine the exact impact on the coagulation system. Oral preparations seem to have more pronounced effects than transdermal preparations.

Only limited information is available on the effect of HRT on the coagulation factors II, V, VIII, IX, X and XI. Several studies have focused on the effects of HRT on factor VII and fibrinogen. The interest in these coagulation factors, which increase substantially during oral contraceptive use and pregnancy, is presumably due to the fact that they have been implicated in causing an increased risk of arterial thrombosis[66,67]. Oral estrogen-only therapy appears to be associated with increased levels of factor VII[68-71], whereas combined HRT or transdermal estrogens have no effect or even lower the plasma level of factor VII[69-72]. In contrast to oral contraceptive use and pregnancy, HRT use with both estrogen-only and combined preparations causes a reduction of fibrinogen[68,73-77]. Since high factor VII and fibrinogen levels are associated with an increased risk of cardiovascular disease[66,67], the lowering of the plasma levels of these proteins during HRT may have a beneficial effect on the risk. These beneficial effects may, however, be counteracted by decreases of the plasma levels of the anticoagulant proteins antithrombin[76,78-83], protein C[82] and protein S[83-85]. We would like to mention, however, that there are also studies in which increases of protein C[68,83,86] and protein S[87] were reported. Like oral contraceptive users and pregnant women, users of HRT develop acquired APC resistance[59,88], the extent of which is, however, much less pronounced than during oral contraceptive use and pregnancy.

HRT also affects the fibrinolytic system. Users of HRT in general have higher plasminogen[85] and lower PAI-1[71,77,85,89-91] and t-PA[77,85,89,90] levels than women who do not use HRT. The decrease of PAI-1 is particularly observed after oral administration of estrogen and not after transdermal administration[79,84,92,93].

Markers of ongoing coagulation, such as F1 + 2[83,85,91], fibrinopeptide A[83] and soluble fibrin[91], are increased during HRT. Despite modest effects of HRT on the levels of individual coagulation factors, this is indicative of activation of the coagulation system. Increased D-dimer[91] and plasmin-antiplasmin[71] levels show that not only the coagulation system but also fibrinolysis are enhanced during HRT. However, there are also studies in which no changes of F1 + 2[71], TAT complexes[85] or D-dimer[71] were observed. In the cases in which increased coagulant and fibrinolytic activities were observed there appeared to be no correlation between the elevation of markers of coagulation and fibrinolysis[92,93]. This suggests that the potentiation of fibrinolysis during HRT is not a response to enhanced activation of coagulation.

SUMMARY AND CONCLUSIONS

The overview of the literature given in this paper indicates that both the coagulation and the fibrinolytic systems are in an activated state during HRT, oral contraceptive use and pregnancy. Increased levels of coagulation factors (prothrombin, factor VIII) and a diminished activity of the protein C system (acquired APC resistance and decreased plasma levels of protein S) are particularly observed in pregnant women and women who use oral contraceptives. These changes are indicative of a prothrombotic state and may explain the increased risk of venous thromboembolism during pregnancy and oral contraceptive use. The observation that HRT has less pronounced effects on procoagulant and anticoagulant parameters is in agreement with the lower risk of venous thrombosis during HRT use.

References

1. Nordstrom M, Lindblad B, Bergqvist D, Kjellstrom T. A prospective study of the incidence of deep-vein thrombosis within a defined urban population. *J Intern Med* 1992;232:155-60
2. Rosendaal FR. Thrombosis in the young: epidemiology and risk factors. A focus on venous thrombosis. *Thromb Haemost* 1997;78:1-6
3. Rosendaal FR. Venous thrombosis: a multicausal disease. *Lancet* 1999;353:1167-73
4. Simioni P, Sanson BJ, Prandoni P, Tormene D, Friederich PW, *et al*. Incidence of venous thromboembolism in families with inherited thrombophilia. *Thromb Haemost* 1999;81:198-202
5. Bertina RM, Koeleman BP, Koster T, Rosendaal FR, Dirven RJ, *et al*. Mutation in blood coagulation factor V associated with resistance to activated protein C. *Nature (London)* 1994;369:64-7
6. Poort SR, Rosendaal FR, Reitsma PH, Bertina RM. A common genetic variation in the 3′-untranslated region of the prothrombin gene is associated with elevated plasma prothrombin levels and an increase in venous thrombosis. *Blood* 1996;88:3698-703
7. de Visser MC, Rosendaal FR, Bertina RM. A reduced sensitivity for activated protein C in the absence of factor V Leiden increases the risk of venous thrombosis. *Blood* 1999;93:1271-6
8. Rodeghiero F, Tosetto A. Activated protein C resistance and factor V Leiden mutation are independent risk factors for venous thromboembolism. *Ann Intern Med* 1999;130:643-50
9. van Hylckama Vlieg A, van der Linden IK, Bertina RM, Rosendaal FR. High levels of factor IX increase the risk of venous thrombosis. *Blood* 2000;95:3678-82
10. Kraaijenhagen RA, in't Anker PS, Koopman MM, Reitsma PH, Prins MH, *et al*. High plasma concentration of factor VIIIc is a major risk factor for venous thromboembolism. *Thromb Haemost* 2000;83:5-9
11. Meijers JC, Tekelenburg WL, Bouma BN, Bertina RM, Rosendaal FR. High levels of coagulation factor XI as a risk factor for venous thrombosis. *N Engl J Med* 2000;342:696-701
12. Dahlbäck B, Carlsson M, Svensson PJ. Familial thrombophilia due to a previously unrecognized mechanism characterized by poor anticoagulant response to activated protein C: prediction of a cofactor to activated protein C. *Proc Natl Acad Sci USA* 1993;90:1004-8
13. Greengard JS, Sun X, Xu X, Fernandez JA, Griffin JH, Evatt B. Activated protein C resistance caused by Arg506Gln mutation in factor Va. *Lancet* 1994;343:1361-2
14. Voorberg J, Roelse J, Koopman R, Büller H, Berends F, *et al*. Association of idiopathic venous thromboembolism with single-point mutation at Arg506 of factor V. *Lancet* 1994;343:1535-6
15. Koster T, Rosendaal FR, de Ronde H, Briët E, Vandenbroucke JP, Bertina RM. Venous thrombosis due to poor anticoagulant response to activated protein C: Leiden Thrombophilia Study. *Lancet* 1993;342:1503-6
16. Svensson PJ, Dahlbäck B. Resistance to activated protein C as a basis for venous thrombosis. *N Engl J Med* 1994;330:517-22
17. Rosendaal FR, Koster T, Vandenbroucke JP, Reitsma PH. High risk of thrombosis in patients homozygous for factor V Leiden (activated protein C resistance). *Blood* 1995;85:1504-8
18. Gerstman BB, Piper JM, Tomita DK, Ferguson WJ, Stadel BV, Lundin FE. Oral contraceptive estrogen dose and the risk of deep venous thromboembolic disease. *Am J Epidemiol* 1991;133:32-7
19. World Health Organization. Effect of different progestagens in low-oestrogen oral contraceptives on venous thromboembolic disease. World Health Organization Collaborative Study of Cardiovascular Disease and Steroid Hormone Contraception. *Lancet* 1995;346:1582-8
20. Jick H, Jick SS, Gurewich V, Myers MW, Vasilakis C. Risk of idiopathic cardiovascular death and nonfatal venous thromboembolism in women using oral contraceptives with differing progestagen components. *Lancet* 1995;346:1589-93
21. Bloemenkamp KWM, Rosendaal FR, Helmerhorst FM, Büller HR, Vandenbroucke JP. Enhancement by factor V Leiden mutation of risk of deep-vein thrombosis associated with oral contraceptives containing third-generation progestagen. *Lancet* 1995;346:1593-6
22. Spitzer WO, Lewis MA, Heinemann LA, Thorogood M, MacRae KD. Third-generation oral contraceptives and risk of venous thromboembolic disorders: an international case-control study. Transnational Research Group on Oral Contraceptives and the Health of Young Women. *Br Med J* 1996;312:83-8
23. Farmer RD, Williams TJ, Simpson EL, Nightingale AL. Effect of 1995 pill scare on rates of venous thromboembolism among women taking combined oral contraceptives: analysis of general practice research database. *Br Med J* 2000;321:477-9
24. Jick H, Kaye JA, Vasilakis-Scaramozza C, Jick SS. Risk of venous thromboembolism among users of third-generation oral contraceptives compared with users of oral contraceptives with levonorgestrel before and after 1995: cohort and case-control analysis. *Br Med J* 2000;321:1190-5
25. Skegg DCG. Pitfalls of pharmacoepidemiology. *Br Med J* 2000;321:1171-2

26. Newton JR. Classification and comparison of oral contraceptives containing new-generation progestagens. *Hum Reprod Update* 1995;1:231–63

27. Speroff L. Oral contraceptives and venous thromboembolism. *Int J Gynaecol Obstet* 1996;54:45–50

28. Kluft C, Lansink M. Effects of oral contraceptives on haemostasis variables. *Thromb Haemost* 1997;78:315–26

29. Tans G, Curvers J, Middeldorp S, Thomassen MCLGD, Meijers JCM, et al. A randomized cross-over study on the effects of levonorgestrel- and desogestrel-containing oral contraceptives on the anticoagulant pathways. *Thromb Haemost* 2000;84:15–21

30. Middeldorp S, Meijers JCM, van den End AE, van Enk A, Bouma BN, et al. Effects on coagulation of levonorgestrel- and desogestrel-containing low-dose oral contraceptives: a cross-over study. *Thromb Haemost* 2000;84:4–8

31. Meijers JCM, Middeldorp S, Tekelenburg W, van den Ende AE, Tans G, et al. Increased fibrinolytic activity during use of oral contraceptives is counteracted by an enhanced factor XI-independent downregulation of fibrinolysis: a randomized cross-over study of two low-dose oral contraceptives. *Thromb Haemost* 2000;84:9–14

32. van Tilburg NH, Rosendaal FR, Bertina RM. Thrombin activatable fibrinolysis inhibitor and the risk for deep vein thrombosis. *Blood* 2000;95:2855–9

33. Rosing J, Tans G, Nicolaes GAF, Thomassen MCLGD, van Oerle R, et al. Oral contraceptives and venous thrombosis: different sensitivities to activated protein C in women using second- and third-generation oral contraceptives. *Br J Haematol* 1997;97:233–8

34. Rosing J, Middeldorp S, Curvers J, Christella M, Thomassen LG, et al. Low-dose oral contraceptives and acquired resistance to activated protein C: a randomised cross-over study. *Lancet* 1999;354:2036–40

35. Lindqvist PG, Svensson PJ, Marsaal K, Grennert L, Luterkort M, Dahlbäck B. Activated protein C resistance (FV:Q506) and pregnancy. *Thromb Haemost* 1999;81:532–7

36. Rosendaal FR. Risk factors for venous thrombosis: prevalence, risk and interaction. *Semin Hematol* 1997;34:171–87

37. Walker ID. Inherited coagulation disorders and thrombophilia and pregnancy. In Bonnar J, ed. *Recent Advances in Obstetrics and Gynaecology*, Vol. 20. London: Churchill-Livingstone, 1998

38. Rutherford S, Montoro M, McGhee W, Strong T. Thromboembolic disease associated with pregnancy: an 11-years review. *Am J Obstet Gynecol* 1991;164(Suppl):286

39. Macklon NS, Greer IA. Venous thromboembolic disease in obstetrics and gynaecology: the Scottish experience. *Scott Med J* 1996;41:83–6

40. Letsky E, de Swiet M. Annotation. Thromboembolism in pregnancy and its management. *Br J Haematol* 1984;57:543–52

41. Bonnar J, Green R, Norris L. Inherited thrombophilia and pregnancy: the obstetric perspective. *Semin Thromb Hemost* 1998;24:49–53

42. Stirling Y, Woolf L, North WR, Seghatchian MJ, Meade TW. Haemostasis in normal pregnancy. *Thromb Haemost* 1984;52:176–82

43. van Wersch JW, Ubachs JM. Blood coagulation and fibrinolysis during normal pregnancy. *Eur J Clin Chem Clin Biochem* 1991;29:45–50

44. Bremme K, Ostlund E, Almqvist I, Heinonen K, Blomback M. Enhanced thrombin generation and fibrinolytic activity in normal pregnancy and the puerperium. *Obstet Gynecol* 1992;80:132–7

45. Levine AB, Teppa J, McGough B, Cowchock FS. Evaluation of the prethrombotic state in pregnancy and in women using oral contraceptives. *Contraception* 1996;53:255–7

46. Mercelina-Roumans PE, Ubachs JM, van Wersch JW. Coagulation and fibrinolysis in smoking and nonsmoking pregnant women. *Br J Obstet Gynaecol* 1996;103:789–94

47. Kjellberg U, Andersson NE, Rosen S, Tengborn L, Hellgren M. APC resistance and other haemostatic variables during pregnancy and puerperium. *Thromb Haemost* 1999;81:527–31

48. Clark P, Brennand J, Conkie JA, McCall F, Greer IA, Walker ID. Activated protein C sensitivity, protein C, protein S and coagulation in normal pregnancy. *Thromb Haemost* 1998;79:1166–70

49. Comeglio P, Fedi S, Liotta AA, Cellai AP, Chiarantini E, et al. Blood clotting activation during normal pregnancy. *Thromb Res* 1996;84:199–202

50. Schlit AF, Col-De Beys C, Moriau M, Lavenne-Pardonge E. Acquired activated protein C resistance in pregnancy. *Thromb Res* 1996;84:203–6

51. Montes R, Paramo JA, Angles-Cano E, Rocha E. Development and clinical application of a new ELISA assay to determine plasmin-alpha2-antiplasmin complexes in plasma. *Br J Haematol* 1996;92:979–85

52. Comp PC, Thurnau GR, Welsh J, Esmon CT. Functional and immunologic protein S levels are decreased during pregnancy. *Blood* 1986;68:881–5

53. Faught W, Garner P, Jones G, Ivey B. Changes in protein C and protein S levels in normal pregnancy. *Am J Obstet Gynecol* 1995;172:147–50

54. Cumming AM, Tait RC, Fildes S, Yoong A, Keeney S, Hay CR. Development of resistance to activated protein C during pregnancy. *Br J Haematol* 1995;90:725–7

55. Mathonnet F, de Mazancourt P, Bastenaire B, Morot M, Benattar N, et al. Activated protein C sensitivity ratio in pregnant women at delivery. *Br J Haematol* 1996;92:244–6

56. Bokarewa MI, Wramsby M, Bremme K, Blomback M. Variability of the response to activated protein

C during normal pregnancy. *Blood Coagul Fibrinolysis* 1997;8:239-44

57. Meinardi JR, Henkens CM, Heringa MP, van der Meer J. Acquired APC resistance related to oral contraceptives and pregnancy and its possible implications for clinical practice. *Blood Coagul Fibrinolysis* 1997;8:152-4

58. Nicolaes GA, Thomassen MC, Tans G, Rosing J, Hemker HC. Effect of activated protein C on thrombin generation and on the thrombin potential in plasma of normal and APC-resistant individuals. *Blood Coagul Fibrinolysis* 1997;8:28-38

59. Thomassen MCLGD, Curvers J, Rimmer JE, Preston FE, van Wersch JWJ, *et al.* Influence of hormone replacement therapy, oral contraceptives and pregnancy on APC resistance. *Thromb Haemost* 1999;82(Suppl):770-1

60. Sugimura M, Kobayashi T, Kanayama N, Terao T. Detection of marked reduction of sensitivity to activated protein C prior to the onset of thrombosis during puerperium as detected by endogenous thrombin potential-based assay. *Thromb Haemost* 1999;82:1364-5

61. Petitti DB, Wingerd J, Pellegrin F, Ramcharan S. Risk of vascular disease in women. Smoking, oral contraceptives, noncontraceptive estrogens, and other factors. *J Am Med Assoc* 1979;242:1150-4

62. Nachtigall LE, Nachtigall RH, Nachtigall RD, Beckman EM. Estrogen replacement therapy II: a prospective study in the relationship to carcinoma and cardiovascular and metabolic problems. *Obstet Gynecol* 1979;54:74-9

63. Devor M, Barrett-Connor E, Renvall M, Feigal D Jr, Ramsdell J. Estrogen replacement therapy and the risk of venous thrombosis. *Am J Med* 1992;92:275-82

64. Daly E, Vessey MP, Hawkins MM, Carson JL, Gough P, Marsh S. Risk of venous thromboembolism in users of hormone replacement therapy. *Lancet* 1996;348:977-80

65. Jick H, Derby LE, Myers MW, Vasilakis C, Newton KM. Risk of hospital admission for idiopathic venous thromboembolism among users of postmenopausal oestrogens. *Lancet* 1996;348:981-3

66. Ernst E, Resch KL. Fibrinogen as a cardiovascular risk factor: a meta-analysis and review of the literature. *Ann Intern Med* 1993;118:956-63

67. Thomas DP, Roberts HR. Hypercoagulability in venous and arterial thrombosis. *Ann Intern Med* 1997;126:638-44

68. Nabulsi AA, Folsom AR, White A, Patsch W, Heiss G, Wu KK, Szklo M. Association of hormone-replacement therapy with various cardiovascular risk factors in postmenopausal women. The Atherosclerosis Risk in Communities Study Investigators. *N Engl J Med* 1993;328:1069-75

69. Lobo RA, Pickar JH, Wild RA, Walsh B, Hirvonen E. Metabolic impact of adding medroxyprogesterone acetate to conjugated estrogen therapy in postmenopausal women. The Menopause Study Group. *Obstet Gynecol* 1994;84:987-95

70. Medical Research Council. Randomised comparison of oestrogen versus oestrogen plus progestogen hormone replacement therapy in women with hysterectomy. Medical Research Council's General Practice Research Framework. *Br Med J* 1996;312:473-8

71. Cushman M, Meilahn EN, Psaty BM, Kuller LH, Dobs AS, Tracy RP. Hormone replacement therapy, inflammation, and hemostasis in elderly women. *Arterioscler Thromb Vasc Biol* 1999;19:893-9

72. Scarabin PY, Vissac AM, Kirzin JM, Bourgeat P, Amiral J, Agher R, Guize L. Population correlates of coagulation factor VII. Importance of age, sex, and menopausal status as determinants of activated factor VII. *Arterioscler Thromb Vasc Biol* 1996;16:1170-6

73. The Writing Group for the PEPI Trial. Effects of estrogen or estrogen/progestin regimens on heart disease risk factors in postmenopausal women. The Postmenopausal Estrogen/Progestin Interventions (PEPI) Trial. *J Am Med Assoc* 1995;273:199-208

74. Folsom AR, Wu KK, Davis CE, Conlan MG, Sorlie PD, Szklo M. Population correlates of plasma fibrinogen and factor VII, putative cardiovascular risk factors. *Atherosclerosis* 1991;91:191-205

75. Lee AJ, Lowe GD, Smith WC, Tunstall-Pedoe H. Plasma fibrinogen in women: relationships with oral contraception, the menopause and hormone replacement therapy. *Br J Haematol* 1993;83:616-21

76. Meilahn EN, Kuller LH, Matthews KA, Kiss JE. Hemostatic factors according to menopausal status and use of hormone replacement therapy. *Ann Epidemiol* 1992;2:445-55

77. Andersen LF, Gram J, Skouby SO, Jespersen J. Effects of hormone replacement therapy on hemostatic cardiovascular risk factors. *Am J Obstet Gynecol* 1999;180:283-9

78. Lindberg UB, Crona N, Stigendal L, Teger-Nilsson AC, Silfverstolpe G. A comparison between effects of estradiol valerate and low-dose ethinyl estradiol on haemostasis parameters. *Thromb Haemost* 1989;61:65-9

79. Kroon UB, Silfverstolpe G, Tengborn L. The effects of transdermal estradiol and oral conjugated estrogens on haemostasis variables. *Thromb Haemost* 1994;71:420-3

80. Gordon EM, Williams SR, Frenchek B, Mazur CA, Speroff L. Dose-dependent effects of postmenopausal estrogen and progestin on antithrombin III and factor XII. *J Lab Clin Med* 1988;111:52-6

81. Boschetti C, Cortellaro M, Nencioni T, Bertolli V, Della Volpe A, Zanussi C. Short- and long-term effects of hormone replacement therapy (transdermal estradiol vs. oral conjugated equine estrogens, combined with medroxyprogesterone acetate) on blood coagulation factors in postmenopausal women. *Thromb Res* 1991;62:1-8

82. Sporrong T, Mattsson LA, Samsioe G, Stigendal L, Hellgren M. Haemostatic changes during continuous oestradiol-progestogen treatment of postmenopausal women. *Br J Obstet Gynaecol* 1990;97:939–44

83. Caine YG, Bauer KA, Barzegar S, ten Cate H, Sacks FM, *et al*. Coagulation activation following estrogen administration to postmenopausal women. *Thromb Haemost* 1992;68:392–5

84. Gilabert J, Estelles A, Cano A, Espana F, Barrachina R, *et al*. The effect of estrogen replacement therapy with or without progestogen on the fibrinolytic system and coagulation inhibitors in postmenopausal status. *Am J Obstet Gynecol* 1995;173:1849–54

85. van Baal WM, Emeis JJ, van der Mooren MJ, Kessel H, Kenemans P, Stehouwer CD. Impaired procoagulant-anticoagulant balance during hormone replacement therapy? A randomised, placebo-controlled 12-week study. *Thromb Haemost* 2000;83:29–34

86. Clarkson TB, Shively CA, Morgan TM, Koritnik DR, Adams MR, Kaplan JR. Oral contraceptives and coronary artery atherosclerosis of cynomolgus monkeys. *Obstet Gynecol* 1990;75:217–22

87. De Mitrio V, Marino R, Cicinelli E, Galantino P, Di Bari L, *et al*. Beneficial effects of postmenopausal hormone replacement therapy with transdermal estradiol on sensitivity to activated protein C. *Blood Coagul Fibrinolysis* 2000;11:175–82

88. Marcucci R, Abbate R, Fedi S, Gori AM, Brunelli T, *et al*. Acquired activated protein C resistance in postmenopausal women is dependent on factor VIII:c levels. *Am J Clin Pathol* 1999;111:769–72

89. Gebara OC, Mittleman MA, Sutherland P, Lipinska I, Matheney T, *et al*. Association between increased estrogen status and increased fibrinolytic potential in the Framingham Offspring Study. *Circulation* 1995;91:1952–8

90. Shahar E, Folsom AR, Salomaa VV, Stinson VL, McGovern PG, *et al*. Relation of hormone replacement therapy to measures of plasma fibrinolytic activity. Atherosclerosis Risk in Communities (ARIC) Study Investigators. *Circulation* 1996;93:1970–5

91. Teede HJ, McGrath BP, Smolich JJ, Malan E, Kotsopoulos D, Liang YL, Peverill RE. Postmenopausal hormone replacement therapy increases coagulation activity and fibrinolysis. *Arterioscler Thromb Vasc Biol* 2000;20:1404–9

92. Scarabin PY, Alhenc-Gelas M, Plu-Bureau G, Taisne P, Agher R, Aiach M. Effects of oral and transdermal estrogen/progesterone regimens on blood coagulation and fibrinolysis in postmenopausal women. A randomized controlled trial. *Arterioscler Thromb Vasc Biol* 1997;17:3071–8

93. Koh KK, Horne MK III, Cannon RO III. Effects of hormone replacement therapy on coagulation, fibrinolysis, and thrombosis risk in postmenopausal women. *Thromb Haemost* 1999;82:626–33

Lipoprotein-associated estrogen: the role of lecithin : cholesterol acyltransferase and cholesteryl ester transfer protein

16

M. J. Tikkanen, H. Helisten, A. Höckerstedt, K. Wähälä, A. Tiitinen, H. Adlercreutz and M. Jauhiainen

INTRODUCTION

It is generally assumed that ovarian estrogens contribute to the protection of menstruating women against atherosclerotic disease. Part of this protection may be mediated by lower serum concentrations of low-density lipoprotein (LDL) cholesterol and higher high-density lipoprotein (HDL) cholesterol concentrations in women compared to men, both of which differences have been attributed to the effects of endogenous estrogens. However, although administration of exogenous estrogen is known to effectively lower LDL cholesterol and elevate HDL cholesterol concentrations[1], the effect of endogenous ovarian estrogen production on lipoprotein concentrations is less clear. For example, several studies have been unable to detect consistent changes in serum lipids associated with fluctuations in serum estradiol levels during the menstrual cycle[2-4]. Comparisons between hypoestrogenic, amenorrheic and eumenorrheic female athletes with normal serum estrogen levels have yielded conflicting results. One study reported no differences between serum lipids[5], while another reported higher concentrations of total and LDL cholesterol and triglycerides in amenorrheic athletes[6]. However, in the latter study, hypoestrogenic females also had higher, not lower, HDL and HDL_2 cholesterol concentrations.

It is possible that, in addition to effects on plasma lipoprotein risk factor levels, estrogens act through other protective mechanisms. These might involve favorable effects on vascular endothelial function, or antioxidative mechanisms. The latter possibility will be considered here. Many human estrogen metabolites exhibit marked antioxidative efficacy in lipid–aqueous systems in vitro[7-9], and similar findings have been reported for phytoestrogens with isoflavonoid structure[10,11]. The antioxidant effect appears to depend on the presence of an unsubstituted hydroxyl group at carbon-3 in the aromatic A ring of the estrogen molecule[12-15]. The detection of very lipophilic estrogen derivatives in the form of fatty acid esters present in human blood[16,17] has provided a possible mechanism by which such substances could protect lipoproteins against oxidation and exert an antiatherogenic effect not based on modifications of serum lipoprotein concentrations. Since the oxidation of LDL occurs mainly in the arterial intima where LDL particles have been sequestered from most of the water-soluble antioxidants present in plasma, lipophilic antioxidant substances that remain incorporated in lipoprotein particles probably provide important protection.

PROTECTION OF LIPOPROTEIN PARTICLES AGAINST OXIDATION BY ESTROGEN IN VITRO

Our initial studies demonstrated that incubation of estradiol (E_2) and E_2 17 fatty acid esters with plasma resulted in incorporation of esterified E_2, but not free E_2, in both LDL and HDL particles[18]. However, the amounts of E_2 17 fatty acid esters incorporated were small and no antioxidant efficacy could be demonstrated in Cu^{2+}-induced LDL oxidation experiments in vitro. In order to improve incorporation efficacy, we set up a Celite 545 transfer system which allowed transfer of relatively large amounts of E_2 fatty acid esters[18]. This system enables transfer of E_2 esters directly from Celite particle surfaces to lipoproteins, without exposure to organic solvents commonly used for solubilization of estrogen derivatives. This was necessary in order to avoid delipidation and denaturation of the apolipoprotein B of LDL particles, which could have confounded the oxidation experiments. In short, the estrogen derivative solubilized in an organic solvent was added to a test tube containing Celite dispersion, followed by evaporation of the solvent to dryness under nitrogen. After this, LDL or HDL was added to the Celite dispersion in an aqueous buffer and this mixture was incubated for 22 h at 37°C in a shaking water bath. Following this, the lipoprotein was reisolated by centrifugation, filtered through a Millipore filter and purified further by gel filtration on Sephadex G25 and subjected to oxidation experiments[18]. This improved incorporation efficacy of the E_2 esters and increased oxidation resistance of lipoproteins, in contrast to incubation with plasma which did not alter oxidation susceptibility. Unesterified E_2 did not become incorporated in lipoproteins under any incubation conditions, nor did it provide any protection against oxidation *in vitro*. This is demonstrated in Figure 1 showing typical oxidation curves for HDL following incubation with Celite containing labelled E_2 and E_2 17-ester.

ESTROGEN TRANSFER BETWEEN LIPOPROTEINS

The preliminary incubation experiments had suggested, in line with previous studies by others[19], that esterification of E_2 was a prerequisite for its incorporation in lipoproteins, as well as for its antioxidant efficacy. We were particularly interested in the role of lecithin : cholesterol acyltransferase (LCAT), the enzyme catalyzing formation of cholesteryl esters. This enzyme is known to be present in human ovarian follicular fluid, which is the richest source of E_2 17-esters[17] and where it catalyzes the formation of these esters[20]. Interestingly, follicular fluid contains one lipoprotein species, HDL, but no apolipoprotein B-containing lipoproteins. We therefore explored the incorporation of estrogen in HDL by incubating labeled E_2 with follicular fluid, followed by isolation of HDL by ultracentrifugation, and further analysis of the radioactivity contained in this lipoprotein[21]. Using hydrophobic column chromatography on Sephadex LH20[22], complete separation of the labeled E_2 17-ester from the free E_2 label was achieved. The results indicated, as expected, that only esterified E_2, but no free E_2, had been incorporated in HDL. Moreover, addition of the LCAT inhibitor 5,5'-dithio-*bis*-(2-nitrobenzoic acid) (DTNB) to the incubation mixture completely inhibited incorporation of the label in

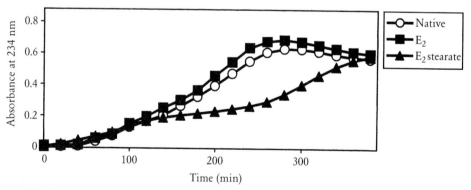

Figure 1 Cu^{2+}-induced oxidation of HDL isolated from Celite dispersion, following incubation with Celite particles pretreated with free E_2, E_2 17-stearic acid ester, or no hormone (native control). E_2 17-stearic acid ester, but not free E_2, had been incorporated in HDL and caused a shift of the oxidation curve to the right, indicating increased oxidation resistance. Adapted from reference 18

HDL. These results confirmed the LCAT-mediated production of E$_2$ 17-esters in human follicular fluid[20] and demonstrated that these esters were completely taken up by the HDL particles, the only lipoprotein available[21].

One of the findings in the initial plasma incubation studies was the presence of E$_2$ 17-esters also in LDL particles[18], despite the fact that LCAT is known to associate mainly with HDL particles. We asked the question whether or not the cholesterol ester transfer protein (CETP), the transfer protein involved in transporting cholesterol esters from HDL to LDL, might be contributing to the transfer of E$_2$ 17-esters from HDL to LDL. We designed incubation experiments in which HDL particles containing labeled E$_2$ 17-esters produced during plasma incubations were co-incubated with native LDL particles isolated from the same individual. Purified exogenous CETP was added to some of the incubations. Analysis of the radioactivity following reisolation of the lipoproteins indicated that, with increasing incubation time, the label in HDL decreased and started to appear in LDL, and the shift was accelerated when exogenous CETP was added to the incubation mixture[21]. On the other hand, 'washing' of the HDL by an additional ultracentrifugation before incubation resulted in a reduction of transfer of the label. This was taken to reflect partial removal of the endogenous HDL-associated CETP from the lipoprotein surface during ultracentrifugation, causing loss of transfer activity. These results seemed consistent with the hypothesis that the same factors that esterified and transported cholesterol, LCAT and CETP, also esterified and transported E$_2$ 17-esters.

DO LIPOPROTEIN-CARRIED ESTROGEN DERIVATIVES HAVE A PHYSIOLOGICAL ROLE?

Because the oxidation of LDL is regarded as an essential step in the initiation and formation of the atherosclerotic plaque[23], the possible role of estrogens as lipoprotein-associated antioxidants has received attention. It is well known that direct addition of supraphysiological amounts of estrogen to LDL mixtures invariably causes inhibition of oxidation *in vitro*[8,9,24]. While we had been unable to demonstrate increased LDL oxidation resistance following incubations with E$_2$ in plasma, Schwaery and colleagues[25], using different conditions, reported that incubations *in vitro* with physiologically relevant concentrations of E$_2$ in male plasma protected LDL against oxidation, and that LCAT was necessary for this protection. The same authors showed in another study that estrone (E$_1$) which was not esterified by LCAT did not protect LDL from oxidation, although it became incorporated in LDL[19]. On this basis, one can speculate that the carbon side-chain created by fatty acid esterification of E$_2$ is somehow responsible for the antioxidant activity. Significantly, E$_2$ is esterified at carbon-17 in the D ring[20,26], at the opposite end of the molecule from the esterification site of cholesterol (hydroxyl at C-3, ring A). Lipid peroxidation presumably starts in the polyunsaturated fatty acids of the phospholipids in the surface layer of LDL, and then propagates to the core lipids[27]. E$_2$ 17-esters are probably aligned on the lipoprotein surface, with the hydrophobic carbon side-chain directed towards the lipid core and the part containing the ring structure with the free hydroxyl group reaching the lipoprotein surface. It is not known whether such positioning of the antioxidative structure (aromatic A ring with free hydroxyl at carbon-3) might be necessary for antioxidant activity. The fact, that E$_1$ containing the same structure but incorporated in LDL without esterification by LCAT did not exhibit antioxidant activity, gives some support for the importance of the positioning of the molecules in the lipoprotein structure.

In theory, transport of estrogen derivatives in lipoproteins could have an endocrine role. Clearly, such derivatives could enter cells via lipoprotein receptors such as the LDL receptor. These aspects have not been studied using estrogen but they have been explored with a number of delta-5-3β-hydroxysteroid fatty acid esters which are formed by LCAT and carried exclusively by lipoproteins in blood[28]. These studies indicated that steroid esters could be taken up into cells by lipoprotein receptors, following which they were hydrolyzed into free steroid[29-31]. Whether or not the lipoprotein system constitutes a circulating reservoir for estrogen and other steroid esters with an endocrine role remains to be clarified.

COMMENT

It is likely that oxidative modification of LDL particles occurs in the subendothelial space in the arterial intima, where it is not protected by the various antioxidants present in plasma. Under such circumstances, the antioxidant content of LDL may play an important role in preventing LDL oxidation. Vitamin E, β-carotene and ubiquinone are such endogenous antioxidants contained in LDL in man. A lipophilic drug, probucol, has been shown to accumulate in LDL and to exert a powerful antioxidant effect, protecting LDL against oxidation *in vitro*[32]. It is not yet known whether human estrogen derivatives incorporated in LDL have a physiological role related to their antioxidant properties detectable *in vitro*. If further studies confirm that physiologically relevant concentrations of E_2 17-esters influence LDL oxidation susceptibility, this is of great importance. Our studies have indicated that E_2 17-esters produced by HDL-associated LCAT activity can be transported to LDL, in a process at least partially dependent on CETP. It is somewhat unexpected that the same mechanisms of esterification and transfer are shared by cholesterol and E_2, although these molecules differ in many respects, including different esterification sites.

Estrogen esters, as well as other steroid esters, could also have a role in maintaining a circulating hormone reservoir. These extremely non-polar substances differ from all other hormones in that they are exclusively carried in lipoproteins and they appear to be more resistant to catabolism than the free steroids[16]. There is now preliminary evidence that the esters of pregnenolone and dehydroepiandrosterone could act as lipoprotein-associated prohormones, enter the cells *via* lipoprotein receptors, become hydrolyzed and serve as precursors for progesterone and testosterone, respectively[29-31]. Tissue-specific hydrolysis could determine targeting of the hormone effect. Both the possible antioxidative and endocrine functions of the estrogen (and other steroid) esters need further studies, as they have important preventive and therapeutic implications.

ACKNOWLEDGEMENTS

This work received support from EVO research grants 0062 and 0337.

References

1. Tikkanen MJ. Sex hormones. In Betteridge J, Illingworth R, Shepherd J, eds. *Lipoproteins in Health and Disease*. London: Hodder and Stoughton Publishers, 1999:967–84
2. Woods M, Schaefer EJ, Morrill A, *et al.* Effect of menstrual cycle phase on plasma lipids. *J Clin Endocrinol Metab* 1987;65:321–3
3. Tikkanen MJ, Kuusi T, Nikkilä EA, *et al.* Variations of postheparin plasma hepatic lipase by menstrual cycle. *Metabolism* 1986;35:99–104
4. Demacker PMN, Schade RWB, Stalenhoef AFH, *et al.* Influence of contraceptive pill and menstrual cycle on serum lipids and high-density lipoprotein cholesterol concentrations. *Br Med J* 1982;284:1212–15
5. Lamon-Fava S, Fisher EC, Nelson ME, *et al.* Effect of exercise and menstrual cycle status on plasma lipids, low density lipoprotein particle size and apolipoproteins. *J Clin Endocrinol Metab* 1989;68:17–21
6. Friday KE, Drinkwater BL, Bruemmer B, *et al.* Elevated plasma low-density lipoprotein and high-density lipoprotein levels in amenorrheic athletes: effects of endogenous hormone status and nutrient intake. *J Clin Endocrinol Metab* 1993;77:1605–9
7. Ayres S, Tang M, Subbiah MT. Estradiol-17beta as an antioxidant: some distinct features when compared with common fat-soluble antioxidants. *J Lab Clin Med* 1996;128:367–75
8. Rifici VA, Khachadurian AK. The inhibition of low-density lipoprotein oxidation by 17-beta estradiol. *Metabolism* 1992;41:1110–14
9. Maziere C, Auclair M, Ronveaux MF, *et al.* Estrogens inhibit copper and cell-mediated modification of low density lipoprotein. *Atherosclerosis* 1991;89:175–82

10. Tikkanen MJ, Wahala K, Ojala S, *et al*. Effect of soybean phytoestrogen intake on low density lipoprotein oxidation resistance. *Proc Natl Acad Sci USA* 1998;95:3106-10

11. Meng Q-H, Lewis P, Wähälä K, *et al*. Incorporation of esterified soybean isoflavones with antioxidant activity into low density lipoprotein. *Biochim Biophys Acta* 1999;1438:369-76

12. Nakano M, Sugioka K, Naito I, *et al*. Novel and potent biological antioxidants on membrane phospholipid peroxidation: 2-hydroxy estrone and 2-hydroxy estradiol. *Biochem Biophys Res Commun* 1987;142:919-24

13. Ruiz-Larrea MB, Leal AM, Liza M, *et al*. Antioxidant effects of estradiol and 2-hydroxyestradiol on iron-induced lipid peroxidation of rat liver microsomes. *Steroids* 1994;59:383-8

14. Miller CP, Jirkovsky I, Hayhurst DA, *et al. In vitro* antioxidant effects of estrogens with a hindered 3-OH function on the copper-induced oxidation of low density lipoprotein. *Steroids* 1996;61:305-8

15. Mukai K, Daifuku K, Yokoyama S, *et al*. Stopped-flow investigation of antioxidant activity of estrogens in solution. *Biochim Biophys Acta* 1990;1035:348-52

16. Hochberg RB. Biological esterification of steroids. *Endocr Rev* 1998;19:331-48

17. Larner JM, Pahuja SL, Shackleton CH, *et al*. The isolation and characterization of estradiol-fatty acid esters in human ovarian follicular fluid. Identification of an endogenous long-lived and potent family of estrogens. *J Biol Chem* 1993;268:13893-9

18. Meng QH, Hockerstedt A, Heinonen S, *et al*. Antioxidant protection of lipoproteins containing estrogens: *in vitro* evidence for low- and high-density lipoproteins as estrogen carriers. *Biochim Biophys Acta* 1999;55492:1-10

19. Shwaery GT, Vita JA, Keaney JF, Jr. Antioxidant protection of LDL by physiologic concentrations of estrogens is specific for 17-beta-estradiol. *Atherosclerosis* 1998;138:255-62

20. Pahuja SL, Kim AH, Lee G, Hochberg RB. Origin of estradiol fatty acid esters in human ovarian follicular fluid. *Biol Reprod* 1995;52:625-30

21. Helisten H, Höckerstedt A, Wähälä K, *et al*. Accumulation of high-density lipoprotein-derived estradiol-17β fatty acid esters in low-density lipo-

protein particles. *J Clin Endocrinol Metab* 2001;28: in press

22. Adlercreutz H, Fotsis T, Heikkinen R. In Görög S, ed. *Advances in Steroid Analysis. Proceedings of the Symposium on the Analysis of Steroids*. Budapest: Akademiai Kiado, 1981:3-33

23. Steinberg D, Parthasarathy S, Carew TE, *et al*. Beyond cholesterol. Modifications of low-density lipoprotein that increase its atherogenicity. *N Engl J Med* 1989;320:915-24

24. Tang M, Abplanalp W, Ayres S, *et al*. Superior and distinct antioxidant effects of selected estrogen metabolites on lipid peroxidation. *Metabolism* 1996;45:411-14

25. Shwaery GT, Vita JA, Keaney JF, Jr. Antioxidant protection of LDL by physiological concentrations of 17 beta-estradiol. Requirement for estradiol modification. *Circulation* 1997;95:1378-85

26. Kanji SS, Kuohung W, Labaree DC, Hochberg RB. Regiospecific esterification of estrogens by lecithin : cholesterol acyltransferase. *J Clin Endocrinol Metab* 1999;84:2481-8

27. Witztum JL. The oxidation hypothesis of atherosclerosis. *Lancet* 1994;344:793-5

28. Lavallee B, Provost PR, Belanger A. Formation of pregnenolone- and dehydroepiandrosterone-fatty acid esters by lecithin : cholesterol acyltransferase in human plasma high density lipoproteins. *Biochim Biophys Acta* 1996;1299:306-12

29. Provencher PH, Roy R, Belanger A. Pregnenolone fatty acid esters incorporated into lipoproteins: substrates in adrenal steroidogenesis. *Endocrinology* 1992;130:2717-24

30. Roy R, Belanger A. Elevated levels of endogenous pregnenolone fatty acid esters in follicular fluid high density lipoproteins support progesterone synthesis in porcine granulosa cells. *Endocrinology* 1992;131:1390-6

31. Roy R, Belanger A. ZR-75-1 breast cancer cells generate nonconjugated steroids from low-density lipoprotein-incorporated lipoidal dehydroepiandrosterone. *Endocrinology* 1993;133:683-9

32. Witztum JL, Steinberg D. Role of oxidized low density lipoprotein in atherogenesis. *J Clin Invest* 1991;88:1785-92

17

Cardiovascular effects of hormone replacement therapy: what factors may influence risk?

P. de Vane

INTRODUCTION

Coronary heart disease (CHD) is the leading killer of both men and women in the USA, accounting for more deaths each year than the next five major causes of mortality combined[1]. Although men typically comprise the majority of patients in randomized, controlled prevention trials, in part because cardiovascular disease (CVD) typically manifests at earlier ages in men, CHD is a major health issue for women, particularly those who have reached menopause. By one estimate[2], this is a rapidly expanding population sector: 50 million American women will pass the age of 50 years in the year 2000. CHD-specific mortality rates rise sharply with each succeeding decade in women aged 45 years and over: from < 0.1% between ages 45 and 54 years to approximately 0.5% between ages 65 and 74 years, 1.7% between 75 and 84 years, and 6.1% above 85 years[3].

Various lines of evidence support the premise that estrogen confers cardioprotective and possibly vasculoprotective biological effects on all women in all phases of the life cycle, whether the reproductive hormone is produced endogenously or administered exogenously as estrogen replacement therapy (ERT) or hormone replacement therapy (HRT) (estrogen in combination with a progestin) after the cessation of menses. Not only are women with premature menopause typically much more prone to CHD[4], but current users of ERT or HRT have an approximately 35% lower CHD risk than postmenopausal women who do not receive such treatment, according to a recent meta-analysis of prospective observational studies[5].

With one exception[6], major population-based trials have demonstrated that postmenopausal ERT or HRT users have a significantly reduced risk of CVD[7,8], myocardial infarction[9-12], stroke[13], mortality from CVD[8,14,15] and all-cause mortality[16,17]. Relative risk (RR) reductions ranged from 35 to 50% in these trials[7-20].

Currently, there are no data from large randomized clinical trials that have investigated the influence of ERT or HRT on the primary prevention of CHD. Several randomized trials discussed below have investigated the impact of ERT and/or HRT on the secondary prevention of CHD in postmenopausal women[21,22]. These studies have not reported the consistent benefit seen in the observational studies for primary prevention of CHD. This paper addresses the current literature investigating the cardiovascular effects of ERT/HRT and proposes possible mechanisms to explain why the cardioprotective effects of estrogens may not be available to all postmenopausal women.

HRT IN THE SECONDARY PREVENTION OF CHD: THE HEART AND ESTROGEN/PROGESTIN REPLACEMENT STUDY (HERS)

The first prospective, double-blind, placebo-controlled trial of its kind, the Heart and Estrogen/progestin Replacement Study (HERS)[21] was designed to assess the influence of HRT on recurrent myocardial infarction or CHD death in postmenopausal women with existing heart disease at baseline (i.e. secondary prevention). A total of 2763 women meeting these entry criteria were treated with either oral conjugated equine estrogens (CEE, 0.625 mg/day) combined with medroxyprogesterone acetate (MPA, 2.5 mg/day; n = 1380) or matching placebo (n = 1383) and followed for an average of 4.1 years. Secondary outcome variables included hospitalization for unstable angina, congestive heart failure, cardiac arrest, need for revascularization and stroke[21].

Entry characteristics

At baseline, the manifestations of CHD in the study population included signs of congestive heart failure (treatment group 10%, placebo 9%), myocardial infarction (17%), coronary artery bypass grafting (treatment group 42%, placebo 41%) and percutaneous transluminal coronary angioplasty (45%). The HRT and placebo groups were well matched at baseline. The mean age at entry was 67 ± 7 years, the average time since cessation of menses was 18 ± 8 years, and 89% of the population were Caucasians. The mean educational attainment was 13 ± 3 years[21].

In addition to a history of CHD, the study population exhibited a number of cardiovascular risk factors: 55% had a body mass index (BMI) of more than 27 kg/m^2, 18% had diabetes mellitus, 13% were current smokers and fewer than 40%

reported exercising more than three times each week. Cardiovascular medication use was also common at baseline: 78% of patients were taking aspirin, nearly 33% β-blockers, 45% (treatment group) and 47% (placebo) lipid-lowering medications, 55% calcium channel blockers, 28% diuretics, and 17% angiotensin-converting enzyme inhibitors. Approximately one-quarter of all women had been ERT users prior to baseline[21].

Results

HRT with CEE plus MPA did not significantly affect the incidence of either the primary composite outcome – myocardial infarction or CHD death – or the various secondary outcome variables, over the 4.1-year follow-up interval. However, statistically significant ($p \leq 0.01$) time trends were observed for HRT versus placebo differences in rates of both the primary outcome as well as in non-fatal myocardial infarction considered in isolation (Figure 1). Within the first year of the study, the risks of CHD events and non-fatal myocardial infarction alone were increased by nearly 50% in the HRT group. In contrast, years 3–5 of treatment witnessed significantly diminished CHD risk in

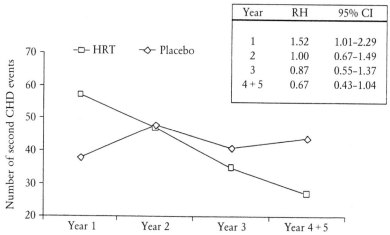

Year	RH	95% CI
1	1.52	1.01–2.29
2	1.00	0.67–1.49
3	0.87	0.55–1.37
4 + 5	0.67	0.43–1.04

Figure 1 The number of second coronary heart disease (CHD) events over the course of the Heart and Estrogen/progestin Replacement Study (HERS) is shown for women with documented CHD administered hormone replacement therapy (HRT) or placebo for an average of 4.1 years. The relative hazards (RH) estimates and 95% confidence intervals (CI) are shown over time in the insert. A statistically significant ($p = 0.009$) time trend was noted, with more CHD events in the HRT group than in the placebo group in year 1 and fewer events in years 3–5. Adapted from reference 21

the HRT group versus placebo controls – by 13–33% for total CHD event rates and 30–42% for the myocardial infarction rate as compared with placebo (Figure 1)[21].

The somewhat equivocal findings from the HERS may be ascribed, in part, to certain methodological issues. First, the HERS investigators estimated that 2340 postmenopausal women were needed to demonstrate – with 90% power and at an α of 0.05 – a 24% HRT-versus-placebo difference in the primary outcome variable over a planned follow-up of 4.75 years (on an intent-to-treat basis). Although 2763 women were enrolled, exceeding the foregoing estimate by 18%, the observed event rate in the placebo group was only 3.3%, or 34% lower than the projected 5%. Second, the follow-up interval was only 4.1 years, a shorter period than in landmark statin trials demonstrating significant clinical benefits in the secondary prevention setting. In conclusion, the HERS investigators stated that, 'given the favorable pattern of CHD events after several years of therapy, it could be appropriate for women already receiving hormone treatment to continue'[21]. Although some have suggested that the findings from HERS raise concern about the data from observational studies[23], the HERS, by design, evaluated the influence of HRT on prevention of recurrent CHD in postmenopausal women with CVD at baseline, not their healthy counterparts (i.e. secondary vs. primary prevention). Nevertheless, despite its limitations, HERS has proved instrumental in revealing a potential disparity between the short- and long-term effects of HRT in secondary prevention of CHD. For the most part, observational studies are not designed to observe any potential adverse effects at the onset of HRT. Further investigation is clearly necessary to establish the relative risks and benefits of HRT in these women.

THE 'HEALTHY ENDOTHELIUM' CONCEPT

Findings from the HERS can be explained to a large extent in relation to a pathophysiological formulation, the 'healthy endothelium'. Based on both clinical and experimental evidence, this concept holds that many of the cardioprotective and anti-atherogenic effects of estrogen are receptor-mediated and endothelium-dependent. Both estrogen receptor populations and endothelial function are influenced markedly by advancing age and the progression of atherosclerotic injury. Clinically, the term 'healthy endothelium' may be applied to individuals lacking evidence or symptoms of CHD, which does not imply that there is no plaque formation.

In this context, women in the HERS had a mean age of about 67 years and a history of CHD. At least two lines of evidence suggest that estrogen receptor expression in the arterial wall is sharply diminished with increasing age. First, an *ex vivo* study[24] showed significant age-related rises in methylation (inactivation) of the promoter region of the estrogen receptor-α (ERα) gene within the right atria of both men and women 34–88 years of age. Second, endothelial cells explanted from coronary atheromata in 19 patients undergoing directional coronary atherectomy displayed significant increases in ERα gene methylation compared with grossly normal segments of the proximal aorta[24].

Clinical and observational evidence

Nurses' Health Study

The premise that postmenopausal women with a healthy endothelium derive more pronounced cardioprotective benefits from ERT or HRT than do women with CHD is supported by data from the Nurses' Health Study[25]. This observational trial involved postmenopausal women who were both free of CVD at baseline and considerably younger than typical patients in the HERS.

Among nearly 86 000 women aged 34–59 years at entry, the risk of developing CVD was 40% lower in ERT users and 61% lower in HRT users as compared with non-users[25]. In addition, the proportion of postmenopausal women taking HRT increased by 175% from 1980 to 1992, and postmenopausal hormone use accounted for 9% of the significant, age-adjusted 31% decline in the coronary event rate among women during this interval[25].

On the other hand, coronary events among postmenopausal ERT or HRT users screened for the Nurses' Health Study who did have a history of myocardial infarction exhibited a pattern qualitatively similar to women in the HERS. In a prospective study involving a subset of 2245 women with prior myocardial infarction, the RR of recurrent events increased during the first 2 years of ERT or HRT use. After 2 years, however, the RR was reduced by 44% and by 35% overall for hormone users (Figure 2)[26].

Finally, women with prior CHD but no history of myocardial infarction experienced a 50% decline in the risk of CHD during both short- and long-term ERT or HRT. The foregoing findings can be explained by the 'healthy endothelium' concept if myocardial infarction is construed as evidence of relatively advanced atherosclerosis or an unhealthy endothelium, in contrast to an endothelium with no clinical manifestations of CHD.

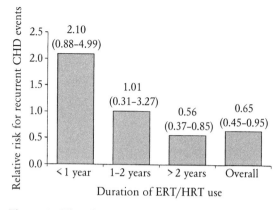

Figure 2   The relative risk (RR) for recurrent coronary heart disease (CHD) events with duration of use is shown in a subset of 2245 women with prior myocardial infarction from the prospective Nurses' Health Study. The RR increased during the first 2 years of estrogen replacement therapy (ERT) or hormone replacement therapy (HRT). After 2 years, however, the RR was reduced by 44% and by 35% overall for hormone users. Adapted from reference 26

Estrogen Replacement and Atherosclerosis trial

Further support for the contention that postmenopausal women without a healthy endothelium derive less clinical benefit from ERT or HRT than their healthy counterparts emerged from the recent Estrogen Replacement and Atherosclerosis (ERA) trial[22]. In this randomized, double-blind, angiographic study, 309 postmenopausal women with baseline CHD were treated with unopposed CEE (0.625 mg/day), CEE 0.625 mg/day together with MPA (2.5 mg/day), or placebo, for a mean follow-up of 3.2 years. The primary outcome variable was the change in minimum lumen diameter, a surrogate marker for CHD events. Secondary endpoints included percentage stenosis in the coronary arteries, development of new atherosclerotic lesions, lipoprotein levels and coronary events.

In addition to being about the same mean age (66 years) as patients enrolled in the HERS, women in the ERA trial were also at considerable baseline cardiovascular risk. Of individuals randomly allocated to the control group ($n = 105$), 30% had diabetes, 69% had hypertension, 53% had BMI exceeding 27.5 kg/m^2 and only 50% reported at least some physical activity. A total of 80% of patients ($n = 248$) had evaluable angiograms at follow-up.

Among these women, who manifested considerable evidence suggestive of relatively 'unhealthy endothelia' at study entry, neither ERT nor HRT significantly decreased baseline-adjusted percentage stenosis or minimum lumen diameter as compared with placebo (Figure 3). These trends in minimum lumen diameter persisted irrespective of compliance with ERT or HRT, smoking, or a history of diabetes, myocardial infarction or hypertension. Neither form of hormonal therapy elicited significant declines in total mortality, coronary event rates, or the occurrence of stroke or transient ischemic attack.

One potentially intriguing result from the ERA trial was that the only baseline-adjusted changes in atherosclerotic progression approaching statistical significance (vs. placebo) occurred among postmenopausal women treated with CEE/MPA. As shown in Figure 3, only 20% of women randomized to this regimen developed at least one new lesion over the 3.2-year follow-up interval, as compared to 33% of placebo controls ($p = 0.06$). Furthermore, as compared with data in placebo controls, baseline-adjusted changes in MLD reached or approached statistical significance in CEE/MPA-treated women who did not take aspirin ($n = 65$) or statins ($n = 160$). The 'healthy endothelium' formulation would lead one to expect that non-users of statins, which are time-tested cardioprotective and vasculoprotective agents, would have poorer endothelial function and thus derive less-pronounced clinical benefits

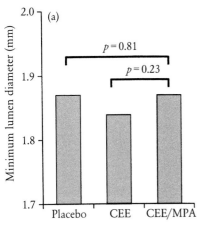
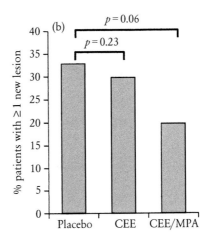

Figure 3 Mean values for minimum lumen diameter (a) and percentage of patients developing one or more new lesions (b) are shown for the 309 women with coronary artery disease who participated in the 3.2-year Estrogen Replacement and Atherosclerosis (ERA) trial. No differences were noted among the women treated with placebo (*n* = 84), conjugated equine estrogens (CEE, 0.625 mg/day; *n* = 79), or CEE plus medroxyprogesterone acetate (MPA, 2.5 mg/day; *n* = 85), although a non-significant trend (*p* = 0.06) was seen with fewer patients with new lesions in the CEE/MPA treatment group

from HRT. Although the foregoing trends were based on sub-analyses involving relatively modest numbers of women, they clearly do not support the contention made following the HERS that the progestin component of the CEE/MPA regimen opposed the cardiovascular effect of the estrogen component.

Aside from the advanced age and risk status of the study population – which were also features of the HERS population – the ERA trial had other limitations that could have restricted its overall implications. First, in both the ERA trial and the HERS, follow-up intervals may have been insufficient to reverse long-standing atherosclerotic disease[2]. In this context, HRT was initiated an average of 23 years after the cessation of menses in women enrolled in a study by Herrington and co-workers[22]. Second, the primary outcome in the ERA trial was an intermediate endpoint, and changes in angiographic lesion size may be discordant with the occurrence of ischemic coronary events[27].

Women's Health Initiative

The Women's Health Initiative[28] (WHI) is evaluating the effects of HRT (as well as low-fat dietary patterns) on the risk of CHD in postmenopausal women without evidence of baseline disease. This study, which has clinical and observational phases involving 64 500 and 100 000 participants, respectively, involves women aged 50 to 79 years who are treated with HRT and will be followed-up for an average of 9 years.

Women enrolled in the WHI were recently informed that a small increase (< 1%) in the occurrence of myocardial infarction, stroke and/or venous thrombosis had been observed in the study within 2 years of initiation of treatment with CEE (0.625 mg/day) alone or combined with MPA (2.5 mg/day). Study participants were also advised that this mild increase in risk is reduced or abolished over time, and the Data and Safety Monitoring Board (DSMB) has recommended that the study continue. These data, combined with the early risk of recurrent events observed in the HERS and the Nurses' Health Study, raise the possibility that for a susceptible group of women, estrogen therapy may initially increase the risk of thrombosis.

CARDIOPROTECTIVE PHYSIOLOGICAL EFFECTS OF HRT

Brachial artery models

Although results from the WHI and other large, randomized, controlled trials are eagerly awaited in order to evaluate the 'healthy endothelium' model, considerable scientific evidence already supports the beneficial effects of hormone replacement on endothelial function, coronary vasodilator reserve, myocardial perfusion, low- and high-density lipoprotein cholesterol, emerging inflammatory mediators, and other novel, putative CHD risk markers.

For instance, a recent non-randomized study[29] that included 23 women with a mean age of 58 years and 11 healthy premenopausal women demonstrated that treatment with either HRT or ERT progressively enhanced brachial artery vasomotor responses, one index of endothelial dysfunction within the coronary vasculature. Within 1 month, women treated with various regimens, including CEE, CEE/MPA and/or 17β-estradiol, exhibited a significant 4.8% rise in post-ischemic vasodilatation as compared with baseline. The baseline-adjusted increase at 6 months (8.3%) was, in turn, significantly greater than the improvement observed at 1 month[29]. On the other hand, neither HRT nor ERT influenced nitroglycerin-induced vasodilatation, which is independent of endothelial function.

Consistent with the 'healthy endothelium' concept, this small observational study showed that vasodilator responses to hyperemic flow were nearly an order of magnitude higher in premenopausal women (mean age 33 years) than in their postmenopausal counterparts. The fact that the 6-month improvement in the vasodilator response to hyperemia was particularly robust in women with the most pronounced abnormalities at baseline does not necessarily contradict the 'healthy endothelium' model. The mean age and time since the onset of menopause of these women – 58 and 11 years, respectively – might be associated with more readily reversible endothelial dysfunction than seen in HERS or ERA trial participants, who were nearly a decade older on average.

A double-blind cross-over trial[30] involving 12 healthy postmenopausal women with a mean age of 55 years showed that 7–14 days of therapy with continuous oral CEE/MPA (0.625 mg/ 2.5 mg/day) enhanced flow-mediated dilation (flow-mediated dilation) and diminished resistance in the brachial artery. As compared with baseline, this regimen increased flow-mediated dilation

by 12% ($p < 0.01$) and decreased arterial resistance by 15%. On the other hand, treatment with 17β-estradiol (2 mg/day) plus norethisterone acetate (1 mg/day) showed opposite trends, decreasing flow-mediated dilation by 20% and elevating arterial resistance by 16% ($p < 0.01$).

Finally, a recent randomized, double-blind, cross-over trial[31] involving 24 women with CHD at baseline demonstrated that short-term treatment with CEE/MPA, either alone or together with lovastatin (20 mg/day), significantly increased brachial artery vasodilator response, as well as the duration of this effect (area under the curve) as compared with baseline. Indeed, the HRT-induced increase (63%) during a 6-week interval was more pronounced than that elicited by combination HRT/lovastatin (46%) over a similar period, although this difference did not reach statistical significance.

Both the HRT and low-dose statin regimens significantly decreased circulating low-density lipoprotein (LDL) cholesterol and augmented high-density lipoprotein (HDL) cholesterol as compared with baseline. Statin-induced declines in LDL cholesterol (30%) and the atherogenic LDL : HDL ratio (35%) were significantly greater than corresponding changes during the HRT treatment interval (14.5% and 26%). The combined HRT/lovastatin regimen decreased the LDL : HDL ratio to the greatest extent (43%) of the three evaluated ($p < 0.05$ vs. lovastatin or HRT alone). Addition of the statin also tended to attenuate a modest 9% HRT-induced increase in triglycerides ($p > 0.05$) from baseline.

Coronary artery measures

Preliminary data from a recent $^{13}NH_3$-positron emission tomography (PET) study on myocardial blood flow within the myocardium gave further support to the 'healthy endothelium' concept[32]. Vasodilator capacity within the coronary arteries was assessed by PET scanning as the percentage rise in myocardial blood flow in response to the cold pressor test. Four groups of women were studied, including 16 postmenopausal HRT users (mean age 60 years) with CHD risk factors (e.g. obesity, cigarette smoking, hypercholesterolemia), and 11 HRT users (mean age 56 years) without such risk factors. Serving as controls were 11 postmenopausal women (mean age 55 years) not on HRT and seven young, healthy women whose mean age was 22 years.

Among controls, postmenopausal women exhibited a similar mean rate–pressure product but a significantly lower myocardial blood flow response to the cold pressor test than did young, healthy women: approximately 29% vs. 54% ($p < 0.05$) (Figure 4). Hormone replacement for at least 6 months restored the myocardial blood flow vasodilator response to nearly the level seen in young healthy volunteers (52%), but only among postmenopausal women without CHD risk factors. Postmenopausal women at advanced risk for CHD appeared to derive less marked benefits from HRT than did chronic HRT users without risk factors, exhibiting a vasodilator response to cold stress of only 22% ($p < 0.05$ vs. young women).

Further support for the 'healthy endothelium' formulation was derived from a study[33] evaluating the effects of ERT on coronary vasomotor responses to a different form of challenge. In patients with intact endothelial function in epicardial segments of coronary conductance vessels, intracoronary infusion of acetylcholine caused vasodilatation through endothelium-dependent generation of nitric oxide, also termed endothelium-derived relaxing factor[34]. The acetylcholine-induced changes in vasomotor function parallel those occurring daily in response to physical activity or mental stress[35,36].

In an angiographic study[33] of postmenopausal women referred for coronary angiography on the basis of stable angina, atypical chest pain, or abnormal electrocardiogram responses to exercise, intravenous administration of ethinylestradiol (35 µg) enhanced basal coronary tone in resistance vessels, increasing coronary blood flow by 23% ($p < 0.01$) while inducing a 15% decline in resistance ($p < 0.01$). In conductance vessels, ethinylestradiol administration increased epicardial cross-sectional area by 20% ($p = 0.02$). Placebo exerted no significant effects on hemodynamic parameters in 11 healthy, postmenopausal controls, and the significant effects of ethinylestradiol administration on vasomotor tone within coronary resistance vessels were not accompanied by changes in blood pressure.

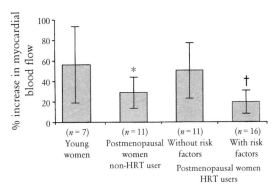

Figure 4 Mean ± SD values for the percentage increase in myocardial blood flow following a cold pressor test are shown for healthy premenopausal women ($n = 7$), postmenopausal women without risk factors for coronary heart disease (CHD) not on hormone replacement therapy (HRT; $n = 11$), postmenopausal women without risk factors for CHD on HRT ($n = 11$), and postmenopausal women with risk factors for CHD (hypertension, obesity, cigarette smoking, hypercholesterolemia and diabetes) on HRT ($n = 16$). *$p < 0.05$ versus young women; †$p < 0.01$ versus postmenopausal women without risk factors on HRT. Adapted from reference 32

Of 15 consecutive subjects who received an acetylcholine challenge, seven exhibited a paradoxical 33.5% decline in coronary blood flow ($p < 0.01$) and a nearly 39% increase in coronary resistance ($p = 0.05$), which were associated with certain angiographic abnormalities. Acetylcholine challenge also induced a 14% decline in epicardial cross-sectional area within conductance vessels in these patients with diseased arteries ($p = 0.04$). Although ethinylestradiol significantly attenuated these abnormal responses to acetylcholine challenge in patients with diseased arteries, the related increases in coronary blood flow and diameter were decidedly less pronounced than in persons with angiographically normal arteries (Figure 5).

Effects on lipid profiles

Unopposed estrogen and CEE/MPA regimens consistently decreased LDL cholesterol while increasing HDL cholesterol in three studies involving women with various degrees of baseline risk. Of these, two studies – the HERS[21] and the ERA[22] trial – involved women with baseline CHD, whereas the Postmenopausal Estrogen/Progestin

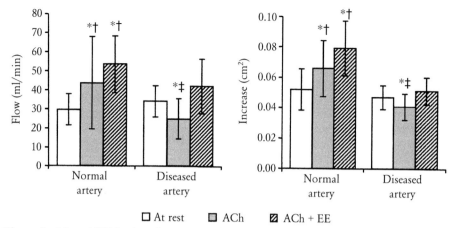

Figure 5 Mean ± SEM values for coronary blood flow (left) and coronary diameter changes (right) at rest, after an acetylcholine (ACh) challenge, and after a combined ethinylestradiol (EE) plus ACh challenge are shown for postmenopausal women who presented with normal coronary resistance vessel endothelial function ($n = 8$) or coronary resistance vessel endothelial dysfunction ($n = 7$). *$p < 0.05$ for change in flow versus rest; †$p < 0.05$ for change in flow versus diseased artery; ‡$p < 0.05$ for change in flow versus ACh plus EE. Adapted from reference 33

Interventions (PEPI) trial[37] was performed in 875 healthy postmenopausal women.

As compared with the placebo control group, women treated with CEE/MPA for 4.1 years in the HERS exhibited an 11% lower serum LDL-cholesterol concentration and 10% higher HDL-cholesterol level ($p < 0.001$ for both comparisons). Differences in LDL cholesterol between actively treated patients and placebo seen for 3.2 years in the ERA trial were 8.1% for unopposed estrogen and 15.2% for CEE/MPA; corresponding placebo-adjusted changes from baseline in HDL cholesterol were 12% and 7.4%.

Similar effects were observed in the PEPI trial[37], which evaluated the effect on CHD risk factors of a wider range of ERT and HRT regimens. These therapies were unopposed estrogen (CEE, 0.625 mg/day), or the same daily dose of CEE combined with: cyclic MPA at a daily dose of 10 mg for 12 days each month; consecutive MPA (2.5 mg/day); or cyclic micronized progesterone at a daily dose of 200 mg for 12 days per month.

In short, all active treatments elicited significantly greater increments in mean HDL cholesterol, as well as declines in mean LDL cholesterol, as compared with placebo. These changes reached maximum values within the first 6–12 months of treatment in the PEPI trial. However, women

randomly allocated to treatment with either unopposed estrogen or CEE/micronized progesterone exhibited significantly greater increases in HDL-cholesterol levels (9% and 6.5%) than did those randomized to either cyclic or continuous MPA-containing regimens (1.9% and 2.5%). Decreases in LDL cholesterol did not differ significantly among these regimens, averaging 15.9 mg/dl in all actively treated study arms, as compared with 4.3 mg/dl for placebo. All hormone replacement regimens significantly increased triglycerides, by 12.9% on average ($p < 0.001$ vs. placebo).

Effects on putative coronary risk factors

According to follow-up data from the Lipid Research Clinics Coronary Prevention Trial, the cardioprotective effects of ERT were more pronounced than would have been expected on the basis of attendant lipid-lowering effects alone[38]. Estrogens also decrease lipoprotein(a)[37,39] and blunt LDL oxidation[40,41]. By one estimate[42], non-lipid-dependent mechanisms account for only 25–35% of the cardioprotective benefits of estrogens.

Other potential barometers of vascular occlusion risk include total homocysteine, as well as indices of fibrinolytic function, such as tissue-type plasminogen activator (t-PA) and plasminogen activator inhibitor-1 (PAI-1), inflammatory markers, which include fibrinogen, intercellular or vascular cell fibrinogen adhesion molecule (ICAM or VCAM), C-reactive protein, and certain interleukins[43], and coagulation factors V and VII.

The effect of fibrinogen VII levels on degree of myocardial infarction risk in patients with CHD may have a genetic basis. A recent study[44] showed significantly higher frequencies of homozygotes and heterozygotes for the A2 and R353Q alleles in 175 patients with angiographically verified CHD who experienced myocardial infarction than in 110 patients free of myocardial infarction despite baseline CHD. These alleles code the factor VII promoter and catalytic regions, respectively. Genotypes for these polymorphisms in the factor VII gene also correlated significantly with circulating levels of activated factor VII. In summary, certain genotypes may help to protect patients from major adverse cardiovascular events despite advanced CHD. Whether the women administered HRT in HERS who exhibited an increase in recurrent events in the first year had an alteration in their factor VII genotype remains unknown.

Inflammatory mediators

Various forms of hormone replacement significantly influence at least five of the above putative risk markers. In a randomized, double-blind, cross-over study involving 28 healthy postmenopausal women, carried out by Koh and colleagues[45], 6 weeks of treatment with CEE (0.625 mg/day), but not vitamin E alone (800 IU/day), significantly diminished levels of three adhesion molecules that have been implicated in the atherosclerotic cascade. As against baseline circulating levels, ERT decreased E-selectin by 14.2% ($p < 0.0001$), ICAM-1 by 8.6% ($p < 0.05$), and VCAM-1 by 8.2% ($p < 0.01$). Furthermore, in a setting of much longer-term HRT for primary prevention, the PEPI trial[37] demonstrated that all forms of ERT and HRT left mean fibrinogen levels significantly lower than in the placebo group.

Estrogen receptor ligands may act at the gene level to attenuate inflammatory events that contribute to the progression of atherosclerosis. In an *in vitro* model of human umbilical endothelial cells engineered to express ERα selectively, introduction of estradiol to a culture medium significantly blunted interleukin-1β (IL-1β)-induced up-regulation of genes for several inflammatory mediators, including VCAM-1 and E-selectin[46].

Using a C57BL/6 ovariectomized mouse model, the same investigators reported further, but somewhat indirect, evidence in support of the concept that estrogen is less effective in blunting inflammation in a setting of endothelial dysfunction. When fed to ovariectomized mice, an atherogenic diet induced the proinflammatory transcription factor NF-κB as compared with animals fed a normal diet[47]. Although daily subcutaneous injections of ethinylestradiol for 5 weeks blunted expression of NF-κB-dependent genes, this effect did not occur at the DNA-binding level. The data suggested for the first time a reciprocal inhibition of both estrogen receptor and NF-κB activity, such that estrogen activity is impaired by inflammation, in part perhaps by virtue of cross-talk between the receptor and inflammatory transcription factor.

Homocysteine

In a double-blind, randomized, placebo-controlled trial involving 390 healthy postmenopausal women studied by Walsh and co-workers[48], 8 months of treatment with either CEE/MPA or the selective estrogen receptor modulator (SERM) raloxifene significantly reduced homocysteine levels in healthy postmenopausal women as compared with placebo controls. Changes were 8% or less with these forms of hormone replacement, and there was no dose–response effect with raloxifene. The effect of raloxifene in postmenopausal women with CHD is being assessed in the ongoing Raloxifene Use for The Heart (RUTH) trial[49].

Considerable debate surrounds the relative efficacy of these and other potential markers of atherothrombotic risk (e.g. thrombin, coagulation factors, insulin sensitivity and high-sensitivity C-reactive proteins (CRPs)) in populations. For high-sensitivity CRPs, a standardized assay is available, and findings on predictive value from prospective epidemiological trials have been reported[50]. These data also established an interaction between the high-sensitivity CRPs and the total cholesterol : HDL cholesterol ratio in estimating the RR for future myocardial infarction.

On the basis of a multivariate analysis from the Physicians' Health Study[50], a case–control trial that included nearly 15 000 apparently healthy men followed for approximately 9 years, models that included both CRPs and lipid levels were superior to one based on lipids alone. The RR for myocardial infarction among patients with high levels of both CRPs (> 1.69 mg/l) and total cholesterol (> 223 mg/dl) was 5.0, which is greater than the product of the RR for high levels of either parameter in isolation: 1.5 for high CRPs and 2.3 for high total cholesterol. According to tertile analyses illustrated in Figure 6, myocardial infarction risk increases most steeply among patients with high high-sensitivity CRP levels across increasing total cholesterol : HDL cholesterol ratios, reaching a peak of 4.4 when both CRP levels and the total cholesterol : HDL cholesterol ratio were in the highest tertile.

Fibrinolytic function

In their study of 28 healthy postmenopausal women, Koh and colleagues[45] reported that levels of PAI-1 were nearly 30% lower after CEE treatment than at baseline ($p < 0.05$). Significantly enhanced systemic fibrinolysis also resulted from 1 month of treatment with CEE, either alone or combined with MPA, in 50 postmenopausal

women seen in a prior trial conducted by Koh and colleagues[45]. In this randomized, cross-over study, both CEE and CEE/MPA decreased plasma PAI-1 levels from baseline by more than 50%, from 32 to 14 ng/ml ($p < 0.001$) and 31 to 15 ng/ml ($p = 0.003$), respectively. These effects were more pronounced in women with higher levels of PAI-1 at baseline.

A group from the UK[51] also reported that 6 weeks of ERT tended to enhance cardiovascular hemodynamics and coagulation status. Among 27 women who underwent hysterectomy with bilateral salpingo-oophorectomy, unreplaced premature menopause was associated with non-significant rises in D-dimer and PAI-1 that were reversed by administration of unopposed CEE therapy. In addition, such treatment also significantly reduced levels of soluble thrombomodulin, von Willebrand factor and t-PA – three putative markers of endothelial injury and other vascular functions – as compared with baseline[51]. Finally, 6 months of hormonal therapy with oral cyclic estradiol combined with micronized progesterone also increased global fibrinolytic capacity by 63% as against baseline ($p = 0.001$) and diminished both PAI-1 antigen (24%; $p = 0.02$) and PAI activity (54%; $p = 0.004$) in 45 healthy postmenopausal women[52].

CONCLUSIONS

ERT or HRT has been clinically demonstrated to improve the health and well-being of postmenopausal women in a number of major areas, including in reducing the incidence of hot flushes and/or sweating in peri- and postmenopausal women[53], alleviating osteoporosis[54,55], and relieving manifestations of vaginal atrophy[56-59].

In addition to the above, a sound, internally consistent body of clinical, preclinical and observational data supports the beneficial effects of ERT and HRT on CVD in postmenopausal women. Moreover, randomized, cross-over trials have shown that HRT can act synergistically with therapies designed for cardioprotection. Specifically, HRT in combination with statins produces greater benefits on lipoprotein profiles and vasodilatation than either therapy alone[31,60].

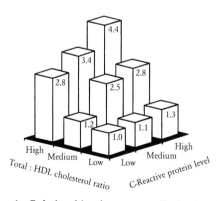

Figure 6 Relationships between tertile levels of the total cholesterol : high-density lipoprotein (HDL) cholesterol ratio in determining the risk of myocardial infarction. From reference 50, with permission

The beneficial effects of ERT and HRT on CVD depend largely on the integrity and functional status of the coronary artery endothelium. Therefore, the timing of the initiation of ERT/HRT plays a key role in its impact. In healthy postmenopausal women, ERT and HRT augment endothelial function significantly as assessed by vasodilator response, enhance the overall lipid profile, blunt the expression of inflammatory mediators, and possibly also reduce levels of novel, putative coronary risk markers (e.g. homocysteine).

Advancing age and atherosclerotic injury to the vessel wall can deplete estrogen receptors, compromise endothelial function, and hence diminish the potential cardioprotective and vasculoprotective effects of ERT and HRT. Recent studies demonstrated directly that an advanced inflammatory state evidenced by increases in NF-κB activity can reciprocally inhibit estrogen receptor activity, possibly diminishing the clinical utility of estrogen receptor ligands – for instance, various forms of estrogen replacement – in such patients with unhealthy endothelia. Thus, the earlier treatment with ERT/HRT can be initiated in postmenopausal women, the greater the potential benefit.

The controversy spawned by the HERS can be resolved only through sufficiently powered, randomized, controlled trials, including the WHI[28], the Women's International Study of Long-Duration Oestrogen after Menopause (WISDOM)[61], the Estrogen and Graft Atherosclerosis Research (EAGAR) investigation, the Women's Angiographic Vitamin and Estrogen (WAVE) study and the Women's Estrogen/Progestin and Lipid-Lowering Hormone Atherosclerosis Regression Trial (WELL-HART)[62]. In the interim, convergent evidence strongly supports roles for hormone replacement in relatively young postmenopausal women without evidence of CHD or significant coronary risk factors, as well as those with a history of myocardial infarction who have already been on CEE/MPA for at least 2 years. Irrespective of these findings, efforts to promote a healthy endothelium through lifestyle modifications, including weight management, diet, physical activity and smoking cessation in appropriate patients constitute a central therapeutic aim.

References

1. Hoyert DL, Kochanek KD, Murphy SL. Deaths: final data for 1997. *National Vital Statistics Reports* 1999;47(19)
2. Nabel EG. Coronary heart disease in women – an ounce of prevention [Editorial]. *N Engl J Med* 2000;343:572–4
3. Kramarow E, Lentzner H, Rooks R, *et al. Health and Aging Chartbook. Health, United States, 1999.* Hyattsville, MD: National Center for Health Statistics, 1999
4. Kannel WB. Metabolic risk factors for coronary heart disease in women: perspective from the Framingham Study. *Am Heart J* 1987;114:413–19
5. Barrett-Connor E, Grady D. Hormone replacement therapy, heart disease, and other considerations. *Annu Rev Public Health* 1998;19:55–72
6. Wilson PWF, Garrison RJ, Castelli WP. Postmenopausal estrogen use, cigarette smoking, and cardiovascular morbidity in women over 50: the Framingham Study. *N Engl J Med* 1985;313: 1038–43
7. Grodstein F, Stampfer MJ, Manson J, *et al.* Postmenopausal estrogen and progestin use and the risk of cardiovascular disease. *N Engl J Med* 1996;335: 453–61
8. Sellers TA, Mink PJ, Cerhan JR, *et al.* The role of hormone replacement therapy in the risk for breast cancer and total mortality in women with a family history of breast cancer. *Ann Intern Med* 1997; 127:973–80
9. Henderson BE, Paganini-Hill A, Ross RK. Estrogen replacement therapy and protection from acute myocardial infarction. *Am J Obstet Gynecol* 1988; 159:312–17
10. Psaty BM, Heckbert SR, Atkins D, *et al.* The risk of myocardial infarction associated with the combined use of estrogens and progestins in postmenopausal women. *Arch Intern Med* 1994;154:1333–9

11. Stampfer MJ, Willett WC, Colditz GA, *et al.* A prospective study of postmenopausal estrogen therapy and coronary heart disease. *N Engl J Med* 1985;313:1044-9

12. Falkeborn M, Persson I, Adami H-O, *et al.* The risk of acute myocardial infarction after oestrogen and oestrogen–progestogen replacement. *Br J Obstet Gynaecol* 1992;99:821-8

13. Boysen G, Nyboe J, Appleyard M, *et al.* Stroke incidence and risk factors for stroke in Copenhagen, Denmark. *Stroke* 1988;19:1345-53

14. Bush TL, Barrett-Connor E, Cowan LD, *et al.* Cardiovascular mortality and noncontraceptive use of estrogen in women: results from the Lipid Research Clinics Program Follow-up Study. *Circulation* 1987;75:1102-9

15. Wolf PH, Madans JH, Finucane FF, *et al.* Reduction of cardiovascular disease-related mortality among postmenopausal women who use hormones: evidence from a national cohort. *Am J Obstet Gynecol* 1991;164:489-94

16. Grodstein F, Stampfer MJ, Colditz GA, *et al.* Postmenopausal hormone therapy and mortality. *N Engl J Med* 1997;336:1769-75

17. Criqui MH, Suarez L, Barrett-Connor E, *et al.* Postmenopausal estrogen use and mortality. Results from a prospective study in a defined, homogeneous community. *Am J Epidemiol* 1988; 128:606-14

18. van der Giezen AM, Schopman-Geurts van Kessel JG, Schouten EG, *et al.* Systolic blood pressure and cardiovascular mortality among 13 740 Dutch women. *Prev Med* 1990;19:456-65

19. Petitti DB, Perlman JA, Sidney S. Noncontraceptive estrogens and mortality: long-term follow-up of women in the Walnut Creek Study. *Obstet Gynecol* 1987;70:289-93

20. Folsom AR, Mink PJ, Sellers TA, *et al.* Hormonal replacement therapy and morbidity and mortality in a prospective study of postmenopausal women. *Am J Public Health* 1995;85:1128-32

21. Hulley S, Grady D, Bush T, *et al.* Randomized trial of estrogen plus progestin for secondary prevention of coronary heart disease in postmenopausal women. *J Am Med Assoc* 1998;280:605-13

22. Herrington DM, Reboussin DM, Brosnihan KB, *et al.* Effects of estrogen replacement on the progression of coronary artery atherosclerosis. *N Engl J Med* 2000;343:522-9

23. Petitti DB. Hormone replacement therapy and heart disease prevention. Experimentation trumps observation [Editorial]. *J Am Med Assoc* 1998;280: 650-62

24. Post WS, Goldschmidt-Clermont PJ, Wilhide CC, *et al.* Methylation of the estrogen receptor gene is associated with aging and atherosclerosis in the cardiovascular system. *Cardiovasc Res* 1999;43: 985-91

25. Hu FB, Stampfer MJ, Manson JE, *et al.* Trends in the incidence of coronary heart disease and changes in diet and lifestyle in women. *N Engl J Med* 2000;343:530-7

26. Grodstein F, Manson JE, Stampfer MJ. Postmenopausal hormones and recurrence of coronary events in the Nurses' Health Study [Abstract]. *Circulation* 1999;100(Suppl):I-871

27. Brown BG, Zhao X-Q, Sacco DE, *et al.* Lipid lowering and plaque regression: new insights into prevention of plaque disruption and clinical events in coronary disease. *Circulation* 1993;87:1781-91

28. Women's Health Initiative Study Group. Design of the Women's Health Initiative clinical trial and observational study. *Control Clin Trials* 1998;19: 61-109

29. Bush DE, Jones CE, Bass KM, *et al.* Estrogen replacement reverses endothelial dysfunction in postmenopausal women. *Am J Med* 1998;104:552-8

30. Rosano GMC, Leonardo F, Panina G, *et al.* Comparative effect of continuous combined hormone replacement therapy with either conjugated equine oestrogens plus medroxyprogesterone acetate or 17β-oestradiol plus norethisterone acetate on brachial artery blood flow [Abstract]. *Eur Heart J* 1998;19(Suppl):681

31. Herrington DM, Werbel BL, Riley WA, *et al.* Individual and combined effects of estrogen/progestin therapy and lovastatin on lipids and flow-mediated vasodilation in postmenopausal women with coronary artery disease. *J Am Coll Cardiol* 1999;33: 2030-7

32. Campisi R, Nathan L, Pampaloni MH, *et al.* Effect of chronic hormone replacement therapy on coronary vasomotion in postmenopausal women [Abstract]. *Circulation* 1999;100(Suppl): I-221

33. Reis SE, Gloth ST, Blumenthal RS, *et al.* Ethinyl estradiol acutely attenuates abnormal coronary vasomotor responses to acetylcholine in postmenopausal women. *Circulation* 1994;89:52-60

34. Hodgson JM, Marshall JJ. Direct vasoconstriction and endothelium-dependent vasodilation. Mechanisms of acetylcholine effects on coronary flow and arterial diameter in patients with nonstenotic coronary arteries. *Circulation* 1989;79:1043-51

35. Gordon JB, Ganz P, Nabel EG, *et al.* Atherosclerosis influences the vasomotor response of epicardial coronary arteries to exercise. *J Clin Invest* 1989;83: 1946-52

36. Yeung AC, Vekshtein VI, Krantz DS, *et al.* The effect of atherosclerosis on the vasomotor response of coronary arteries to mental stress. *N Engl J Med* 1991;325:1551-6

37. Writing Group for the PEPI Trial. Effects of estrogen or estrogen/progestin regimens on heart disease risk factors in postmenopausal women: the Postmenopausal Estrogen/Progestin Interventions (PEPI) Trial. *J Am Med Assoc* 1995;273:199-208

38. Barrett-Connor E, Bush TL. Estrogen and coronary heart disease in women. *J Am Med Assoc* 1991;265:1861-7

39. Shlipak MG, Simon J, Vittinghoff E, *et al.* Estrogen and progestin, lipoprotein(a), and the risk of recurrent coronary heart disease events after menopause. *J Am Med Assoc* 2000;283:1845-52

40. Keaney JF Jr, Shwaery GT, Xu A, *et al.* 17 beta-estradiol preserves endothelial vasodilator function and limits low-density lipoprotein oxidation in hypercholesterolemic swine. *Circulation* 1994;89:2251-9

41. Sack MN, Rader DJ, Cannon RO III. Oestrogen and inhibition of oxidation of low-density lipoprotein in postmenopausal women. *Lancet* 1994;343:269-70

42. Clarkson TB, Anthony MS. Effects on the cardiovascular system: basic aspects. In Lindsay R, Dempster DW, Jordan VC, eds. *Estrogens and Antiestrogens: Basic and Clinical Aspects.* Philadelphia: Lippincott-Raven Publishers, 1997:89-117

43. Ridker PM. Evaluating novel cardiovascular risk factors: can we better predict heart attacks? *Ann Intern Med* 1999;130:933-7

44. Girelli D, Russo C, Ferraresi P, *et al.* Polymorphisms in the factor VII gene and the risk of myocardial infarction in patients with coronary artery disease. *N Engl J Med* 2000;343:774-80

45. Koh KK, Blum A, Hathaway L, *et al.* Vascular effects of estrogen and vitamin E therapies in postmenopausal women. *Circulation* 1999;100:1851-7

46. Evans MJ, Lai KY, Adelman SJ. Estrogen receptor-mediated inhibition of inflammatory gene expression in human endothelial cells [Abstract]. *Circulation* 2000;102:II-66

47. Harnish DC, Lai KD, Eckert AM, *et al.* Repression of estrogen-mediated transactivation by inflammatory stimuli *in vivo* and *in vitro* [Abstract]. *Circulation* 2000;102:II-318

48. Walsh BW, Paul S, Wild RA, *et al.* The effects of hormone replacement therapy and raloxifene on C-reactive protein and homocysteine in healthy postmenopausal women: a randomized, controlled trial. *J Clin Endocrinol Metab* 2000;85:214-18

49. Barrett-Connor E, Wenger NK, Grady D, *et al.* Hormone and nonhormone therapy for the maintenance of postmenopausal health: the need for randomized controlled trials of estrogen and raloxifene. *J Women's Health* 1998;7:839-47

50. Ridker PM, Glynn RJ, Hennekens CH. C-reactive protein adds to the predictive value of total and HDL cholesterol in determining risk of first myocardial infarction. *Circulation* 1998;97:2007-11

51. Lip GYH, Blann AD, Jones AF, *et al.* Effects of hormone replacement therapy on hemostatic factors, lipid factors, and endothelial function in women undergoing surgical menopause: implications for prevention of atherosclerosis. *Am Heart J* 1997;134:764-71

52. Scarabin P-Y, Alhenc-Gelas M, Plu-Bureau G, *et al.* Effects of oral and transdermal estrogen/progesterone regimens on blood coagulation and fibrinolysis in postmenopausal women: a randomized controlled trial. *Arterioscler Thromb Vasc Biol* 1997;17:3017-78

53. Casper RF, Dodin S, Reid RL, *et al.* The effect of 20 μg ethinyl estradiol/1 mg norethindrone acetate (Minestrin™), a low-dose oral contraceptive, on vaginal bleeding patterns, hot flashes, and quality of life in symptomatic perimenopausal women. *Menopause* 1997;4:139-47

54. Lindsay R, Aitken JM, Anderson JB, *et al.* Long-term prevention of postmenopausal osteoporosis by oestrogen: evidence for an increased bone mass after delayed onset of oestrogen treatment. *Lancet* 1976;1:1038-41

55. Ettinger B, Genant HK, Cann CE. Long-term estrogen replacement therapy prevents bone loss and fractures. *Ann Intern Med* 1985;102:319-24

56. Berman JR, Berman LA, Werbin TJ, *et al.* Clinical evaluation of female sexual function: effects of age and estrogen status on subjective and physiologic sexual responses. *Int J Impotence Res* 1999;11 (Suppl 1):S31-8

57. Fernandez E, La Vecchia C, Braga C, *et al.* Hormone replacement therapy and risk of colon and rectal cancer. *Cancer Epidemiol Biomarkers Prev* 1998;7:329-33

58. Grodstein F, Martinez ME, Platz EA, *et al.* Postmenopausal hormone use and risk for colorectal cancer. *Ann Intern Med* 1998;128:705-12

59. Calle EE, Miracle-McMahill HL, Thun MJ, *et al.* Estrogen replacement therapy and risk of fatal colon cancer in a prospective cohort of postmenopausal women. *J Natl Cancer Inst* 1995;87:517-23

60. Darling GM, Johns JA, McCloud PI, *et al.* Concurrent use of simvastatin and estrogen–progestin therapy compared with each therapy alone for hypercholesterolemia in postmenopausal women. *Climacteric* 1999;2:181-8

61. Vickers MR, Meade TW, Wilkes HC. Hormone replacement therapy and cardiovascular disease: the case for a randomized controlled trial. *Ciba Found Symp* 1995;191:150-64

62. Blumenthal RS, Zacur HA, Reis SE, *et al.* Beyond the null hypothesis – do the HERS results disprove the estrogen/coronary heart hypothesis? *Am J Cardiol* 2000;85:1015-17

Effects of transdermal hormone replacement therapy on cardiovascular outcomes: epidemiological evidence

18

C. Varas-Lorenzo, S. Pérez-Gutthann, J. Castellsague and L. Gutierrez

INTRODUCTION

Hormone replacement therapy (HRT) remains controversial because diverse information contributes to the overall balance between risks and benefits. There is a very wide range of HRT preparations that can be administered either orally or transdermally. However, most of the studies evaluating known risks and benefits of HRT have been performed in populations using oral preparations.

There is now considerable evidence that estrogens exert non-direct and direct beneficial effects on the cardiovascular system[1]. Evidence from multiple observational studies suggests a marked reduction in the risk of coronary heart disease associated with postmenopausal estrogen use in primary prevention. The latest meta-analysis of published studies suggests 30% and 34% reductions in risk among ever-users of unopposed and opposed therapy, respectively, compared with never-users[2]. However, all these studies were conducted in populations using oral preparations, many of them from the USA. No studies were available on the effects of the transdermal route on the risk of coronary heart disease until we performed a population cohort study. The results of our study were published elsewhere recently[3].

Relatively few epidemiological studies have examined the effect of HRT on the risk of venous thromboembolism. Studies published from 1974 to 1992 failed to show an association between HRT use and the occurrence of venous thromboembolism[4-9]. However, these studies had several methodological limitations. Most of the limitations were addressed in five observational studies published in 1996 and 1997[10-14]. Three of them provided information on the transdermal route of administration[10,13,14].

The objective of this paper is to report on the available epidemiological evidence in relation to the effects of the transdermal route of administration on cardiovascular outcomes, namely risk of venous thromboembolism and primary prevention of myocardial infarction.

HRT AND THE RISK OF VENOUS THROMBOEMBOLISM

In 1998 we reviewed and quantitatively summarized the available epidemiological data and the public health impact of the effects of HRT on the risk of idiopathic venous thromboembolism[15]. The methodological features of each of the studies reviewed are presented in Table 1. Three of the case–control studies used information recorded in automated health databases, including the Group Health Cooperative (GHC) of Puget Sound in Seattle, Washington, USA[12], the General Practice Research Database (GPRD) in the UK[13], and the Friuli-Venezia Giulia Health Databases in Italy[14]. Both the GPRD study and the study from Italy were case–control studies nested in cohorts of 347 253 women and 265 431 women, respectively. The other case–control study interviewed women admitted to hospitals in the area of the Oxford Regional Health Authority in the UK[10]. The cohort study was conducted using data from the ongoing Nurses' Health Study in the USA[11].

All the studies examined the risk of a first occurrence of venous thromboembolism among women without major risk factors such as a history of venous thromboembolism, cancer, hospitalization and recent trauma or surgery. Whereas all four case–control studies examined the risk of either

Table 1 Characteristics of recent epidemiological studies on hormone replacement therapy and the risk of first hospitalization for idiopathic venous thromboembolism

Study	Population	Study period	Design	Age range (years)	Number of cases	End point
Daly et al.[10]	hospitals of the Oxford Regional Health Authority, UK	1993–1994	matched hospital-based case–control	45–64	103	DVT or PE
Grodstein et al.[11]	Nurses' Health Study, USA	1978–1992	cohort of registered nurses	postmenopausal	68	PE
Jick et al.[12]	Group Health Co-operative of Puget Sound, USA	1980–1994	matched population-based case–control	50–74	42	DVT or PE
Pérez-Gutthann et al.[13]	General Practice Research Database, UK	1991–1994	population-based nested case–control	50–79	292	DVT or PE
Varas et al.[14]	Friuli-Venezia Giulia Health Databases, Italy	1991–1995	population-based nested case–control	45–79	171	DVT or PE

DVT, deep venous thrombosis; PE, pulmonary embolism. Adapted from reference 15

deep venous thrombosis or pulmonary embolism, the Nurses' Health Study was limited to the risk of pulmonary embolism.

Risk of venous thromboembolism associated with current HRT use

Time windows used to define current use of HRT were 1 month[10], 6 months[12-14] and up to 24 months[11]. Prevalence of current HRT use varied from 2.3% of controls in Italy to 25% in the populations of Oxford and the GHC of Puget Sound. None of the studies showed an increased risk with past HRT use. In all studies, women currently using HRT were found to be at a moderately higher risk of venous thromboembolism than women not using HRT. Estimates of relative risk varied from 2.1[11] to 3.6[10,12] (Table 2). We calculated a summary estimate of the relative risk, pooling the results from the five studies and weighting each of them by the inverse of the variance of the log relative risk. The summary relative risk of venous thromboembolism for women currently using HRT was 2.6 (95% confidence interval (CI) 1.6–4.2) (Table 2). The summary relative risks of venous thromboembolism for users of unopposed and opposed estrogens were 2.5 (95% CI 1.3–4.8) and 3.1 (95% CI 1.6–5.8), respectively (Table 2).

Effect of administration route and duration of therapy

Estimates of relative risk varied from 2.1 to 4.6 with oral therapy and from 2.0 to 2.3 with transdermal therapy (Table 2). The study conducted in Italy provided information on the transdermal route only[14]. The summary relative risk for users of oral preparations was 2.8 (95% CI 1.6–4.8) and for users of transdermal therapy 2.1 (95% CI 1.0–4.7).

The risk of venous thromboembolism was higher in the first year of therapy. The summary relative risk during the first year of treatment was 4.2 (95% CI 2.3–7.6) and the risk came down to 2.2 (95% CI 1.3–3.8) after that period of time.

Effect of estrogen dose

The risks associated with different doses of estrogen were inconsistent among studies, although there were few women exposed to high doses of estrogen in all of the studies. A dose–response relationship, with a doubling of risk among users of 0.625mg or more of estrogens, was found in two studies[10,12], whereas no dose effect was found in the other two studies[11,13]. Because of the low prevalence of HRT use, the effect of dose was not examined in the Italian study.

Table 2 Relative risk (95% confidence intervals) of venous thromboembolism according to type of hormone replacement therapy (HRT) among current users

Author	Type of current HRT regimen				
	Any	*Unopposed*	*Opposed*	*Oral*	*Transdermal*
Daly et al.[10]	3.6 (1.8–7.3)	3.2 (1.4–7.4)	5.3 (1.9–14.6)	4.6 (2.1–10.1)	2.0 (0.5–7.6)
Grodstein et al.[11]	2.1 (1.2–3.8)*	–	–	2.1 (1.2–3.8)	–
Jick et al.[12]	3.6 (1.6–7.8)*	4.1 (1.8–9.3)	2.4 (0.8–7.3)	3.6 (1.6–7.8)	–
Pérez-Gutthann et al.[13]	2.1 (1.4–3.2)	1.9 (1.0–3.8)	2.2 (1.4–3.5)	2.1 (1.3–3.6)	2.1 (0.9–4.6)
Varas et al.[14]	2.3 (1.0–5.3)†	1.4 (0.4–4.6)	5.0 (1.5–16.7)	–	2.3 (1.0–5.3)
Summary relative risk	2.6 (1.6–4.2)	2.5 (1.3–4.8)	3.1 (1.6–5.8)	2.8 (1.6–4.8)	2.1 (1.0–4.7)

*All exposed women used oral HRT preparations; †79% of exposed women used transdermal therapy. Adapted from reference 15

Biological plausibility

The effects of estrogens in the coagulation system are complex and not fully understood. The interpretation of available studies on HRT effects on blood coagulation is limited by the small size of the studied populations, and the variations between studies in the types of progestins used, the duration of treatment and the hemostatic factors assessed. Oral estrogens may have potentially opposing actions, while transdermal estrogens seem to modify fewer factors, with beneficial reductions in factor VII (FVII) and fibrinogen[16,17]. Overall, HRT appears to have a beneficial effect on the coagulation/fibrinolysis balance.

In all of these five studies, the risk of venous thromboembolism was more prominent in or restricted to the first year of therapy, which suggests that women with some underlying characteristic may be particularly at risk for developing venous thromboembolism. Several studies have shown that the factor V Leiden mutation increases an individual's risk for venous thromboembolism. There is some evidence that in women the estrogenic state may interact with the factor V Leiden mutation[18–20]. No information is currently available about the role of the factor V Leiden mutation, and other inborn abnormalities of the hemostatic system, in the risk of venous thromboembolism among women using HRT.

Conclusions

Evidence from five epidemiological studies published in 1996 and 1997 consistently indicates

that the risk of venous thromboembolism among current users of HRT is about two to three times higher than among women not using HRT. The risk is more prominent in or restricted to the first year of therapy and appears to be estrogen dose-dependent. Users of unopposed estrogens and transdermal therapy might be at lower risk than users of opposed regimens and oral preparations.

The incidence of idiopathic venous thromboembolism in postmenopausal healthy women not using HRT was estimated to be approximately 1 per 10 000 women per year. The estimated incidence in current users of HRT varies from 1.4[11] to 3.2[12] per 10 000 women per year. Therefore, between one and two cases of idiopathic venous thromboembolism per 10 000 women per year can be attributed to current use of HRT.

HRT AND THE INCIDENCE OF FIRST ACUTE MYOCARDIAL INFARCTION

We conducted a population-based nested case-control study in order to evaluate the association between HRT use and the incidence of first myocardial infarction in a European population taking oral and transdermal estrogens[3].

Summary of methods

We identified a cohort of women, aged 50 to 74 years, from the general population in the UK, registered in the GPRD[21] during the period 1991-1995. Women with a history of cardiovascular and cerebrovascular diseases, neoplasms, coagulopathies, vasculitis and alcohol-related diseases were excluded. Overall, 164 769 women were followed until the occurrence of the first myocardial infarction, the occurrence of any of the exclusion criteria, reaching age 75 years, death or study end, whichever occurred first.

A total of 1242 potential cases of first myocardial infarction were identified. To validate cases we adapted the international standardized diagnostic criteria for acute myocardial infarction[22,23]. Cases were classified as non-fatal and fatal acute myocardial infarction and possible acute coronary heart disease death after reviewing all available medical information related to the acute episode. A total of 1013 women were confirmed as cases; 791 of these cases were non-fatal and 222 were fatal. We selected 5000 controls using a time incidence sampling method and matched them by the age-frequency of cases[24].

Time windows to define current recent and past use were established as within the 6-month period prior to the index date and more than 6 months before the index date. Information on estrogen daily dose, type of regimen and route of administration was obtained from the last prescription.

Results

HRT use during the last 6 months was found in 133 cases (13%) and 855 controls (17%). Use of HRT was inversely related to age. In the age group 50–59 years, 38% of controls used the therapy in the last 6 months. Among women aged 60 years or older, this pattern of use was found in 15% of controls.

In our cohort, the absolute risk of all these events per 1000 person-years of follow-up was 1.6. Overall incidence of myocardial infarction was positively associated with established coronary risk

Table 3 Association of myocardial infarction with hormone replacement therapy (HRT) and main risk factors

Risk factor categories	Number of cases (n = 1013)	Number of controls (n = 5000)	Multivariate odds ratio* (95% CI)
Use of HRT			
never	839	3879	1.0
current/recent	133	855	0.72 (0.59–0.89)
past HRT use	41	266	0.73 (0.51–1.03)
Smoking history			
non-smoker	328	2486	1.0
smoker	329	766	3.64 (3.04–4.35)
ex-smoker	66	288	1.77 (1.32–2.39)
unknown	290	1460	1.60 (1.33–1.92)
Diabetes			
no	927	4830	1.0
yes	86	170	2.45 (1.84–3.26)
Hypertension			
no	682	3806	1.0
yes	331	1194	1.59 (1.35–1.88)
Hypercholesterolemia			
no	954	4848	1.0
yes	59	152	1.80 (1.30–2.50)
Family history of CHD			
no	978	4889	1.0
yes	35	111	1.48 (0.99–2.23)

*Odds ratios were estimated from a logistic model including all variables in this table and use of aspirin during the last 30 days with a duration longer than 30 days, surgical menopause, obesity and comorbidity; CI, confidence interval; CHD, coronary heart disease. Adapted from reference 3

Table 4 Myocardial infarction and current/recent use of hormone replacement therapy (HRT) by duration, regimen, route of administration and dose

Type of HRT use	Number of cases	Number of controls	Multivariate odds ratio* (95% CI)
Non-use (reference category)	839	3879	1.0
Current/recent use			
≤ 1 year	41	239	0.81 (0.57–1.14)
1–3 years	54	329	0.75 (0.56–1.02)
> 3 years	38	287	0.59 (0.42–0.85)
Long-term current/recent use[†]			
unopposed	30	248	0.52 (0.35–0.78)
opposed	55	320	0.79 (0.59–1.08)
oral estrogens ≥ 0.625 mg	50	374	0.63 (0.46–0.86)
transdermal estradiol ≥ 50 μg	17	110	0.62 (0.37–1.06)

*Odds ratio adjusted for age, past use of HRT, history of smoking, hypertension, diabetes, obesity, hypercholesterolemia, family history of coronary heart disease, surgical menopause and preventive use of aspirin; [†]long-term current/recent use of HRT was use in the last 6 months prior to the index date with > 1 year duration; CI, confidence interval. Adapted from reference 3

factors (Table 3). The age-adjusted odds ratio and 95% confidence interval for myocardial infarction in current HRT users, as compared to non-users, was 0.72 (95% CI 0.59–0.88) (Table 3). After adjusting for the main coronary risk factors plus obesity, comorbidity, current long-term use of aspirin and surgical menopause, the odds ratio remained unchanged. Narrowing the time period of use to 30 days before the index date yielded an odds ratio of 0.73 (95% CI 0.59–0.91).

The protective effect was observed in users of more than 1 year of therapy (long-term users) with an adjusted odds ratio of 0.68 (95% CI 0.53–0.86) (data not shown). The adjusted odds ratio for more than 3 years of treatment duration was 0.59 (95% CI 0.42–0.85) (Table 4). In addition, we subdivided the first year into shorter periods of time. During the first 4 months the odds ratio was 0.90 (95% CI 0.54–1.50), and thereafter it was 0.72 (95% CI 0.46–1.15).

The use of unopposed therapy was associated with a greater reduction in the risk of myocardial infarction than the use of opposed therapy, with adjusted odds ratios of 0.52 (95% CI 0.35–0.78) and 0.79 (95% CI 0.59–1.08), respectively (Table 4). The majority of women used oral preparations (79%), while 21% used transdermal therapy. The effect of estrogen dose was examined among current recent users of long-term oral estrogens

and transdermal estradiol, either unopposed or opposed. Among them, 51% of cases and 61% of controls used medium doses. The odds ratio associated with ≥ 0.625 mg of oral estrogen was 0.63 (95% CI 0.46–0.86) and with ≥ 50 μg of transdermal estradiol 0.62 (95% CI 0.37–1.06).

The odds ratio associated with past use of HRT was 0.73 (95% CI 0.51–1.03) (Table 3). The benefit on the risk of myorcardial infarction provided by HRT was lost about 2–3 years after the cessation of use.

Conclusion

The results from this large population-based study are consistent with those of prior epidemiological studies, conducted in different populations with different methodologies, which show a 20–70% reduction in the risk of acute coronary heart disease events among current users of HRT in primary prevention[2]. The results of the present study also suggest that oral and transdermal therapy might have similar cardioprotective effect at medium-high doses.

Biological plausibility

The cardioprotective effects of estrogens are explained by changes in serum lipids and blood coagulation factors, and effects on the vasculature and the carbohydrate metabolism. Compared to oral estrogens, transdermal estradiol seems to have similar beneficial effects on total cholesterol and low-density lipoproteins, but also decreases triglycerides with a lesser increase in high-density lipoproteins[25,26]. Medroxyprogesterone acetate given orally may attenuate the effect of estrogens on high-density lipoprotein levels[27]. However, there is no conclusive evidence to suggest that the addition of progestogens attenuates the effects of transdermal estrogen on lipid profiles.

Long-term HRT has been associated with improved arterial endothelial function in healthy postmenopausal women. The percutaneous route of estrogen administration seems to be at least as effective as the oral route in improving peripheral vascular flow velocity, and is not affected by the addition of a progestogen[28,29].

Oral and transdermal estrogens have been reported to increase insulin sensitivity[30]. However, oral conjugated equine estrogen doses of more than 0.625 mg might increase insulin resistance[31]. Estrogen–progestin regimens may decrease insulin sensitivity[32]. The progestin effect seems to be related to the type and dose of progestin.

References

1. Mendelsohn ME, Karas RH. The protective effects of estrogen on the cardiovascular system. *Rev N Engl J Med* 1999;340:1801–11
2. Barrett-Connor E, Grady D. Hormone replacement therapy, heart disease and other considerations. *Annu Rev Public Health* 1998;19:55–72
3. Varas-Lorenzo C, García-Rodriguez LA, Perez-Gutthann S, Duque-Oliart A. Hormone replacement therapy and incidence of acute myocardial infarction. A population-based nested case–control study. *Circulation* 2000;101:2572–8
4. The Boston Collaborative Drug Surveillance Program, Boston University Medical Center. Surgically confirmed gallbladder disease, venous thromboembolism and breast tumors in relation to postmenopausal estrogen therapy. *N Engl J Med* 1974; 290:15–19
5. Pettiti DB, Wingerd J, Pellegrin F, *et al*. Risk of vascular disease in women. Smoking, oral contraceptives, noncontraceptive estrogens, and other factors. *J Am Med Assoc* 1979;242:1150–4
6. Devor M, Barrett-Connor E, Renvall M, *et al*. Estrogen replacement therapy and the risk of venous thrombosis. *Am J Med* 1992;92:275–84
7. Quinn DA, Thompson BT, Terrin ML, *et al*. A prospective investigation of pulmonary embolism in women and men. *J Am Med Assoc* 1992;268:1689–96
8. Hammond CB, Jelovsek FR, Lee KL, *et al*. Effects of long-term estrogen replacement therapy. I: Metabolic effects. *Am J Obstet Gynecol* 1979;133:525–36
9. Nachtigall LE, Nachtigall RH, Nachtigall RD, *et al*. Estrogen replacement therapy. II: A prospective study in the relationship to carcinoma and cardiovascular and metabolic problems. *Obstet Gynecol* 1979;54:74–9
10. Daly E, Vessey MP, Hawkins MM, *et al*. Case-control study of venous thromboembolism disease and use of hormone replacement therapy. *Lancet* 1996;348:977–80
11. Grodstein F, Stampfer MJ, Goldhaber SZ, *et al*. Prospective study of exogenous hormones and risk of pulmonary embolism in women. *Lancet* 1996; 348:983–7
12. Jick H, Derby L. The risk of hospitalization for idiopathic venous thromboembolism among users of postmenopausal estrogens. *Lancet* 1996;348: 981–3
13. Pérez-Gutthann S, García-Rodríguez LA, Castellsague J, Duque A. Hormone replacement therapy and risk of venous thromboembolism: population-based case–control study. *Br Med J* 1997;314:796–800
14. Varas C, García-Rodríguez LA, Castaruzzi C, *et al*. Hormone replacement therapy and the risk of hospitalization for venous thromboembolism: a population-based study in southern Europe. *Am J Epidemiol* 1998;147:387–90
15. Castellsague J, Pérez-Gutthann S, García-Rodríguez LA. Recent epidemiological studies of the association between hormone replacement therapy and venous thromboembolism. *Drug Saf* 1998;18: 117–23

16. Lindoff C, Peterson F, Lecander I, *et al*. Transdermal estrogen replacement therapy: beneficial effects on hemostatic risk factors for cardiovascular disease. *Maturitas* 1996;24:43–50

17. The Writing Group for the Estradiol Clotting Factors Study. Effects on haemostasis of hormone replacement therapy with transdermal estradiol and oral sequential medroxyprogesterone acetate: a 1-year, double-blind placebo-controlled study. *Thromb Haemost* 1996;75:476–80

18. Vandenbroucke JP, Koster T, Briët E, *et al*. Increased risk of venous thrombosis in oral contraceptive users who are carriers of factor V Leiden mutation. *Lancet* 1994;344:1454–7

19. Rosing J, Tans G, Nicolaes GAF, *et al*. Oral contraceptives and venous thrombosis: different sensitivities to activated protein C in women using second and third-generation oral contraceptives. *Br J Haematol* 1997;97:233–8

20. Vandenbroucke JP, Rosendaal FR. End of the line for 'third-generation pill' controversy? *Lancet* 1997;349:1113–14

21. Garcia-Rodriguez LA, Perez-Gutthann S. Use of the UK General Practice Research Database for pharmacoepidemiology. *Br J Clin Pharmacol* 1998;45:419–25

22. World Health Organization Regional Office for Europe. *Myocardial Infarction Community Registers*, Public Health in Europe No. 5: Copenhagen: WHO, 1976

23. Gillum RF, Fortmann SP, Prineas RJ, Kottke TE. International diagnostic criteria for acute myocardial infarction and acute stroke. *Am Heart J* 1984;108:150–8

24. Walker AM. *Observation and Inference*. Newton Lower Falls, MA: Epidemiology Resources Inc., 1991

25. Stevenson JC, Drook D, Godsland IF. Oral versus transdermal hormone replacement therapy. *Int J Fertil* 1994;38(Suppl 1):30–5

26. Rozenberg S, Ylikorkala O, Arrenbrech S. Comparison of continuous and sequential transdermal progestogen with sequential oral progestogen in postmenopausal women using continuous transdermal estrogen: vasomotor symptoms, bleeding patterns and serum lipids. *Int J Fertil* 1997;42 (Suppl 2):376–87

27. Lemay A, Dodin S, Cédrin I, T-Lemay L. Phasic serum lipid excursions occur during cyclical oral conjugated oestrogens but not during transdermal oestradiol sequentially combined with oral medroxyprogesterone acetate. *Clin Endocrinol* 1995; 42:341–51

28. Lau TK, Wan D, Yim SF, *et al*. Prospective, randomized, controlled study of the effect of hormone replacement therapy on peripheral blood flow velocity in postmenopausal women. *Fertil Steril* 1998;70:284–8

29. Cacciatore B, Paakkari I, Toivonen J, Tikkanen MJ, Ylikorkala O. Randomized comparison of oral and transdermal hormone replacement on carotid and uterine artery resistance to blood flow. *Obstet Gynecol* 1998;92:563–8

30. Cagnacci A, Soldani R, Carriero PL, Paoletti AM, Fioretti P, Melis GB. Effects of low doses of transdermal 17-beta-estradiol on carbohydrate metabolism in postmenopausal women. *J Clin Endocrinol Metab* 1992;74:1396

31. Barrett-Connor E, Laasko M. Ischemic heart disease risk in postmenopausal women: effects of estrogen use on glucose and insulin levels. *Arteriosclerosis* 1990;10:531–4

32. Lindheim SR, Vijod MA, Duffy DM, *et al*. The route of administration influences the effect of estrogen on insulin sensitivity in postmenopausal women. *Fertil Steril* 1994;62:1176–80

Pulsed estrogen therapy: Aerodiol® 19

Y. Tsouderos

INTRODUCTION

Achieving plasma estradiol concentrations of mid-follicular phase levels has long been recognized as a goal for hormone replacement therapy. Thresholds were suggested and the need for a flat plateau was generally accepted as a fundamental concept. Marth and Daxenbichler[1] were probably the first to investigate the relative importance of both concentrations and times of exposure. Investigating *in vitro* the proliferative effects of pulsed and continuous exposure on a human breast cancer cell line, these authors concluded that proliferative effects were linearly dependent on the duration of exposure and non-linearly dependent on concentration. A few years later, Otto[2] demonstrated that short exposure to estradiol was able, *in vitro*, to exert proliferative effects on breast cancer cell lines and the transcription of the progesterone receptor nRNA for several days.

PULSED VERSUS CONTINUOUS ESTRADIOL EXPOSURE

Aiming to explore the possible differences between pulsed and continuous exposure, several independent groups carried out *in vitro* experiments using the same principle. They compared a short 1-h estradiol exposure at a 24-unit concentration with a 24-h exposure at a concentration of 1 unit. Vignon and colleagues[3] studied the proliferative effects of estradiol on normal human breast cell lines comparing pulsed and continuous exposure. The results showed that the cell proliferation was stimulated with the same intensity with both the pulsed and continuous exposure after 1 week. The same investigators also studied the proliferative effects of estradiol on the ZR-75-1 and MCF-7 cell lines, two estrogen receptor-positive breast cancer cell lines, over 7 days, comparing pulsed and continuous exposures at several levels of concentration. Clear dose/effect relationships in the proliferation of the cells were observed up to a plateau, but no difference was observed between pulsed and continuous exposure when the 24-h exposure was similar[3].

Finally, Cavailles (unpublished data) was able to show *in vitro* that similar pulsed or continuous 24-h exposures have the same effects 12–48 h after the beginning of the experiments, by checking the activation process of the estrogen receptor and DNA transcription through the expression of estrogen-dependent protein mRNAs, such as progesterone-receptor mRNA, cathepsine D mRNA or protein pS2 mRNA.

PULSED ESTROGEN THERAPY

The Servier Laboratories were able to prepare an aqueous solution of estradiol, using a methylated cyclodextrin as an excipient. This formulation (Aerodiol®) was developed as a nasal spray for estrogen replacement therapy. After a nasal administration of 300 μg Aerodiol (one spray in each nostril) the plasma estradiol concentration time curve shows a quick increase up to 1200pg/ml, then a rapid decrease within a few minutes, indicating an intense tissue distribution with the estradiol concentration ultimately dropping to postmenopausal values within 8–12 h. Obviously, this pulsed kinetic profile is totally different to that observed after a patch or tablet administration[4].

Alleviation of climacteric symptoms

The reproducibility of the pulse was excellent and permitted clinical evaluation of the therapeutic efficacy. This was done in three prospective clinical trials. Aerodiol was firstly assessed in a large multicenter, double-blind controlled study with randomization of the treatments[5]. Four hundred and twenty postmenopausal women were treated for 3 months (unopposed estrogen) in seven parallel groups, either with placebo, one of four active doses (100, 200, 300 or 400 μg/day) of the nasal spray or one of two doses (1 or 2 mg/day) of estradiol valerate. The primary end point was the Kupperman Index[6]. The results showed a placebo effect at 4 weeks with no further decrease in the Kupperman Index at 12 weeks. A dose-dependent decrease in the Kupperman Index was observed in the four Aerodiol-treated groups. The 300- and 400-μg/day treated groups had significantly improved climacteric symptoms at 4 week (67% decrease in the Kupperman Index) in comparison with placebo. With a further decrease at 12 weeks, the 200 μg group showed significant improvement at this time when compared to the placebo group. The positive controls showed a similar decrease in the Kupperman Index as observed after 4 weeks in the 300 μg/day treated group and after 12 weeks with a dose relationship in the 200 μg/day and 300-μg/day groups.

In a multinational, double-blind controlled study, comparing Aerodiol with oral micronized estradiol (2 mg/day), both sequentially combined with dydrogesterone, in 659 early postmenopausal women in two parallel groups treated for 6 months, Mattsson and colleagues[7] demonstrated a statistically significant equivalence in reducing climacteric symptoms after 3 and 6 months of treatment.

Finally, in a third multinational study comparing Aerodiol with Estraderm TTS® 50 for 3 months, Lopes and colleagues[8] showed a statistically significant equivalence in reducing the climacteric symptoms of 358 postmenopausal women randomized in two parallel groups.

Decreased stimulation of reproductive tissues

Mastodynia is a main cause of withdrawal from treatment. There are often signs of overdosing, especially if the mastodynia is moderate or severe in intensity. Using marketed patches with the same strength (Esclim® and Menorest® 50 μg/day), similar incidences of mastodynia have been reported in two recently published clinical trials[9,10], and by Lopes and colleagues[8] with the Estraderm TTS 50, when compared with Aerodiol. In this comparative study, a significantly lower incidence of moderate and severe mastodynia was observed with the pulsed estrogen therapy.

The same observations were made by Mattsson and colleagues[7] comparing Aerodiol with oral estradiol (2 mg/day). There was evidence of a significantly lower incidence of moderate and severe mastalgia. With regard to vaginal bleeding, significantly fewer patients had withdrawal bleeding (46% vs. 69%, $p < 0.05$) or breakthrough bleeding (22.6% vs. 26.6%) with Aerodiol, indicating lower endometrial stimulation.

Cardiovascular risks

Obviously, the nasal route avoids the metabolic consequences of the so-called hepatic first pass effect. Six months of treatment induced a statistically significant decrease in total cholesterol, apolipoprotein B and lipoprotein(a), and no increase in triglycerides or angiotensinogen. The potential effects of pulsed estrogen 3-month treatment therapy were assessed in animals (Doursoult, unpublished data). Intact and ovariectomized dogs were chronically instrumented and conscious when the measures were taken (no anesthesia). Surgical procedures enabled the introduction of catheters into the abdominal aorta and the implantation of probes at the level of the coronary artery, pulmonary artery and myocardiac wall and a microtransducer into the left ventricle. The dogs wore jackets to protect the catheters and wires. Several hemodynamic parameters were assessed: (1) cardiac output, measured with a precalibrated transonic flow probe (transit time blood flow meter) which had been demonstrated to be more suitable in the dog than the Doppler system (cuff type blood flow meter); (2) systemic vascular resistances calculated as mean arterial blood pressure/cardiac output; and (3) mean arterial blood pressures, measured from the catheter inserted into the abdominal aorta via the iliac artery. The results showed, as expected, an increase in systemic vascular resistances and a decrease in cardiac output in the ovariectomized non-treated animals. Normalization of vascular resistances

(−28%) and cardiac output (+30%) was observed in the estradiol-treated animals, with a return to values close to those of non-ovariectomized animals.

CONCLUSIONS

Nasal administration of estradiol leads to a pulsed kinetic profile. A dose-dependent efficacy of the pulsed estrogen therapy has been demonstrated in comparison with placebo. The 300-µg daily dose, in a single administration, is the optimal dose to start treatment in the early postmenopause. Using equivalent total 24-h hormone exposure, comparing pulsed and continuous treatments, the same efficacy on climateric symptoms with a lower stimulation of reproductive tissues (breast and endometrium) was observed in comparison with oral estradiol (2 mg/day) or transdermal devices delivering 50 µg/day. Some differences in lipid profile changes, already observed with other extra-digestive routes, were observed in comparison with the oral route after 6 months of treatment. In contrast, *in vitro* experiments did not show any substantial differences between pulsed and continuous exposure with regard to the proliferative effects of estradiol.

References

1. Marth C, Daxenbichler G. Pulsatile versus continuous estradiol exposure in inducing proliferation of cultured ZR-75-1 human breast cells. *J Steroid Biochem* 1985;23:567–72

2. Otto A. A 1-minute pulse of estradiol to MCF-7 breast cancer cells changes estrogen receptor binding properties and commits cells to induce estrogenic responses. *Steroid Biochem Mol Biol* 1995;54:39–46

3. Vignon F, Gompel A, Siromachkova M, Prébois C, Varin C, Rostène W. Effects of pulsed or continuous estradiol administration on proliferation of normal and tumoral human breast cells. *Menopause* 1999;6:362

4. Devissaguet JP, Brion N, Lhote O, Deloffre P. Pulsed estrogen therapy: pharmacokinetics of intranasal 17β-estradiol (S21400) in postmenopausal women and comparison with transdermal and oral formulations. *Eur J Drug Metab Pharmacokinet* 1999;24:265–71

5. Studd J, Pornel B, Marton I, Bringer J, Varin C, Tsouderos Y, Christiansen CI. Efficacy and acceptability of intranasal 17β-estradiol for menopausal symptoms: randomised dose-response study. *Lancet* 1999;853:1574–8

6. Wiklund I, Karlberg J, Mattsson L. Quality of life of postmenopausal women on a regimen of transdermal estradiol therapy: a double-blind placebo-controlled study. *Am J Obstet Gynecol* 1993;168:824–30

7. Mattsson L, Christiansen CI, Colau J-C, Palacios S, Kenemans P, Bergeron C, Chevallier O, Von Holst T, Gangar K. Clinical equivalence of intranasal and oral 17β-estradiol for postmenopausal symptoms. *Am J Obstet Gynecol* 2000;182:545–52

8. Lopes P, Merkus JHW, Nauman J, Calaf J, Foidart JM, Crosiguani P. Patient acceptability and efficacy of intranasal estradiol: a randomized cross-over comparison with transdermal estradiol. *Obstet Gynecol* 2000;96:906–12

9. Utian WH, Burry KA, Archer DF, Gallagher JC, Boyett RL, Guy MP, Tachon GJ, Chadha-Boreham HK, Bouvet AA. Efficacy and safety of low, standard and high dosages of an estradiol transdermal system (ESCLIM) compared with placebo on vasomotor symptoms in highly symptomatic patients. *Am J Obstet Gynecol* 1999;181:71–9

10. Cooper C, Stakkestad SM, Radowicki S, Hardy P, Pilate P, Dain M, Delmas PD. The international study for Matrix delivery transdermal 17β-estradiol for the prevention of bone loss in postmenopausal women. *Osteoporos Int* 1999;9:358

Cardiovascular effects of raloxifene: data from preclinical studies and clinical trials in postmenopausal women

20

E. Moscarelli and D. A. Cox

INTRODUCTION

Hormone replacement therapy (HRT) has long been the mainstay of treatment for menopausal symptoms. It is indicated for the control of hot flushes and to prevent osteoporosis, but it also reduces low-density lipoprotein (LDL) cholesterol levels and increases high-density lipoprotein (HDL) cholesterol levels. Data from observational studies suggest that HRT may reduce the risk of cardiovascular disease, colon cancer and Alzheimer's disease, although these effects have yet to be confirmed in controlled clinical trials[1]. The use of HRT in postmenopausal women is often associated with the resumption of vaginal bleeding and, in the long term, with an increased risk of breast cancer and endometrial cancer, even if a progestogen is included in the regimen. Thus, compounds that avoid the nuisance of vaginal bleeding and the other potential risks of HRT may be more acceptable and safer for postmenopausal women. The concept of a selective estrogen receptor modulator (SERM) was defined to develop a compound which had the favorable effects of estrogens on bone and on the cardiovascular system, while avoiding the undesired effects on other tissues, especially the breast and uterus.

Raloxifene is a non-steroidal benzothiophene SERM that exerts estrogen-agonistic effects in bone and on lipids, while it functions as an estrogen antagonist in the uterus and breast. Different hypotheses have been put forward to explain the potential mechanisms by which SERMs produce tissue-selective effects[2]. The purpose of this short review is to discuss the main effects of raloxifene on the cardiovascular system.

PRECLINICAL FINDINGS

In vivo studies

In ovariectomized rats, raloxifene lowers serum cholesterol[3], inhibits arterial intimal thickening following balloon injury to the carotid artery[4], and attenuates pressor responses to vasopressin via a mechanism that may involve enhanced vascular expression of nitric oxide synthase[5]. In ovariectomized, cholesterol-fed rabbits, raloxifene inhibits atherogenesis of the aorta, although to a slightly lesser extent than that observed with estrogen[6,7]. In ovariectomized sheep, raloxifene treatment increases angiographically determined coronary artery diameter compared with both placebo and estrogen[8], and increases coronary blood flow via an endothelium-dependent and estrogen receptor-mediated mechanism[9,10]. In contrast, Clarkson and colleagues[11] showed that raloxifene did not attenuate the development of coronary artery atheroma in monkeys fed a moderately atherogenic diet for 2 years, while estrogen inhibited atherosclerosis in this model. Thus, raloxifene has demonstrated favorable cardiovascular effects in most, but not all, *in vivo* animal models studied.

In vitro studies

Potentially favorable cardiovascular effects have also been demonstrated for raloxifene using *in vitro* models. Raloxifene and related SERMs inhibit copper-mediated oxidation of isolated human LDL cholesterol to a greater extent than estrogen[12,13]. Consistent with *in vivo* studies described above, raloxifene acutely increases availability of nitric oxide in cultured human endothelial cells[14]. In coronary arteries from both male and female rabbits, raloxifene induced acute arterial relaxation by an endothelium-dependent and estrogen receptor-dependent mechanism involving nitric oxide, and by an endothelium-independent mechanism involving calcium antagonism[15]. In the same model, estrogen induced only endothelium-independent coronary arterial relaxation[15].

Finally, raloxifene diminishes the expression of adhesion molecules and the binding of monocytes in cultured human endothelial cells[16]. Thus, the body of evidence suggests that raloxifene has favorable cardiovascular effects both in animal models and *in vitro*.

CLINICAL FINDINGS

While the results from animal and *in vitro* models may provide preliminary information as to the usefulness of a pharmaceutical compound, it is obvious that these must be followed and supplemented by studies in humans.

Effect on risk factors for cardiovascular disease

The acute and long-term effects of raloxifene on lipids have been evaluated in several clinical trials.

In patients at risk for osteoporosis, randomized to different doses of raloxifene or placebo, reductions in total and LDL cholesterol levels were evident with the dose of 60 mg/day after as soon as 3 months of therapy and were sustained up to 24 months (Figure 1)[17]. In patients with osteopenia, raloxifene significantly decreased serum total and LDL cholesterol levels over 3 years of treatment, whereas HDL cholesterol and triglyceride concentrations were unchanged[18]. When the population was divided into tertiles, based on the baseline total cholesterol levels, the effect of raloxifene in lowering LDL cholesterol was greatest among women with the highest LDL cholesterol at baseline (Figure 2).

Lipids and coagulation factors were the main objectives of a further 6-month study in healthy postmenopausal women randomized to two doses of raloxifene (60 mg/day and 120 mg/day), HRT (0.625 mg/day conjugated equine estrogen and 2.5 mg/day medroxyprogesterone acetate) or placebo[19]. At the end-point, LDL cholesterol levels were lowered by 12% with both raloxifene doses and by a comparable 14% with HRT. Interestingly, serum levels of apolipoprotein B, the apolipoprotein associated with LDL cholesterol, were reduced significantly by raloxifene but not by HRT in this study. Total HDL cholesterol levels were unchanged with raloxifene therapy, but were significantly increased by HRT. However, raloxifene increased HDL_2 cholesterol, a sub-fraction

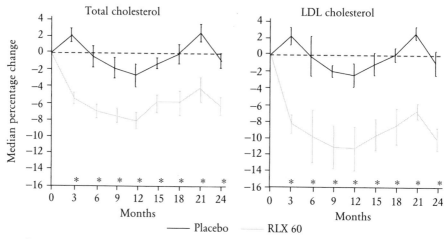

Figure 1 Median percentage change in serum total and LDL cholesterol concentrations in postmenopausal women treated with raloxifene 60 mg/day (RLX 60) or placebo for 2 years

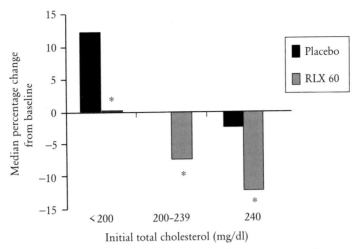

Figure 2 Median percentage change in LDL cholesterol concentrations in postmenopausal women treated with raloxifene 60 mg/day (RLX 60) or placebo for 2 years and different LDL cholesterol concentrations at baseline. $^*p < 0.05$ compared with placebo

that is postulated to account for the majority of HDL's cardioprotective effect. Triglyceride levels were not changed by either raloxifene dose, but were significantly increased by 20% with HRT. Lipoprotein(a) levels were also significantly reduced by both doses of raloxifene (7% and 8%, respectively), but to a lesser extent than that observed with HRT (19%). Fibrinogen levels were significantly lowered by raloxifene (10%) but were unaffected by HRT. Plasminogen activator inhibitor-1 (PAI-1) levels were not changed by raloxifene, but were significantly reduced by 29% with HRT.

The effects of raloxifene and HRT on non-lipid risk factors for cardiovascular disease have also been compared. Serum homocysteine, an independent risk factor for the development of cardiovascular disease, and serum tumor necrosis factor-α, a pro-inflammatory cytokine, were both decreased by raloxifene and HRT to comparable extents in postmenopausal women[20,21]. C-reactive protein (CRP), a systemic marker of inflammation and an independent risk factor for cardiovascular events in postmenopausal women[22], was unaffected by raloxifene but was dramatically increased with HRT, even after women with acute infection and/or elevated CRP level prior to the treatment were excluded from the analysis[20] (Figure 3). Finally, both raloxifene and HRT significantly lowered serum levels of certain adhesion

molecules (E-selectin and ICAM-1), but only HRT significantly increased serum levels of matrix metalloproteinase-9 (MMP-9)[23], an enzyme thought to be involved in atherosclerotic plaque rupture[24].

The information summarized in this section indicates that, although raloxifene probably exerts its effects through the estrogen receptor, the influences of raloxifene on lipids, coagulation or fibrinolysis factors, inflammatory markers, and other markers of cardiovascular risk may be different from those exerted by HRT. These include the effects on HDL cholesterol, triglycerides, apolipoprotein B, fibrinogen, PAI-1, C-reactive protein and MMP-9.

Effects on body systems other than cardiovascular

As a SERM, raloxifene has effects on body systems in addition to the cardiovascular system that play an important role in its clinical profile. Oral once-daily raloxifene (60 mg/day) consistently increases bone mineral density in the lumbar spine, femoral neck, total hip and total body in postmenopausal women, with or without calcium supplementation[17,18]. More importantly, in postmenopausal women with osteoporosis (low bone mineral density or with a prevalent vertebral

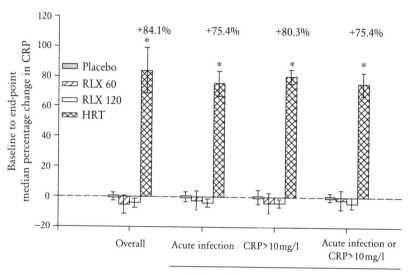

Figure 3 Changes in serum C-reactive protein (CRP) concentration in postmenopausal women assigned to placebo, two different doses of raloxifene (RLX), or HRT, observed after 6 months. Data are expressed as the median percentage change ± SE of the median. HRT was conjugated equine estrogen (0.625 mg/day) and medroxy-progesterone acetate (2.5 mg/day). Data are presented for the overall population and for subsets of women, excluding those with clinical history of acute infection, elevated CRP at baseline, or both conditions. * $p < 0.001$ compared with placebo

fracture), up to 3 year's follow-up, raloxifene increases bone mineral density in the spine and in the femoral neck and reduces the risk of new vertebral fractures[25].

Data collected in postmenopausal women with osteoporosis, followed for a median of 40 months, suggest that raloxifene treatment is associated with a significantly reduced risk (76%) of invasive breast cancer[26]. In the same trial, raloxifene decreased the risk of estrogen receptor-positive invasive breast cancer by 90%, without affecting the incidence of estrogen receptor-negative breast cancer[26].

Finally, it is worth mentioning that raloxifene therapy is associated with a 2–3-fold increased risk of venous thromboembolic disease (deep vein thrombosis, pulmonary embolism or retinal vein thrombosis)[26], comparable to the risk previously reported for HRT[27]. Raloxifene treatment does not control hot flushes and it may be associated with an increased occurrence of leg cramps.[28] However, unlike estrogen, raloxifene does not increase the incidence of uterine bleeding[28] or the risk of endometrial cancer[26].

Effects on acute coronary events

Though favorable effects of raloxifene on risk factors for cardiovascular disease have been clinically observed, the most important area that needs to be investigated is the effect of long-term raloxifene therapy on the clinical outcomes of atherosclerosis. A clinical trial, Raloxifene Use in The Heart (RUTH), has been designed to provide answers to three very important questions regarding postmenopausal women's health:

(1) Is raloxifene able to reduce the incidence of acute coronary events?

(2) Is raloxifene able to reduce the risk of invasive breast cancer?

(3) What is the safety profile of raloxifene in a wider population of postmenopausal women?

THE RUTH TRIAL

The RUTH trial is a double-blind, placebo-controlled, long-term assessment of cardiovascular and breast cancer outcomes in 10 101 postmenopausal women with documented history of coronary artery disease or a combination of risk factors for developing acute coronary events. The primary end-point of the study is a composite coronary end-point, which includes hospitalized acute coronary syndrome other than myocardial infarction, non-fatal myocardial infarction and coronary death. Invasive breast cancer is a co-primary end-point. Secondary end-points include the individual components of the coronary primary end-point, cardiovascular disease death, myocardial and non-coronary arterial revascularization, stroke, venous thromboembolism, all breast cancers (invasive or otherwise), fractures, and all causes of death or hospitalization. Biochemical risk factors will be examined in parallel. Enrollment into the trial began in 1998 and was completed in August 2000. There will be a minimum follow-up of 5 years.

CONCLUSIONS

The concept of raloxifene as a SERM in postmenopausal women has been demonstrated with respect to its estrogen-agonist effects on bone and lipids, its lack of uterine stimulation, and its potentially favorable effect to reduce the risk of invasive breast cancer in postmenopausal women. The results of the RUTH study will help to confirm and extend this hypothesis, to include the impact of raloxifene on acute clinical events associated with coronary artery disease, as well as to provide a risk/benefit assessment of the compound in a larger population of postmenopausal women.

References

1. Barrett-Connor E. Hormone replacement therapy. *Br Med J* 1998;317:457-61
2. Khovidhunkit W, Shoback DM. Clinical effects of raloxifene hydrochloride in women. *Ann Intern Med* 1999;130:431-9
3. Kauffman RF, Bensch WR, Roudebush RE, *et al.* Hypocholesterolemic activity of raloxifene (LY139481): pharmacological characterization as a selective estrogen receptor modulator. *J Pharmacol Exp Ther* 1997;280:146-53
4. Kauffman RF, Bean JS, Fahey KJ, Cullinan GJ, Cox DA, Bensch WR. Raloxifene and estrogen inhibit neointimal thickening after balloon injury in the carotid artery of male and ovariectomized female rats. *J Cardiovasc Pharmacol* 2000;36:459-65
5. Pavo I, Laszlo F, Morschl E, *et al.* Raloxifene, an oestrogen-receptor modulator, prevents decreased constitutive nitric oxide and vasoconstriction in ovariectomized rats. *Eur J Pharmacol* 2000;410:101-4
6. Bjarnason NH, Haarbo J, Byrjalsen I, Kauffman RF, Christiansen C. Raloxifene inhibits aortic accumulation of cholesterol in ovariectomized, cholesterol-fed rabbits. *Circulation* 1997;96:1964-9
7. Bjarnason NH, Haarbo J, Byrjalsen I, Kauffman RF, Knadler MP, Christiansen C. Raloxifene reduces atherosclerosis: studies of optimized raloxifene doses in ovariectomized, cholesterol-fed rabbits. *Clin Endocrinol (Oxf)* 2000;52:225-3
8. Gaynor JS, Monnet E, Selzman C, *et al.* The effect of raloxifene on coronary arteries in aged ovariectomized ewes. *J Vet Pharmacol Ther* 2000;23:175-9
9. Zoma WD, Baker RS, Clark KE. Coronary and uterine vascular responses to raloxifene in the sheep. *Am J Obstet Gynecol* 2000;182:521-8
10. Clark KE, Zoma WD, Baker RS, Friedman A. Effect of chronic raloxifene on cardiovascular responses. *J Soc Gynecol Invest* 2000;7:187A
11. Clarkson TB, Anthony MS, Jerome CP. Lack of effect of raloxifene on coronary artery atherosclerosis of postmenopausal monkeys. *J Clin Endocrinol Metab* 1998;83:721-6
12. Zuckerman SH, Bryan N. Inhibition of LDL oxidation and myeloperoxidase dependent tyrosyl radical formation by the selective estrogen receptor modulator raloxifene (LY139481 HCl). *Atherosclerosis* 1996;126:65-75
13. Rattan AK, Arad Y. Inhibition of LDL oxidation by a new estradiol receptor modulator compound LY-139478: comparative effect with other steroids. *Atherosclerosis* 1998;136:305-14
14. Simoncini T, Genazzani AR. Raloxifene acutely stimulates nitric oxide release from human endothelial cells via an activation of endothelial nitric oxide synthase. *J Clin Endocrinol Metab* 2000;85:2966-9
15. Figtree GA, Lu YQ, Webb CM, Collins P. Raloxifene acutely relaxes rabbit coronary arteries

in vitro by an estrogen receptor-dependent and nitric oxide-dependent mechanism. *Circulation* 1999;100:1095–101

16. Simoncini T, De Caterina R, Genazzani AR. Selective estrogen receptor modulators: different actions on vascular cell adhesion molecule-1 (VCAM-1) expression in human endothelial cells. *J Clin Endocrinol Metab* 1999;84:815–18

17. Delmas PD, Bjarnason NH, Mitlak BH, *et al.* Effects of raloxifene on bone mineral density, serum cholesterol concentrations, and uterine endometrium in postmenopausal women. *N Engl J Med* 1997;337:1641–7

18. Johnston CC Jr, Bjarnason NH, Cohen FJ, *et al.* Long-term effects of raloxifene on bone mineral density, bone turnover, and serum lipipds in early postmenopausal women. 3-year data from two double-blind, randomized, placebo-controlled trials. *Arch Intern Med* 2000;160:3444–50

19. Walsh BW, Kuller LH, Wild RA, *et al.* Effects of raloxifene on serum lipids and coagulation factors in healthy postmenopausal women. *J Am Med Assoc* 1998;279:1445–51

20. Walsh BW, Paul S, Wild RA, *et al.* The effects of hormone replacement therapy and raloxifene on C-reactive protein and homocysteine in healthy postmenopausal women: a randomized, controlled trial. *J Clin Endocrinol Metab* 2000;85:214–18

21. Cox DA, Sashegyi A, Paul S, *et al.* Effects of raloxifene and hormone replacement therapy on markers of inflammation in healthy postmenopausal women. *Circulation* 1999;100:I-826

22. Ridker PM, Hennekens CH, Buring JE, Rifai N. C-reactive protein and other markers of inflammation in the prediction of cardiovascular disease in women. *N Engl J Med* 2000;342:836–43

23. Blum A, Schenke WH, Hathaway L, *et al.* Effects of estrogen and the selective estrogen receptor modulator raloxifene on markers of inflammation in postmenopausal women. *Am J Cardiol* 2000;86:892–5

24. Lee RT, Libby P. The unstable atheroma. *Arterioscler Thromb Vasc Biol* 1997;17:1859–67

25. Ettinger B, Black DM, Mitlak BH, *et al.* Reduction of vertebral fracture risk in postmenopausal women with osteoporosis treated with raloxifene: results from a 3-year randomized clinical trial. *J Am Med Assoc* 1999;282:637–45

26. Cummings S, Eckert S, Krueger K, *et al.* The effect of raloxifene on risk of breast cancer in postmenopausal women. *J Am Med Assoc* 1999;281:2189–97

27. Grady D, Wenger NK, Herrington D, *et al.* Postmenopausal hormone therapy increases risk for venous thromboembolic disease. The Heart and Estrogen/progestin Replacement Study. *Ann Intern Med* 2000;132:689–96

28. Davies GC, Huster WJ, Lu Y, Plouffe L, Lakshmanan M. Adverse events reported by postmenopausal women in controlled trials with raloxifene. *Obstet Gynecol* 1999;93:558–65

21

Cardiovascular risk assessment for postmenopausal hormone replacement therapies such as tibolone (Livial®)

D. Crook

INTRODUCTION

Tibolone (Org OD14, Livial®) is a steroid hormone with a progestin-like structure (Figure 1). Following oral administration, tibolone undergoes metabolic conversions that generate two estrogenic derivatives (3α-hydroxy and 3β-hydroxy) as well as a Δ^4 isomer that displays both progestogenic and androgenic activities in receptor binding and other assays[1] (Figure 1). As the split between conversions to the two types of metabolite differs between tissues, tibolone is sometimes referred to as a 'tissue-specific' steroid. For example, the isomerase required to convert the parent molecule to the Δ^4 metabolite (progestogenic/androgenic) is localized in endometrial tissue[2].

The therapeutic role of tibolone emerged when a dose of 2.5 mg/day was shown to relieve climacteric symptoms in many women and to have positive effects on mood and libido[1]. Tibolone maintains bone mineral density (BMD) in postmenopausal women[3] although, as with many other therapies, this effect on this biophysical surrogate has yet to be validated using bone fracture as the primary endpoint. Tibolone induces amenorrhea in many women and the incidence of breakthrough bleeding is less than that seen with continuous combined therapy[4]. Clinical trials often find less breast tenderness in women randomized to tibolone as opposed to estrogen-based forms of hormone replacement therapy (HRT)[4], and there

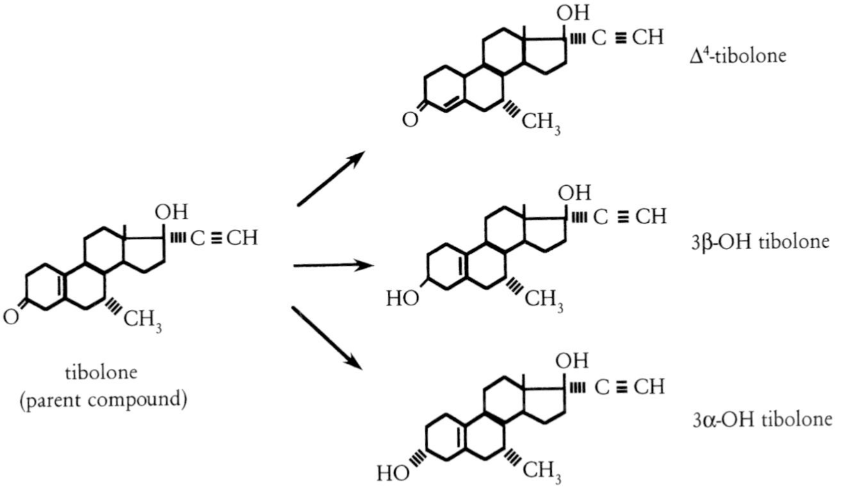

Figure 1 Structure of tibolone ((7α,17α)-17-hydroxy-7-methyl-19-norpregn-5(10)-en-20-yn-3-one) and its three major metabolites

is experimental evidence that this steroid does not stimulate breast tissue[5], perhaps due to specific effects on the activity of enzymes involved in endogenous estradiol metabolism[6]. In the absence of a formal clinical trial, any claims for a clinical benefit in breast disease must be treated with caution.

One of the more controversial aspects of this intriguing postmenopausal therapy is the cardiovascular risk profile. In 1983, Crona and colleagues[7] noted that tibolone reduced plasma concentrations of high-density lipoproteins (HDL) by 30%, a typically 'androgenic' effect that they considered out of keeping with the profile of this steroid in traditional bioassays. As the increased HDL concentrations induced by oral estrogen were held at that time to contribute to the lower incidence of coronary heart disease (CHD) seen in HRT users compared with those choosing not to use HRT, such a change was a concern.

The intention of this report is to summarize the cardiovascular risk profile of tibolone as it is currently understood. What may have been a straightforward assumption 20 years ago – that, based on the HDL effect, tibolone would increase CHD risk whereas estrogens would reduce this risk – is now an immeasurably more complex issue. Recent developments include:

(1) The repeated failure of recent randomized clinical trials to find any benefit of HRT over placebo in terms of myocardial infarction or other clinical cardiovascular endpoints;

(2) Increasing realization of the complexity of the atherosclerotic process, with an emphasis away from bulk transport of plasma components (such as lipids) to the microenvironment of the endothelium;

(3) Increasing awareness of the complexity of HDL metabolism;

(4) A frustration that conventional risk factor profiling may not after all provide net estimates of CHD risk with steroid hormones.

HISTORICAL BACKGROUND

The risk/benefit balance of postmenopausal HRT drugs, initially developed to relieve climacteric symptoms such as hot flushes and night sweats, was transformed by the claim that they may protect women from long-term diseases such as CHD. As arterial diseases are the major cause of morbidity and mortality in older women, this potential benefit came to dominate the development of postmenopausal HRT. In particular, the choice of a progestin to partner the estrogen component of HRT in women with a uterus became largely dictated by the issue of 'metabolic side-effects' such as the effect on cardiovascular risk markers, in particular the plasma HDL concentration. Biochemical changes, or the relative lack of them, also became an issue when evaluating the merits of transdermal administration of HRT.

A consensus emerged during the 1980s that oral estrogen therapy reduced CHD risk by 50% (perhaps more in women with pre-existing disease) and that the primary mechanism was by an increase in plasma HDL concentrations. This action was assumed – not proven – to accelerate 'reverse cholesterol transport', the process by which cellular cholesterol is transported centripetally to the liver for excretion. HRT was also claimed by some to protect through mechanisms such as glucose and insulin metabolism, but such theories could not compete with the huge amount of interest in HDL at that time.

The rather derogatory concept of progestin 'androgenicity', introduced in the context of oral contraceptive reformulation, was soon applied to postmenopausal HRT. As with oral contraceptives, there was uncertainty over the precise definition of this term: some progestins were classified on the basis of receptor or bioassay studies as being more androgenic than others, even though their clinical side-effect profiles (acne, hirsutism, etc.) were often quite similar when considering the low-dose therapies used in modern prescribing practice. Progestins oppose the estrogenic increase in plasma HDL concentrations, according to their type and dose (but not their route of administration), and eventually the plasma HDL concentration became used as the primary index of progestin androgenicity.

The 1990s witnessed an explosion of interest in 'direct' actions of estrogen on the arterial wall. HRT at last began to attract the interest of cardiologists, a profession previously suspicious of HRT due to the publicity surrounding the adverse vascular effects of oral contraceptives in the 1970s. As the role of estrogen in endothelial function began to unravel, there was a commensurate downgrading of the importance of HDL in the risk factor profile of HRT. Indeed, when epidemiologists began to compare CHD risk in women taking combined (estrogen–progestin) HRT, they were pleasantly surprised to see that co-administration of a progestin such as medroxy-progesterone acetate (MPA) did not appear to compromise the low CHD risk seen in women treated with estrogen alone compared with those who did not take HRT[8]. This single observation argues strongly against the primacy of the plasma HDL concentration as a determinant of the cardiovascular risk of HRT, especially as the issue of 'compliance bias' that haunts observational epidemiology in this area is unlikely to be operating when one compares different types of HRT.

The process of 'ranking' different steroids, initially by impact on plasma HDL concentrations, was repeated using endpoints derived from non-invasive measurement of arterial function and from fat-fed animal models. The results were not as clear-cut as with HDL: researchers often disagreed about the merits of one estrogen or progestin over another. As more and more cardiovascular endpoints became established, it became harder and harder to predict whether a specific HRT formulation would be better or worse than another. By the late 1990s, the limitations of surrogate studies had been reached: such data are relatively easy to generate but at present they cannot give an assessment of *net* risk.

Investigation of the effects of HRT on cardiovascular disease often involves varied approaches, such as biochemistry, the study of fat-fed animal models, and studies of vascular function and cell culture, but these data cannot be consolidated to give a point estimate of risk. Personal opinion becomes overpowering: the hypothetical scientist who works on HRT and plasma homocysteine feels that his is the most important way of assessing CHD risk, whereas the scientist who treats fat-fed animals with steroid hormones would counterclaim to be measuring 'real' arterial disease. Formal, randomized, placebo-controlled trials of different HRT formulations would be needed to resolve these controversies. If such studies confirmed the 'risk factor' approach to predicting cardiovascular risk in HRT users, then this would validate their use with steroids such as transdermal estradiol or tibolone.

Primarily for reasons of cost, the first of these studies were conducted in women with pre-existing CHD, a population that could be relied on to generate a high event rate. When these studies were designed, the climate of opinion derived from epidemiological, cardiological and animal model studies was that HRT was especially beneficial in damaged arteries. Consequently, the use of heart disease patients was considered to be an acceptable short-cut to understanding the effects in healthy women. A second and potentially vexatious decision was for some investigators to test not estrogen alone but a combination of estrogen and progestin.

Within the past few years, the findings of some of these formal clinical trials have been reported, although the results of others remain unpublished. Following over 40 years of perception of post-menopausal estrogen therapy as an anti-atherosclerotic drug, the utter failure of these studies to prove that any form of HRT is better than placebo in terms of clinical endpoints such as myocardial infarction forces us to regroup and rethink[9]. Such failure compounds the disappointment seen when cardiological endpoints such as coronary angiography[10], aortic distensibility[11] and carotid intima–media thickness (CIMT)[12] were used to search for evidence of a beneficial effect of HRT over placebo.

Indeed, a pattern of *increased* risk of cardiovascular events such as myocardial infarction and stroke (in addition to the predicted increase in venous thromboembolism), particularly in the early years, is emerging. These developments have led to a concern that the surrogate endpoints used for decades may have been misleading[13,14]. Furthermore, these negative results have emerged at the time that the traditional perception of oral HRT as an anti-atherosclerotic drug was marred by the discovery of a potentially adverse effect of estrogen on C-reactive protein, suggesting that estrogen may be pro-inflammatory[15]. Even the impressive evidence that estrogen reduces atherosclerosis in fat-fed animal models is now undergoing a process of re-evaluation.

Others are unimpressed by these developments and maintain that the clinical trial findings are simply freak occurrences or have been subject to misinterpretation[16,17]. The critical evidence to resolve these disputes will come from the randomized, controlled trial elements of the Women's Health Initiative (WHI), subgroups of which include healthy women randomized not just to combined therapy but, in some cases, to estrogen alone or placebo. This landmark clinical trial should be able to tell us whether, as claimed, the failure of the current studies is related to the progestin component or to the health status of the participants (or both). Initial reports from the WHI would seem to argue against both these possibilities and once again raise the issue of a subgroup of women who react adversely to estrogen[18], regardless of their baseline health status or the concomitant use of progestin.

This mismatch between observed and expected results for estrogen-based HRT in the prevention of CHD is so serious that risk profiling of therapies such as tibolone must proceed cautiously. Historically, the CHD risk profiles of different HRT have been evaluated using estrogen as a 'gold standard'. The current concerns over estrogen and CHD mean that a simple comparison of metabolic risk profiles may no longer be appropriate. The emphasis now must be to move away from blood measurements and towards rigorous, placebo-controlled, non-invasive evaluation of arterial disease, with the long-term aim of evaluating the quality of atherosclerotic plaques – in other words, their likelihood of fissuring – rather than just their size.

TIBOLONE AND THE RISK OF CARDIOVASCULAR DISEASE

In terms of venous disease, there is a suggestion, based on very small patient numbers, that tibolone may not increase the risk of venous thromboembolism, unlike both estrogen and raloxifene[19]. This intriguing observation is supported by the NV Organon clinical trial and adverse events reporting database (data on file). In terms of stroke, tibolone implants (but not oral administration) were better than estradiol in preventing experimentally induced rat brain infarcts[20]. This was an extraordinarily complex study and the extrapolation of results from this model to postmenopausal women is questionable. As with other forms of HRT, the effect on stroke is likely to remain a puzzle for many years.

Adverse event reporting systems and pooled clinical trial data do not support either a positive or a negative effect of tibolone on arterial disease (data on file). Such approaches to understanding the impact of a drug on CHD events may be unreliable and are no substitute for a program of placebo-controlled investigation.

VASCULAR ENDPOINTS

Blood pressure is unchanged in women using tibolone[1,21], even when they are hypertensive prior to therapy[22]. Non-randomized studies using biophysical measurement of aortic distensibility[23] and CIMT[24] found no effect of long-term tibolone use. A multicenter, randomized, double-blind, parallel-group, placebo-controlled trial ('OPAL') of the effects of tibolone on CIMT (with BMD as a secondary endpoint) is due to be completed in 2001. This is a 3-year study in which 756 healthy postmenopausal women have been randomized to placebo, tibolone 2.5 mg/day or continuous combined therapy (conjugated equine estrogens (CEE) 0.625 mg/day plus MPA 2.5 mg/day), all plus calcium 500 mg/day.

Tibolone increases blood flow, as measured by both nail-fold capillaroscopy[25] and venous occlusion plethysmography[26]. Tibolone has been claimed to increase stroke volume, cardiac output and flow velocity over the aortic valve in non-insulin-dependent diabetics[27], although there was no placebo arm to this study. Such an effect would be consistent with the ability of tibolone to reduce plasma concentrations of the potent vasoconstrictor endothelin (compared with women randomized to placebo) and also to increase those of vascular endothelial growth factor (VEGF)[28,29].

Doren and colleagues[30] randomized 100 healthy postmenopausal women to tibolone 2.5 mg/day or continuous combined therapy (2 mg/day estradiol plus 1 mg/day norethisterone acetate (NETA)) and used transvaginal color Doppler ultrasound of pelvic arteries to assess the response to therapy over 1 year. Neither therapy affected flow in the internal iliac arteries, but resistance and pulsatility indices in arcuate arteries fell with combined therapy but not with tibolone. In the uterine artery, both therapies reduced resistance and pulsatility indices, perhaps more so with continuous combined therapy. The low activity of tibolone in this study is disappointing, given the earlier studies in which improvements in blood flow were evident, and given the effects on endothelin and VEGF. Interpretation of such data is problematical: it is not at all certain whether biophysical evaluation of the pelvic vasculature can be extrapolated to an effect on CHD events.

In postmenopausal women with angina, tibolone improved their ability to exercise as monitored by their electrocardiographic profile[31]. A follow-up study, double-blind and placebo-controlled, will start in 2001. In fat-fed rabbits, tibolone at various doses almost totally blocks atherosclerosis – more so than does estradiol – and restores vascular reactivity[32]. The results of similar studies in fat-fed Cynomolgus macaque monkeys should be reported soon.

Simoncini and Genazzani[33] found that tibolone reduced the expression of vascular cell adhesion molecule-1 (VCAM-1) by endothelial cells in culture. This effect was mediated through estrogen receptors and so was only seen with the 3α- and 3β-hydroxy metabolites of tibolone. As VCAM-1 is involved in the tethering of blood monocytes to the endothelial surface prior to their recruitment into the inner layers of the artery, such an action – shared with both estradiol and raloxifene – is in theory anti-atherosclerotic. To date, there are no published data on the influence of tibolone on C-reactive protein or other markers of an inflammatory response.

GLUCOSE AND INSULIN METABOLISM

Despite an early report of impaired glucose tolerance in women using tibolone[7], recent work by Cagnacci and colleagues[34] suggests that tibolone increases tissue sensitivity to the action of insulin by over 60%, an effect that could be pre-dicted to reduce the risk of both CHD and diabetes mellitus. Confirmation of this extraordinary finding is clearly needed; the results of a prospective study of insulin dynamics in response to tibolone will soon be available (I.F. Godsland, personal communication).

COAGULATION AND FIBRINOLYSIS

Interpretation of the hemostasis profile of tibolone, as with other steroids, is impeded by the use of different endpoints by different researchers and indeed differences in methodology even when measuring the same endpoint. In many cases, the clinical significance of changes in these laboratory measurements is unknown or in dispute. From the earliest study[35] to the most recent[36], the single most striking finding has been that tibolone increases fibrinolytic activity. This potentially desirable effect has been linked to a 30% fall in the activities of tissue plasminogen activator (tPA) and plasminogen activator inhibitor (PAI-1)[37]. In some studies, plasma fibrinogen concentrations and factor VII activity are slightly reduced by tibolone[21]; such changes might be expected to reduce the risk of arterial disease.

Winkler and co-workers[36] have recently published hemostasis data on 60 women randomized to tibolone or continuous combined therapy (oral estradiol/norethisterone) for 3 months. Tibolone reduced factor VII activity by 21% but had no effect on fibrinogen concentrations. Markers of coagulation and fibrinolytic balance (F_{1+2}, D-dimer and fibrin degradation products (FDP)) were increased by tibolone but less so than with continuous combined therapy. Tibolone had no effect on protein C activity but reduced protein S activity and increased activated protein C (APC) resistance at 6 months but not at 12 months. These changes in the protein C/S system need further study, although the relevance to arterial, as opposed to venous, disease is unclear.

PLASMA LIPOPROTEIN METABOLISM

Following the original observation of a fall in plasma HDL concentrations[7], some argued that this fall was transient. This phase has passed (although it remains possible that certain geographical groups react in such a way) and the majority of studies find a sustained decrease of 20–25%. Such an effect might be considered undesirable, although one that might be countered by other positive actions of this steroid. Alternatively, the fall in plasma HDL concentrations may not translate into a fall in HDL function. The ability of HDL to accept cholesterol from cells in culture ('cholesterol efflux') is not impaired in women treated with tibolone[38]; other functions of HDL, such as the regulation of triglyceride-rich lipoprotein metabolism, do not appear to be impaired. These new data add to the questions over the wider area of steroid hormones, 'androgenicity' and atherosclerosis.

It is worth noting that testosterone itself is currently undergoing a re-evaluation as a potentially beneficial hormone in terms of cardiovascular disease[39,40]. Just as attention is now being drawn to the potentially undesirable effects of oral estrogen on the plasma lipoprotein profile, such as the increase in fasting triglyceride levels[13], many 'androgenic' changes in cardiovascular risk markers would be predicted to reduce, not increase, risk. As with all androgenic steroids, tibolone reduces plasma concentrations of fasting triglycerides and lipoprotein(a)[41]. This latter change is of interest as re-analysis of data from a placebo-controlled trial of combined HRT[42] extracted a subgroup with high plasma lipoprotein(a) concentrations in whom therapy has been claimed to reduce CHD risk.

Most studies find a neutral effect of tibolone on plasma concentrations of low-density lipoproteins (LDL)[21], but two recent studies[43,44] claim to see a reduction. The resistance of LDL to oxidation *in vitro* is increased by tibolone[45], although the clinical significance of such changes is itself under question[46].

CONCLUSIONS

Over a period of at least 20 years, tibolone has emerged as a useful treatment option for many postmenopausal women. In some countries, the positive aspects in the clinical profile of this steroid have needed to compete with concern over the 'androgenic' CHD risk profile, by which is meant a reduction in plasma HDL concentrations (and nothing else). Recent evidence suggests that the manner in which steroids such as tibolone reduce HDL concentrations may not have the expected clinical significance. Other aspects of this 'androgenic' lipoprotein profile, such as reduced concentrations of fasting triglycerides and lipoprotein(a), would be considered beneficial by current concepts of risk. Plasma HDL aside, many other aspects of the cardiovascular risk profile of tibolone are encouraging.

As with all forms of HRT, the net effect on CHD in women using tibolone is difficult to predict from the existing database. This is the major issue facing those interested in CHD risk in HRT users: can such 'surrogate' studies ever estimate the net effect on risk? In the current atmosphere of doubt and self-questioning, one could argue that all HRT formulations should be considered neutral until they have been proven to be better than placebo in terms of myocardial infarction or other clinical endpoints.

References

1. Rymer JM. The effects of tibolone. *Gynecol Endocrinol* 1998;12:213–20
2. Tang B, Markiewicz L, Kloosterboer HJ, Gurpide E. Human endometrial 3 beta-hydroxysteroid dehydrogenase/isomerase can locally reduce intrinsic estrogenic/progestagenic activity ratios of a steroidal drug (Org OD14). *J Steroid Biochem Mol Biol* 1993;45:345–51.3
3. Gambacciani M, Ciaponi M. Postmenopausal osteoporosis management. *Curr Opin Obstet Gynecol* 2000;12:189–97

4. Hammar M, Christau S, Nathorst-Boos J, Rud T, Garre K. A double-blind, randomised trial comparing the effects of tibolone and continuous combined hormone replacement therapy in postmenopausal women with menopausal symptoms. *Br J Obstet Gynaecol* 1998;105:904-11

5. Gompel A, Siromachkova M, Lombet A, Kloosterboer HJ, Rostene W. Tibolone actions on normal and breast cancer cells. *Eur J Cancer* 2000; 36(Suppl 4):76-7

6. Pasqualini JR, Chetrite GS. Estrone sulfatase versus estrone sulfotransferase in human breast cancer: potential clinical applications. *J Steroid Biochem Mol Biol* 1999;69:287-92

7. Crona N, Silfverstolpe G, Samsioe G. A double-blind cross-over study on the effects of ORG OD14 compared to oestradiol valerate and placebo on lipid and carbohydrate metabolism in oophorectomized women. *Acta Endocrinol (Copenh)* 1983;102:451-5

8. Grodstein F, Stampfer MJ. The impact of progestin on the cardiovascular benefits of estrogen. In Neves-e-Castro M, Birkhauser M, Clarkson TB, Collins P, eds. *Menopause and the Heart*. Carnforth, UK: Parthenon Publishing, 2000: 89-94

9. Speroff L. Postmenopausal hormone replacement therapy and coronary heart disease: clinical implications of recent randomized trial results. *Maturitas* 2000;35:91-7

10. Herrington DM, Reboussin DM, Brosnihan KB, Sharp PC, Shumaker SA, Snyder TE, *et al*. Effects of estrogen replacement on the progression of coronary artery atherosclerosis. *N Engl J Med* 2000;343:522-9

11. Angerer P, Kothny W, Störk S, von Schacky C. Hormone replacement therapy and distensibility of carotid arteries in postmenopausal women: a randomized, controlled trial. *J Am Coll Cardiol* 2000;36:1789-96

12. Mackay R, Kuller L, Matthews K, Sutton-Tyrell K, Evans R. Does HRT affect associations between carotid atherosclerosis and lipoprotein subclasses? The Healthy Women's Study. Presented at *AHA Council of Epidemiology & Prevention Meeting*, San Diego, March 2000

13. Dayspring T. Estrogen and atherothrombosis. *Am J Cardiol* 2000;86:482-3

14. Mosca L. The role of hormone replacement therapy in the prevention of postmenopausal heart disease. *Arch Intern Med* 2000;160:2263-72

15. Ridker PM, Hennekens CH, Rifai N, Buring JE, Manson JE. Hormone replacement therapy and increased plasma concentration of C-reactive protein. *Circulation* 1999;100:713-16

16. Rosano GM, Graziottin A, Fini M. Cardioprotective effects of ovarian hormones and the HERS in perspective. *Maturitas* 2000; 34(Suppl 2):S3-S10

17. Bush TL. Lessons from HERS: the null and beyond. *J Womens Health* 1998;7:781-3

18. Rossouw J. Interview with New York Times; 2000. http://www.nytimes.com/

19. Daly E, Vessey MP, Hawkins MM, Carson JL, Gough P, Marsh S. Risk of venous thromboembolism in users of hormone replacement therapy. *Lancet* 1996;348:977-80

20. Vergouwen MD, Anderson RE, Meyer FB. Gender differences and the effects of synthetic exogenous and non-synthetic estrogens in focal cerebral ischemia. *Brain Res* 2000;878:88-97

21. Moore RA. Livial: a review of clinical studies. *Br J Obstet Gynaecol* 1999;106(Suppl 19):1-21

22. Lloyd G, McGing E, Cooper A, Patel N, Lumb PJ, Wierzbicki AS, *et al*. A randomised, placebo-controlled trial of the effects of tibolone on blood pressure and lipids in hypertensive women. *J Hum Hypertens* 2000; 14:99-104

23. Lehmann ED, Hopkins KD, Parker JR, Turay RC, Rymer J, Fogelman I, *et al*. Aortic distensibility in post-menopausal women receiving tibolone. *Br J Radiol* 1994;67:701-5

24. Morris EP, Denton ERE, Robinson J, MacDonald LM, Rymer J. High resolution ultrasound assessment of the carotid artery: its relevence in postmenopausal women and the effects of tibolone on carotid artery ultrastructure. *Climacteric* 1999;2: 13-20

25. Haenggi W, Linder HR, Birkhaeuser MH, Schneider H. Microscopic findings of the nail-fold capillaries – dependence on menopausal status and hormone replacement therapy. *Maturitas* 1995; 22:37-46

26. Hardiman P, Nihoyannopoulos P, Kicovic P, Ginsburg J. Cardiovascular effects of Org OD 14 – a new steroidal therapy for climacteric symptoms. *Maturitas* 1991;13:235-42

27. Prelevic GM, Beljic T, Ginsburg J. The effect of tibolone on cardiac flow in postmenopausal women with non-insulin-dependent diabetes mellitus. *Maturitas* 1997;27:85-90

28. Haenggi W, Bersinger NA, Mueller MD, Birkhaeuser MH. Decrease of serum endothelin levels with postmenopausal hormone replacement therapy or tibolone. *Gynecol Endocrinol* 1999; 13:202-5

29. Agrawal R, Prelevic G, Conway GS, Payne NN, Ginsburg J, Jacobs HS. Serum vascular endothelial growth factor concentrations in postmenopausal women: the effect of hormone replacement therapy. *Fertil Steril* 2000;73:56-60

30. Doren M, Rubig A, Coelingh Bennink HJ, Holzgreve W. Resistance of pelvic arteries and plasma lipids in postmenopausal women: comparative study of tibolone and continuous combined estradiol and norethindrone acetate

replacement therapy. *Am J Obstet Gynecol* 2000;183:575–82

31. Lloyd GW, Patel NR, McGing EA, Cooper AF, Kamalvand K, Jackson G. Acute effects of hormone replacement with tibolone on myocardial ischaemia in women with angina. *Int J Clin Pract* 1998;52:155–7

32. Zandberg P, Peters JL, Demacker PN, Smit MJ, de Reeder EG, Meuleman DG. Tibolone prevents atherosclerotic lesion formation in cholesterol-fed, ovariectomized rabbits. *Arterioscler Thromb Vasc Biol* 1998;18:1844–54

33. Simoncini T, Genazzani AR. Tibolone inhibits leukocyte adhesion molecule expression in human endothelial cells. *Mol Cell Endocrinol* 2000;162: 87–94

34. Cagnacci A, Mallus E, Tuveri F, Cirillo R, Setteneri AM, Melis GB. Effect of tibolone on glucose and lipid metabolism in postmenopausal women. *J Clin Endocrinol Metab* 1997;82:251–3

35. Walker ID, Davidson JF, Richards A, Yates R, McEwan HP. The effect of the synthetic steroid Org OD14 on fibrinolysis and blood lipids in postmenopausal women. *Thromb Haemostat* 1985; 53:303–5

36. Winkler UH, Altkemper R, Kwee B, Helmond FA, Coelingh Bennink HJ. Effects of tibolone and continuous combined hormone replacement therapy on parameters in the clotting cascade: a multicenter, double-blind, randomized study. *Fertil Steril* 2000;74:10–19

37. Bjarnason NH, Bjarnason K, Haarbo J, Bennink HJ, Christiansen C. Tibolone: influence on markers of cardiovascular disease. *J Clin Endocrinol Metab* 1997;82:1752–6

38. Crook D, Von Eckardstein A, Dieplinger H, Ragoobir J, Elbers J, Helmond F, *et al*. Tibolone lowers HDL concentrations but does not impair

cholesterol efflux from cells. *Maturitas* 2000;35: S7–8

39. Alexandersen P, Haarbo J, Christiansen C. The relationship of natural androgens to coronary heart disease in males: a review. *Atherosclerosis* 1996;125:1–13

40. Rosano GM. Androgens and coronary artery disease. A sex-specific effect of sex hormones? *Eur Heart J* 2000;21:868–71

41. Rymer J, Crook D, Sidhu M, Chapman M, Stevenson JC. Effects of tibolone on serum concentrations of lipoprotein(a) in post-menopausal women. *Acta Endocrinol (Copenh)* 1993;128:259–62

42. Shlipak MG, Simon JA, Vittinghoff E, Lin F, Barrett-Connor E, Knopp RH, *et al*. Estrogen and progestin, lipoprotein(a), and the risk of recurrent coronary heart disease events after menopause. *J Am Med Assoc* 2000;283:1845–52

43. Castelo-Branco C, Casals E, Figueras F, Sanjuan A, Vicente JJ, Balasch J, *et al*. Two-year prospective and comparative study on the effects of tibolone on lipid pattern, and behavior of apolipoproteins AI and B. *Menopause* 1999; 6:92–7

44. Farish E, Barnes JF, Fletcher CD, Ekevall K, Calder A, Hart DM. Effects of tibolone on serum lipoprotein and apolipoprotein levels compared with a cyclical estrogen/progestogen regimen. *Menopause* 1999;6:98–104

45. Farish E, Barnes JF, O'Donoghue F, Hart DM. A comparison of the effects of two 'no-bleed' HRT regimens on cardiovascular risk factors. *Climacteric* 1999;2(Suppl 1):231

46. Parthasarathy S, Santanam N, Ramachandran S, Meilhac O. Oxidants and antioxidants in atherogenesis: an appraisal. *J Lipid Res* 1999; 40:2143–57

Hormone replacement therapy and myocardial infarction

22

L. Mosca

INTRODUCTION

Compelling data from surrogate endpoint studies and epidemiological observations have suggested a role for estrogen replacement therapy (ERT) in the prevention of myocardial infarction, yet confirmatory data from randomized clinical trials are lacking. It is not known if ERT combined with a progestin to prevent endometrial hyperplasia, or hormone replacement therapy (HRT), has a different clinical impact on risk of myocardial infarction compared to unopposed ERT. Recent data have suggested that some women may be at increased risk of myocardial infarction upon initiation of HRT, although predictors of adverse coronary events among subpopulations of women have been difficult to elucidate. ERT has established benefits (relief of menopausal symptoms and prevention of osteoporosis) and established risks (venous thromboembolism and gallbladder disease). Defining the impact of ERT/HRT on coronary heart disease risk is of major importance because coronary heart disease is the single leading cause of death in women in most of the developed and developing world. The purpose of this chapter is to review clinical endpoint studies that have evaluated the association between ERT/HRT and myocardial infarction among women with established coronary heart disease (secondary prevention) and without pre-existing cardiovascular disease (primary prevention).

SECONDARY PREVENTION

The Heart and Estrogen/progestin Replacement Study (HERS) was the first large-scale, randomized clinical trial to evaluate the impact of HRT on clinical cardiovascular disease events in postmenopausal women[1]. The effect of conjugated equine estrogen (CEE) 0.625 mg/day plus medroxy-progesterone acetate (MPA) 2.5 mg/day on the combined incidence of non-fatal myocardial infarction and coronary heart disease death was compared to placebo in women with a prior history of myocardial infarction, coronary revascularization, or angiographic evidence of coronary heart disease. After an average of 4.1 years of follow-up, there was no difference in the primary outcome of non-fatal myocardial infarction and coronary death between the HRT and placebo arms. A post-hoc time trend analysis revealed an increased risk of cardiovascular events of 52% in the first year in the HRT group compared to placebo. However, there was a significant trend towards fewer events in the treatment arm compared to placebo in later years.

The unexpected null result of HERS may reflect chance, an adverse effect of MPA that offset a beneficial effect of ERT, or inadequate duration of follow-up. Moreover, the women studied may have been too old, or their coronary heart disease too advanced to benefit from therapy (their average age was 66.7 years). A long-term follow-up of the HERS cohort may provide additional information. The finding of an early increase in myocardial infarction risk may be due to an unusually low placebo event rate in year one or, alternatively, is biologically compatible with proinflammatory and/or procoagulant effects of ERT[2].

Prior to HERS, there were no large-scale epidemiological studies that evaluated the role of HRT on cardiovascular events among women with established coronary heart disease. Recently, the Nurses' Health Study reported a similar pattern of early coronary heart disease risk and late benefit associated with HRT, in a subset of women with prior myocardial infarction or atherosclerosis[3]. A non-significant increased relative risk of 2.1 (95%

confidence interval (CI), 0.88–4.99) was observed for current users of HRT for less than 1 year compared to non-users, and a significant trend for benefit over time was observed, with a nearly 50% reduced risk of major coronary heart disease in women taking hormones for more than 2 years. Although the overall 35% reduced risk of coronary heart disease among HRT users in this study is consistent with previous epidemiological reports, the small number of events, possible selection bias and residual confounding limit the data.

Recently, the Papworth HRT Atherosclerosis Study (PHASE) reported findings from a randomized study of postmenopausal women with angiographically proven coronary heart disease, which compared the effect of transdermal ERT, with or without norethisterone, to no HRT on cardiovascular disease events[4]. Over a 4-year period, the HRT group had a non-significant increased risk of cardiovascular disease events, with rates highest in the first 2 years of the study. Each year, the HRT group had a non-significant increase in the risk of thromboembolic complications. These data do not support the hypothesis that transdermal ERT, which does not undergo a first-pass effect in the liver, in contrast to oral ERT, has a differential effect on coronary heart disease events.

Data from the Coronary Drug Project (CDP), a randomized trial conducted in the 1960s in men with documented myocardial infarction, lend support for possible adverse effects of estrogen on coronary heart disease risk[5]. The study compared two doses of estrogen (2.5 and 5.0 mg/day) vs. placebo on major coronary heart disease events. A re-analysis of the CDP data showed a significant increase in primary coronary heart disease events at 0–4 months (relative hazard, 1.58; 95% CI, 1.04–2.40) associated with estrogen. The early increase in coronary heart disease risk in men was similar to that observed in the HERS trial, over a similar time frame (non-significant 2.3-fold increased risk for HRT vs. placebo). While these data are randomized and minimize bias, they are limited by the questionable generalizability of the findings of high-dose estrogen in men to the relevance of the results in women.

The Estrogen Replacement and Atherosclerosis (ERA) trial, an angiographic endpoint trial that randomized postmenopausal women with docu-

mented coronary stenosis to CEE 0.625 mg, with or without MPA 2.5 mg/day, or placebo showed no benefit of ERT/HRT on the angiographic progression of disease, lending support to the HERS findings[6]. These data suggest that the null result of HRT was not due to adverse effects of MPA. Because the mean age of women in the ERA trial was 65.8 years and the average length of time since menopause before ERT/HRT was instituted was 23.1 years, the results may not be generalizable to women earlier in the course of menopause. Previous observational studies using angiographic endpoints showed a consistent inverse association between ERT/HRT use and the extent of coronary atherosclerosis, but these studies were not randomized in design[7]. Ongoing angiographic trials in additional populations will provide further data regarding the impact of HRT on the progression of coronary disease.

The totality of evidence from secondary prevention studies does not support initiation of ERT/HRT to reduce the risk of recurrent myocardial infarction or coronary heart disease death or to slow the progression of coronary heart disease among women with existing coronary heart disease. Data are insufficient to determine if coronary heart disease risk will be altered if therapy is continued after 1 or more years of treatment. No data have evaluated the role of ERT/HRT in acute coronary syndromes; however, it may be prudent to discontinue therapy at the time of admission to the hospital in order to minimize the risk of thromboembolic complications associated with HRT and immobilization[8]. Established non-coronary benefits and risks should guide the decision to re-institute therapy among women with coronary heart disease. Alternatively, anticoagulation for immobilized women with coronary heart disease on HRT could be considered, unless contraindicated.

PRIMARY PREVENTION

Numerous observational epidemiological studies have evaluated the association between use of ERT/HRT and fatal and non-fatal myocardial infarction among women without known cardiovascular disease; however, data from randomized clinical trials are not yet available. Two large-scale trials are now in progress (Women's Health Initiative (WHI) in the US and WISDOM in Europe) and will provide more definitive answers regarding the role of ERT/HRT in the primary prevention of coronary heart disease. The Estrogen in the Prevention of Atherosclerosis Trial (EPAT) randomized 222 women without clinical evidence of cardiovascular disease to 17β-estradiol vs. placebo, and showed that ERT significantly slowed the rate of progression of subclinical atherosclerosis of the carotid arteries to the same extent as lipid-lowering therapy[9]. The findings are not consistent with the ERA trial and may represent differences in methodology or may suggest that ERT is more likely to retard the progression of atherosclerosis of relatively healthy vessels rather than those with advanced disease.

Meta-analyses of epidemiological studies show a 35% reduction in risk of coronary heart disease among current ERT/HRT users compared to non-users[10]. The large reduction in risk may be due, in part, to 'healthy women selection bias', as women who use HRT have improved risk factor profiles, higher levels of socioeconomic status and have more frequent preventive evaluations[2].

Recent data from the Group Health Cooperative examined the association between new use of HRT and risk of first myocardial infarction in a population-based case–control study[11]. Among new users of HRT (< 6 months), the odds ratio for myocardial infarction was 1.39 (95% CI, 0.52–3.72) compared to non-users. After 4 years of therapy, a reduced risk of myocardial infarction-associated HRT became evident (odds ratio, 0.66;

95% CI, 0.47–0.92), consistent with the pattern of early risk and late benefit that was observed in the HERS trial. Preliminary data reported from the WHI are consistent with these findings. An early increased risk of cardiovascular events was observed among predominantly healthy women randomized to ERT alone (CEE 0.625 mg/day) or HRT (CEE 0.625 mg/day plus MPA 2.5 mg/day), compared to women randomized to placebo. During the first 2 years of the trial, there was an excess of venous thromboembolism, non-fatal myocardial infarction and stroke. The difference between the treatment and placebo groups diminished over time. These data suggest that women without known cardiovascular disease may be susceptible to early adverse effects of ERT/HRT; however, it should be noted that the absolute risk of early cardiovascular disease events in the WHI was less than 1%.

As the results of ongoing studies are awaited, clinicians should consider the wealth of biological data, epidemiological observations and preliminary data from randomized studies in primary prevention to make recommendations regarding HRT to prevent incident myocardial infarction/coronary heart disease death. The decision to use HRT should be guided by established benefits and risks of HRT in postmenopausal women, as well as consideration of possible benefits and risks of HRT related to coronary heart disease. The need to more uniformly apply in women consensus recommendations for preventive strategies that are widely underutilized should be emphasized in practice[12].

References

1. Hulley S, Grady D, Bush T, *et al*. Randomized trial of estrogen plus progestin for secondary prevention of coronary heart disease in postmenopausal women. *J Am Med Assoc* 1998;280:605–12
2. Mosca L. The role of hormone replacement therapy in the prevention of postmenopausal heart disease. *Arch Intern Med* 2000;160:2263–72
3. Grodstein F, Manson JE, Stampfer MJ. Postmenopausal hormones and recurrence of coronary events in the Nurses' Health Study. *Circulation* 1999;100 (Suppl):871(abstr)
4. Clarke S, Kelleher J, Lloyd-Jones H, *et al*. Transdermal hormone replacement therapy for the secondary prevention of coronary artery disease in

Hormonal replacement therapy, venous thromboembolism and stroke

23

F. Grodstein

INTRODUCTION

The Nurses' Health Study (NHS) has generated one of the world's largest accessible databases for examining the long-term effects of hormone replacement therapy (HRT) on cardiovascular outcomes[1-3]. Started in the USA in 1976, it is based on a cohort of 121 700 women, all of whom are registered nurses. At inclusion, the subjects were aged 30–55 years, so that that now, after nearly 25 years' follow-up, they range in age from about 55 to 80 years. Most are now postmenopausal.

Most data for the study are obtained by means of questionnaires mailed every 2 years, but this is also backed up by supplementary information. For example, when subjects report a recent diagnosis of any kind of cardiovascular disease, permission is requested to review their medical records. Only cases of cardiovascular disease which have been confirmed are included in the NHS analyses.

This paper will review the major NHS findings on links between HRT, venous thromboembolism (VTE) and stroke, and will compare these data with those of other relevant studies.

IMPLICATIONS OF STUDY DESIGN

The design of any study in any area of medicine largely determines both its power and its limitations. The advantages of being able to run observa-tional studies like the NHS over very long periods of time need to be balanced against the advantages of obtaining randomized data from clinical trials. Equally, mechanistic studies can provide key insights into fundamental processes at work.

A primary problem in observational studies is confounding; however, the extent of this problem may be different in different studies. For example, the Study of Osteoporotic Fractures (SOF)[4], which is a general population study of users and non-users of estrogen therapy, has demonstrated (Table 1) a number of differences between the two groups, probably because the users tend to be better educated than non-users. This is due to the fact that HRT in the USA is only available to those with adequate funds to pay for access to health care and the costs of prescriptions. Hence, the potential for confounding may be high in the SOF study because of differences in the socioeconomic status of users and non-users of HRT. In contrast, the NHS is not based on a general population, since all of its participants are registered nurses. Consequently, they all have a good standard of education, all have good access to health care, and all have an excellent knowledge of HRT and related matters. Hence, in the NHS there are fewer significant socioeconomic differences between the users and non-users of HRT, which reduces the

Table 1 Prevalence of risk factors in the study populations for the Study of Osteoporotic Fractures[4] and the Nurses' Health Study[2], comparing users and non-users of hormone replacement therapy

Characteristic	Study of Osteoporotic Fractures		Nurses' Health Study	
	Users	Non-users	Users	Non-users
Less than high-school education	16%	27%	–	–
Physical activity	76%	63%	48%	42%
Alcohol intake	76%	66%	8 grams	7 grams
Blood pressure	–	–	23%	22%

potential for confounding. Users and non-users in the study are also well matched for general factors such as physical activity, alcohol intake and blood pressure (Table 1), making it more likely that analysis of the differences between the two groups will provide meaningful conclusions that reflect genuine differences in treatment outcomes.

HRT AND VENOUS THROMBOEMBOLISM

Association of the use of oral contraceptives with increased risks of VTE and pulmonary embolism is well established[3]. The possible analogous links between the use of HRT, which involves estrogen doses about 15% of those of oral contraceptives, and VTE are now also well established. It has long been suspected that VTE is more common in current users of HRT than non-users, but, until the results of the NHS[3], simultaneously published with two other large-scale studies, all previous investigations had been based on small numbers of patients, and the largest of these[5] documented only six cases of pulmonary embolism.

The association between pulmonary embolism and hormone use apparent in the observational studies was confirmed in the Heart and Estrogen/progestin Replacement Study (HERS)[6], a randomized clinical trial (RCT) which investigated the secondary prevention of heart disease in a group of 2763 postmenopausal women (mean age 67 years) with an intact uterus, a history of heart disease, but no evidence of prior VTE. They were randomized to receive daily combination hormone therapy (0.625 mg conjugated equine estrogen plus 2.5 mg medroxyprogesterone acetate) or placebo. During 4.1 years of follow-up, HERS documented 47 cases of VTE, 34 in the HRT group and 13 in the placebo group (relative hazard 2.7; 95% confidence interval (CI): 1.4–5.0; $p = 0.003$). The excess risk was calculated to be 3.9 (95% CI: 1.4–6.4) per 1000 woman-years and the number of patients needed to treat for harm was 256 (95% CI: 157-692).

In the cohort of postmenopausal women in the NHS, over the period 1976–92, 68 cases of primary pulmonary embolism were documented[3], giving a relative risk (adjusted for multiple risk factors) for current versus never users of HRT of 2.1 (95% CI: 1.2–3.8), a result which is similar to that found in

the HERS trial. However, the NHS was not able to demonstrate any effect of past use of HRT on risks of pulmonary embolism (relative risk 1.3; 95% CI: 0.7–2.4), thereby suggesting that the increased risk is lost when HRT is stopped.

It is important to emphasize that pulmonary embolism is a very uncommon disease. The HERS trial identified only 47 cases of VTE from both the active and placebo groups, whilst, in the much larger NHS, there were only 68 cases of primary pulmonary embolism. Based on these findings in the NHS, it can be calculated that only five additional cases of pulmonary embolism would result each year from a cohort of 100 000 women receiving HRT.

The extraordinarily low rate of incidence of pulmonary embolism makes it very difficult to study it in a prospective fashion, whether in an observational study like NHS, or in an RCT like HERS. It is much easier to investigate links between hormone therapy and VTE in a case-control study, in which a large number of cases are identified and compared in detail with matched controls. One such study[7], which was based on a British general practice database of 347 253 patients (aged 50–79 years) without major risk factors for VTE, confirmed that the incidence of VTE was raised with HRT, but showed that the effect was restricted to the first year of use. Overall, the study documented 292 cases of pulmonary embolism or deep vein thrombosis admitted to hospital. The cases were compared with a random selection of 10 000 controls from the same database. A detailed examination of medical records for a 10% sample of these VTE patients confirmed the diagnosis in the vast majority of cases. The overall results of the British study were the same as those of the NHS and HERS, namely, a slightly greater than two-fold increased risk of VTE in users (Table 2). Detailed analysis of the British data, however, revealed a strong effect of duration of hormone usage: during the first 6 months of HRT, there was an almost five-fold increase in relative risk of VTE, which decreased after a year to a virtually zero increased risk (Table 3). There appeared to be little effect of estrogen dose on VTE risk (Table 2), though very few women in the study were using high-dose products and the reliability of the result was accordingly small.

Table 2 Relative risks of venous thrombosis from a UK general practice study by estrogen dose[7]

Estrogen dose*	Number of cases	Number of controls	Adjusted odds ratio (95% CI) current users vs non-users
Low	21	704	2.1 (1.2–3.4)
High	6	186	2.4 (1.0–5.6)

*Low and high defined, respectively, as 0.625 or 1.25 mg/day for oral conjugated estrogens and 25 μg and 50 μg or 100 μg for transdermal estradiol

Table 3 Relative risks of venous thrombosis from a UK general practice study by duration of hormone use[7]

Hormone use	Number of cases	Number of controls	Adjusted odds ratio (95% CI) current users vs non-users
Overall			
Current use	37	1179	2.1 (1.4-3.2)
By duration of treatment			
1–6 months	14	195	4.6 (2.5–8.4)
6–12 months	8	176	3.0 (1.4–6.5)
> 1 year	13	773	1.1 (0.6–2.1)

HRT AND STROKE

Following a preliminary analysis of stroke observed in the NHS for data up to 1992[1], we have now been able to extend our observations for additional years, yielding a total of 800 cases of stroke, about 400 of which involve ischemic stroke (as expected in a US population) and 175 hemorrhagic stroke[8]. Looking separately at hormone therapy with estrogen alone and estrogen in combination with progestin, there is, in both cases, a modest increase in risk of stroke with hormone use, with a slightly greater increase in the combined therapy group, for which risks are about 40% greater than in non-users (Figure 1). In the USA, combined hormone therapy is almost always carried out with conjugated estrogens and medroxyprogesterone acetate, and it cannot be concluded with certainty that similar findings would be obtained in countries where a different mix of hormones is in evidence.

The design of the NHS has allowed the effects of estrogen dose on risk of stroke to be determined, thereby demonstrating a striking dose-response effect with oral conjugated estrogens (Figure 2)[8]. At doses of 0.625 mg estrogen or higher, there is a statistically significant increase in risk of stroke with current users.

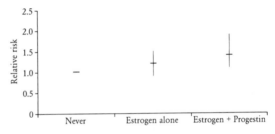

Figure 1 Nurses' Health Study, 1976–96: risk of stroke by hormone use[8]

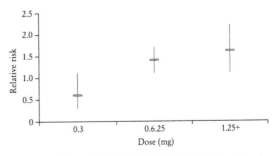

Figure 2 Nurses' Health Study, 1976–96: risk of stroke by estrogen dose[8]

Attempts have been made in the NHS to look separately at the data for hemorrhagic and ischemic strokes. The modest increase with hormone use appeared similar for both types of

Table 4 Hormone therapy and risk of stroke: Danish National Patient Register, based on questionnaires from 1422 stroke cases and 3171 controls[9]

Event	Odds ratio (95% CI), current vs never use	
	Estrogen	*Estrogen + progestin*
Subarachnoid hemorrhage	0.52 (0.23–1.22)	1.22 (0.79–1.89)
Ischemic stroke	1.16 (0.86–1.58)	1.17 (0.92–1.47)

*Termed 'thromboembolic infarction'

stroke, although there are too few hemorrhagic strokes to make firm conclusions.

Turning to other investigations of hormone therapy and stroke in other countries with mainly different types of estrogen products, a Danish case–control study based on 1422 cases of non-fatal, first-ever stroke in women (aged 45–64 years) from the national patient database, and randomly selected matched controls from the national person database, can be interpreted to have shown no effect, or perhaps a small increase of stroke, with estrogen-only or combined hormone therapy (Table 4)[9]. Analysis of the effects of different kinds of estrogens in this study suggests similar effects for varying hormone types. Similar findings were obtained in another Scandinavian study, this time based on a population registry from Uppsala, Sweden, which showed no effect of estriol alone, and only a small effect for a combination of estradiol and conjugated estrogens (Table 5)[10]. Looking separately at acute stroke and sub-arachnoid hemorrhage, the Swedish data show that, for both kinds of event, there appears to be no effect of hormone use, or type of hormone, on risk (Table 6). Recently, we reinvestigated the same population of women using a slightly different method of analysis[11]. In this study, a subgroup of 9236 women from the cohort were mailed a questionnaire asking them directly about their use of hormone therapy. This approach should be con-trasted with that of the earlier Swedish study, in which cross-registry databases were used. The questionnaire generated 289 cases of stroke, which were then analyzed in terms of type of estrogen use: some women were using low-potency estrogens (mainly 1 mg estriol), whilst others were using medium-potency estrogens (mainly 2 mg estradiol or 0.625 mg oral conjugated estrogens). The expec-tation was that low-potency estrogen would have

Table 5 Estrogen-only therapy and risks of all stroke by type of estrogen: Swedish study[10]

Estrogen	Number of cases	Relative risk (95% CI)
Estradiol/conjugated estrogens	169	0.79 (0.67–0.92)
Estriol (termed 'other estrogens')	192	1.02 (0.88–1.17)

Table 6 Estrogen-only therapy and risk of acute stroke and subarachnoid hemorrhage by type of estrogen: Swedish study[10]

Estrogen	Number of cases	Relative risk (95% CI)
Acute stroke		
Estradiol/conjugated estrogens	112	0.72 (0.59–0.86)
Estriol	144	1.00 (0.85–1.18)
Subarachnoid hemorrhage		
Estradiol/conjugated estrogens	33	1.24 (0.85–1.74)
Estriol	9	1.03 (0.47–1.96)

Table 7 Hormone therapy and risk of stroke by type and potency of therapy: re-questioning of Swedish cohort, based on questionnaire mailed to 9236 women, resulting in 289 cases of stroke[11]

Hormone therapy	Relative risk (95% CI)
Estrogen, low potency	1.00[†]
Estrogen, medium potency	0.91 (0.71–1.17)
estrogen alone	1.00 (0.76–1.33)
estrogen and progesterone	0.81 (0.61–1.10)

[†]By definition

no effect on cardiovascular risk, and that there would be less confounding if low-potency users were defined as 'no risk' and compared to

Table 8 Leisure World Study: hormone therapy and stroke mortality by estrogen dose[12]

Estrogen dose (mg/day)	Death rate*	Number of deaths	Follow-up (person-years)	Relative risk (95% CI)
Never used	2.0	43	17 624	1.00[†]
≤ 0.625	1.9	7	6 798	0.73 (0.32–1.66)
≥ 1.25	0.9	5	8 011	0.49 (0.19–1.27)

*Age-adjusted mortality for stroke per 1000 person-years; [†]by definition

medium-potency users. All these women had chosen to take hormone therapy, but in different doses. The results of the study were similar to those of others, namely, little effect on risk of stroke, regardless of whether the women were taking estrogen alone or estrogen in combination with progesterone (Table 7).

There is some evidence that estrogen therapy has some benefits in terms of stroke mortality, as opposed to stroke incidence. The Leisure World Study (LWS)[12], for example, suggests that there is some protection against stroke mortality for higher-dose hormone users (Table 8). Similarly, in the NHS, although there have been few stroke deaths to date, the relative risks for stroke mortality are all lower than for stroke incidence[8].

LIFESTYLE AND PREVENTION OF CORONARY HEART DISEASE

Estrogens are, of course, only one of many factors which may potentially prevent coronary disease. The current uncertainty about whether estrogen therapy is truly cardioprotective has encouraged many physicians to shift the emphasis in patient counselling towards general aspects of a healthy lifestyle. Scientific evidence for the importance of these factors has come from long-term observation over a period of 14 years of an NHS cohort of 84 129 women, all free at the start in 1980 of diagnosed cardiovascular disease, cancer and diabetes. This showed[13] that 82% (95% CI: 58–93%) of coronary events in these women could be attributed to lack of adherence to a menu of lifestyle factors (Table 9). Hence, fairly modest, non-disruptive lifestyle habits, achievable by any average person, have the potential to eliminate more than 80% of coronary events. It is therefore important, in considering the effects of hormone therapy on cardiovascular disease, and in advising patients, to

Table 9 Lifestyle habits leading to 90% fewer cases of heart disease in Nurses' Health Study (compared to women without these habits)[19]

- Modest exercise: one half-hour of brisk walking per day
- Modest weight: body mass index ≤ 25
- Modestly healthy diet: high content of fruit and vegetables, low glycemic load, with a relatively high ratio of polyunsaturated : saturated fats
- Non-smokers
- Some alcohol consumption: 0.5–2.0 glasses per day

emphasize the importance of a healthy lifestyle for preventing heart disease.

CONCLUSIONS

Long-term observational studies such as the NHS complement randomized controlled trials and other kinds of studies. The relative risk of pulmonary embolism in current versus never users of HRT determined in the NHS for the period 1976–92 is 2.1 (95% CI: 1.2–3.8), which compares well with the HERS trial result of 2.7 (95% CI: 1.4–5.0) and the value of 2.1 (95% CI: 1.4–3.2) obtained in a large-scale British case–control study. The case–control study showed that, after 1 year's use of HRT, the excess risk reduces to zero. According to the NHS data, five additional cases of pulmonary embolism can be expected each year from a cohort of 100 000 women using HRT.

The NHS has shown that risks of stroke may be modestly increased with HRT and that there appears to be a dose-response effect with estrogen. At minimum, most data report no benefits of postmenopausal hormones on stroke incidence.

As regards controversies on the effects of HRT on heart disease, the NHS has established that the adoption by women of a range of relatively non-disruptive lifestyle habits can reduce coronary heart disease by more than 80%.

References

1. Grodstein T, Stampfer MJ, Manson JE, *et al*. Post-menopausal estrogen and progestin use and the risk of cardiovascular disease. *N Engl J Med* 1996;335: 453–61

2. Stampfer MJ, Colditz GA, Willett WC, *et al*. Post-menopausal estrogen therapy and cardiovascular disease: ten-year follow-up from the Nurses' Health Study. *N Engl J Med* 1991;325:756–62

3. Grodstein T, Stampfer MJ, Goldhaber SZ, *et al*. Prospective study of exogenous hormones and risk of pulmonary embolism in women. *Lancet* 1996; 348:983–7

4. Cauley JA, Seeley DG, Ensrud K, *et al*. Estrogen replacement therapy and fractures in older women. Study of Osteoporotic Fractures Research Group. *Ann Intern Med* 1995;122:9–16

5. Devor M, Barrett-Connor E, Renvall M, *et al*. Estrogen replacement therapy and the risk of venous thrombosis. *Am J Med* 1992;92:275–82

6. Grady D, Wenger NK, Herrington D, *et al*. Post-menopausal hormone therapy increases risk for venous thromboembolism disease. *Ann Intern Med* 2000;132:689–96

7. Gutthann SP, Rodríguez LAG, Castellsague, *et al*. Hormone replacement therapy and risk of venous thromboembolism: population based case–control study. *Br Med J* 1997;314:796–800

8. Grodstein F. Nurses Health Study. *Ann Intern Med* 2001; in press

9. Pedersen AT, Lidegaard Ø, Kreiner S, Ottesen B. Hormone replacement therapy and risk of non-fatal stroke. *Lancet* 1997;350:1277–83

10. Falkeborn M, Persson I, Terent A, *et al*. Hormone replacement therapy and the risk of stroke: follow-up of a population-based cohort in Sweden. *Arch Intern Med* 1993;153:1201–9

11. Grodstein F, Stampfer MJ, Falkeborn M, *et al*. Postmenopausal hormone therapy and risk of cardiovascular disease and hip fracture in a cohort of Swedish women. *Epidemiology* 1999;10:476–80

12. Paganini-Hill A, Ross RK, Henderson BE. Post-menopausal oestrogen treatment and stroke: a prospective study. *Br Med J* 1988;297:519–22

13. Stampfer MJ, Hu FB, Manson JE, *et al*. Primary prevention of coronary heart disease in women through diet and lifestyle. *N Engl J Med* 2000;343: 16–22

Index